Shoulder Dystocia and Birth Injury

Third Edition

Notice

Medicine is an ever-changing science. As new research and clinical experience broaden our knowledge, changes in treatment and drug therapy are required. The editors and the publisher of this work have checked with sources believed to be reliable in their efforts to provide information that is complete and generally in accord with the standards accepted at the time of publication. However, in view of the possibility of human error or changes in medical sciences, neither the editors nor the publisher, nor any other party who has been involved in the preparation or publication of this work, warrants that the information contained herein is in every respect accurate or complete, and they are not responsible for any errors or omissions or for the results obtained from use of such information. Readers are encouraged to confirm the information contained herein with other sources. For example and in particular, readers are advised to check the product information sheet included in the package of each drug they plan to administer to be certain that the information contained in this book is accurate and that changes have not been made in the recommended dose or in the contraindications for administration. This recommendation is of particular importance in connection with new or infrequently used drugs. Further, this book is not a substitute for legal advice. If you require legal assistance, consult your attorney.

Shoulder Dystocia and Birth Injury

Prevention and Treatment

Third Edition

James A. O'Leary, MD
Editor

Department of Obstetrics and Gynecology
University of South Florida, Tampa, Florida

Foreword by William N. Spellacy, MD

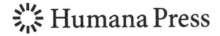 Humana Press

Editor
James A. O'Leary, MD
Department of Obstetrics and
Gynecology
University of South Florida Tampa
Tampa, FL 33620
USA
japoleary@msn.com

ISBN: 978-1-61737-927-7   e-ISBN: 978-1-59745-473-5
DOI 10.1007/978-1-59745-473-5

Cover illustration: From Figure 20 in Chapter 14

Printed on acid-free paper

9 8 7 6 5 4 3 2 1

springer.com

To my wife, Arlene,
for all her love and support,

love to my daughter, Elizabeth (Marc)
and my son, Jim (April),

and to my granddaughters, Sadie, Molly,
and Amy, who bring me great joy and make it
all worthwhile!

The author would very much like to take full
credit for this book, but truthfulness forces
me to admit that only the undiscovered
mistakes were made by me without
assistance from others. Any one of us can
learn from our mistakes; the smart ones learn
from each other.

The philosophy, teachings, concepts, and
much of the clinical data in this book are
those of a very experienced and talented
clinician, James L. O'Leary, MD, often
referred to as Dad.

Foreword

Every obstetrician has a moment of anxiety in the delivery room when there first appears to be some difficulty delivering the anterior shoulder of the infant. Many such cases have predelivery risk factors for shoulder dystocia such as a wide maternal pelvic arch or a macrosomic infant from an obese, postdate, or (especially) diabetic mother. Some, however, are not predictable. Thus, with enough deliveries, everyone will at some time encounter a significant shoulder dystocia. It is important to begin a series of well-tested maneuvers immediately, to successfully deliver a child unharmed, and afterward to clearly enter in the medical record the steps that were taken in the process.

This book reviews the problem of shoulder dystocia in a clear and logical manner, preparing the obstetrician to avoid most cases and to successfully manage the others. It is a timely and important contribution to the modern obstetric literature.

Tampa, Florida, USA   William N. Spellacy, MD

Preface

It is well-known that the intrinsic value of personal experience and the resultant wisdom cause physicians to modify their clinical behavior. However, we cannot expect clinicians to accumulate enough personal experience to fully understand the many nuances of infrequently encountered obstetric problems; one such problem is shoulder dystocia. Here the accumulated experiences of talented clinicians can be valuable to the primary care provider. Any physician can learn from his or her mistakes; intelligent physicians learn from each other.

Our specialty was once largely dependent on manual dexterity. Indeed, it was often stated, "You can best judge an obstetrician by the way he delivers a vaginal breech." Today, we must be knowledgeable and expert in many areas; and we must be skilled surgeons and yet remain compassionate bedside providers rather than foot-of-the-bed doctors clinging to well-indexed charts.

During the past several years, there has been an extensive reappraisal of the physiologic changes of pregnancy and their associated disorders, along with a refinement of diagnostic procedures and a sounder evaluation of the therapeutic approaches that are of primary concern to the physician. An understanding of these physiologic, diagnostic, and therapeutic changes is stressed in this text.

Many of these advances have had an impact on normal obstetrics (which although it is at times routine, is always demanding) and carry with them enormous responsibility. Although our specialty requires intense dedication, it still provides great joy and satisfaction. To meet some of the demands resulting from these changes, I have tried to provide, in an organized manner, information that will be clinically useful to physicians, midwives, and professionals in training.

The proliferation of nonscientific causation articles written by obstetricans for purposes of legal defense will be dealt with. These authors, revisionist historians, have not proved their conclusions. "Then you will know the truth, and the truth will set you free" (John 8:32).1`

Tampa, Florida, USA   James A. O'Leary, MD

Contents

Foreword   vii

Preface   ix

Introduction   xv

Part I   Prevention

1   Preconceptual Risk Factors   3
    James A. O'Leary

2   Antepartum Risk Factors   15
    James A. O'Leary

3   Role of Ultrasound in Shoulder Dystocia   33
    James A. O'Leary

4   Intrapartum Risk Factors   49
    James A. O'Leary

5   Pelvimetry   59
    James A. O'Leary

Part II   Treatment

6   Recognition of Disproportion   71
    James A. O'Leary

7   Delivery Techniques   89
    James A. O'Leary

8   The McRoberts Maneuver   107
    James A. O'Leary

9   Cephalic Replacement: The Gunn-Zavanelli-O'Leary Maneuver   119
    James A. O'Leary

10 Infant Injury...   129
    James A. O'Leary

Part III   Clinical Considerations

11 *In Utero* Causation of Brachial Plexus Injury: Myth or Mystery? ...   147
    James A. O'Leary

12 Recurrent Shoulder Dystocia   163
    James A. O'Leary

13 Predisposing Factors for Shoulder Dystocia-Related Birth
    Injuries: Causation Analysis...............................   169
    Leslie Iffy, Joseph J. Apuzzio, and Vijaya Raju

14 Recognition, Classification, and Management of Shoulder
    Dystocia: The Relationship to Causation of Brachial Plexus Injury ..   179
    Michael S. Kreitzer

15 Minimizing the Risks of Shoulder Dystocia-Related Fetal Injuries ..   209
    Leslie Iffy

16 The Maternal Fetal Medicine Viewpoint: Causation and Litigation ..   227
    Barry S. Schifrin and Wayne R. Cohen

17 Brachial Plexus injury at Cesarean Section   249
    Michael S. Kreitzer and James A. O'Leary

18 Delivery of the Nondiabetic Macrosomic Infant................   257
    Lisa Gittens-Williams

19 The Midwifery View of Shoulder Dystocia...................   269
    Judith S. Mercer and Debra A. Erickson-Owens

20 Recent Research: Relevant and Reliable.....................   285
    James A. O'Leary

21 Observations on the Etiology of Brachial Plexus Birth Palsy Based
    on Radiographic, Intraoperative, and Histologic Findings   289
    Stephen M. Russell, Israel Alfonso, and John A.I. Grossman

Index   295

Contributors

Joseph J. Apuzzio, MD
Professor of Obstetrics and Gynecology, University of Medicine
and Dentistry of New Jersey, New Jersey Medical School, Newark,
New Jersey, USA

Wayne R. Cohen, MD
Chief Academic Officer, North Bronx Healthcare Network, Albert Einstein
College of Medicine, Department of Obstetrics and Gynecology, Jamaica
Hospital and Medical Center, Jamaica, New York, USA; Department of
Obstetrics and Gynecology, Weill Medical College of Cornell University,
New York, New York, USA

Debra A. Erickson-Owens, CNM, MS
Doctoral Student at the University of Rhode Island and Former Director
of the University of Rhode Island Nurse-Midwifery Program, Kingston, Rhode
Island, USA

Lisa Gittens-Williams, MD
Associate Professor, Department of Obstetrics, Gynecology and Women's
Health, New Jersey Medical School, Newark, New Jersey, USA

Leslie Iffy, MD
Professor of Obstetrics and Gynecology, University of Medicine and Dentistry
of New Jersey, New Jersey Medical School, Newark, New Jersey, USA

Michael S. Kreitzer, MD, FACOG
Attending Physician, Overlook Hospital, Summit, NJ, USA; Clin. Assoc. Prof,
OBIYN, University of Medicine and Dentistry of NJ, USA; Senior Risk
Management Consultant, Princeton Insurance Co, Princeton, NJ, USA

Judith S. Mercer, PhD
Certified Nurse Midwife, Cranston, Rhode Island, USA

James A. O'Leary, MD
Professor Obstetrics and Gynecology (retired), University of South Florida,
Tampa, Florida, USA

Vijaya Raju, MD
Assistant Professor of Obstetrics and Gynecology, University of Medicine and
Dentistry of New Jersey, New Jersey Medical School, Newark, New Jersey,
USA

Stephen M. Russell
Department of Neurosurgery, NYU Medical Center, 550 First Avenue,
NY, NY

Barry S. Schifrin, MD
Consulting Obstetrician, Department of Obstetrics and Gynecology, Kaiser
Permanente, Los Angeles Medical Center, Los Angeles, California, USA

Introduction

Overview

Shoulder dystocia, the doctor's dilemma, represents many things to the obstetrician: fear when it occurs; possible frustration when trying to prevent it; and a formidable problem when preparing a legal defense if litigation ensues. The seriousness of shoulder dystocia is a function of the resultant brachial plexus injury. Creasy and Resnik [1] have stated that the brachial plexus is subject to injury when excessive downward traction and lateral flexion or extension of the fetal head and neck occur in an attempt to deliver the anterior shoulder [2].

Strong traction applied on the infant's head during shoulder dystocia is a well-established mechanism of injury to the brachial plexus [3–5]. Brachial plexus injury unrelated to the delivery is a rare phenomenon with little bearing on the overall problem of shoulder dystocia at birth [5]. Successful resolution of this obstetric emergency is dependent on the clinical skill and acumen of the delivering physician [3], use of gentle traction, and other maneuvers. More than 10 years ago [6], the problem of shoulder dystocia was summarized in a publication as follows: "Most of the traditional risk factors for shoulder dystocia have no predictive value, shoulder dystocia itself is an unpredictable event, and infants at risk of permanent injury are virtually impossible to predict. Thus, no protocol should serve to complete substitute for good clinical judgment." This is a very defeatist and potentially dangerous attitude.

This defeatist philosophy has made the implication that the terms *prediction* and *prevention* are interchangeable [6]. Actually, preventive medicine has seldom relied on prediction. The elimination of devastating diseases, such as smallpox, tuberculosis, and puerperal fever, and the teratogenic effects of drugs did not hinge upon prospective identification of individuals who would contract a particular infection or would suffer from the untoward effect of a potentially teratogenic agent. Thus, the numerous publications that confirmed and reconfirmed the unpredictability of shoulder dystocia have not helped to decrease the number of fetal injuries. Instead, orthopedic centers specializing in the surgical repair of Erb's palsy have mushroomed in the United States in recent years [5].

Many obstetricians and midwives have experienced the sudden anxiety, emptiness, and fear at the unexpected and sudden retraction of the infant's head immediately after its delivery. This so-called turtle sign is well-known and can rapidly cause "furor operativum," or operative madness, leading the care provider to take steps he or she would not normally take.

Shoulder dystocia may be considered the obstetrician's Achilles' heel; because it encompasses the entire spectrum of obstetric care, the prepregnancy state, past history, proper prenatal testing, the lost art of clinical pelvimetry, meticulous labor management, and a complete and accurate understanding of the mechanisms of labor. An oversight in any of these areas could lead to the obstetrician's having to deal with this often devastating complication.

Few obstetric events will test the care provider's courage and *sang-froid* as does this challenging situation; hence we use the term *obstetrician distress*. Once dystocia occurs, optimal maternal and fetal outcomes are possible only if the care provider fully understands the nature of the problem and mechanisms involved, has a well-defined management plan, and is able to function without undue haste or the use of excessive physical force.

Shoulder dystocia has replaced breech presentation, and Scanzoni and Kielland forceps rotations, as a major source of injured babies and of medico-legal liability. It is possible that in the future, all shoulder impaction dystocias with a negative outcome will be litigated. McLeod [6] stated that the axiom "shoulder dystocia occurs cataclysmically" must be challenged and that "many, if not the majority, can and should be anticipated." Dignam [7] defined the "absolute essentials" in the management of shoulder dystocia as (1) prior consideration, (2) accurate knowledge, (3) a well-conceived plan of action, and (4) rapidity of execution. A recent edition of *Williams Obstetrics* [8] uses italics to emphasize that the practitioner of obstetrics must be well versed in the management principles of this occasionally devastating complication.

Zuspan and Quilligan [9] emphasized that in most cases, delivery can be accomplished without injury if the obstetrician is familiar with certain manipulative and operative techniques. The use of the word *if* deserves great emphasis because it can have significant legal implications.

Definition

It is not difficult to formulate a definition of shoulder dystocia even though there is a wide variation in the difficulty experienced in delivering the shoulders of an infant after the head has been delivered [7–10]. For some infants, more than the usual amount of pressure is necessary, and thus shoulder dystocia is said to be present. Yet, if the required pressure is not extreme, a formal diagnosis of shoulder dystocia may not be recorded. Recent teachings of the American College of Obstetricians and Gynecologists (ACOG) have defined shoulder dystocia. All standard textbooks emphasize the importance of gentle traction as key to successful outcomes [2].

Definitions of shoulder dystocia may vary slightly among institutions [1,9,11–15]. However, most investigators agree that it has occurred when the standard delivery procedures of gentle downward traction of the fetal head fail to accomplish delivery [16–20]. The problem with this definition is that the qualifier *gentle* lacks precise definition.

When dystocia is marked, the shoulders may be held high in the pelvis. The head may be delivered gradually and with difficulty. Immediately after its delivery, the head is pulled back tightly against the perineum so that even rotation of the head is difficult. This is true and undisputed bilateral shoulder dystocia.

A few other conditions mimic shoulder dystocia. Sometimes, these conditions may be detected by exploration of the uterus above the delivered head, which may reveal contraction ring, fetal abnormalities such as meningocele, tumors of the neck and thorax, or enlargement of the abdomen due to bladder distension, ascites, or tumors of the fetal kidneys, liver, spleen, or gonads. Tumors of the infant's pelvis may also be responsible, and, very rarely, double monsters may be the cause.

An extremely short umbilical cord, or a cord that is somewhat short and also is wrapped several times around the infant's neck, may make it difficult to deliver the shoulders. In either case, traction on the infant may produce marked changes in the fetal heart rate, thereby suggesting the diagnosis.

Recent Developments

Developments in obstetrics over the past 50 years have been largely directed at preventing asphyxia and trauma at the time of birth. These changes have resulted in almost complete elimination of perinatal death (0.6 per 1,000) and permanent cerebral handicap (0.5 per 1,000) caused by peripartum asphyxia and trauma [19]. Neonatal post-asphyxia encephalopathy has also become much less frequent.

Whereas the number of infant deaths and handicaps has decreased, the actual causes of asphyxia and encephalopathy have changed very little. Shoulder dystocia and traumatic deliveries of shoulder impaction appear to be increasing in some institutions. The association between operative and/or difficult deliveries and shoulder dystocia is being more frequently appreciated, and thus operative procedures are being avoided.

It is possible that recently trained obstetricians are less proficient in the use of midforceps and techniques used to deal with shoulder dystocia due to the increase in cesarean section rates. If such is the case, a greater fetal injury rate can be anticipated. The ACOG in 1998 [21] stated that "Brachial plexus injuries result from excessive lateral traction on the fetal head in attempting to dislodge the anterior shoulder." They emphasize that the key to preventing injury is avoidance of excessive traction on the fetal head, avoiding pushing and fundal pressure. In addition, there is much anecdotal evidence of brachial plexus injury occurring without shoulder dystocia. Unfortunately, most of these anecdotes come from deposition testimony [22].

Incidence

As with other infrequent occurrences, the incidence of dystocia may be difficult to establish unless large numbers of obstetric deliveries are considered. Also, there may be different criteria among different reporters and among different populations. It seems clear that the incidence is less than 1% of term deliveries, with 0.3% probably being an accurate determination. However, shoulder dystocia is underreported in the obstetric literature; 71% of *all* injured infants were the product of deliveries where shoulder dystocia was not recognized [23].

Shoulder dystocia has been reported in 0.15% to 1.7% of all vaginal deliveries. Although some observers have reported an apparent increase in the incidence in recent years, others have disputed such a claim [15], believing that the data only reflect increased reporting. Hopwood [24] reported a 1.1% occurrence of this complication in a community hospital. This increased rate is probably a reflection of a general increase in birthweight related to a well-educated clientele, better nutrition, greater maternal weight gain, and more postterm pregnancies. Also, definitions vary, and it is thus inevitable that incidence figures may vary significantly.

Sack [25] noted a 1.7% incidence of shoulder dystocia when fetal weight exceeded 4,500 g. Those infants who weighed more than 4,500 g, and who were born after a second stage of labor that lasted more than 1 hour, had a 35% incidence of shoulder dystocia and a 30% rate of perinatal death. Sack [25] suggested that prolongation of the second stage of labor might serve as a diagnostic point in predicting a large infant and/or subsequent shoulder dystocia. This suggestion was supported by Benedetti and Gabbe [11], who reported an 0.3% incidence of shoulder dystocia in their study. When prolongation of the second stage of labor occurred with midpelvic delivery, the incidence of shoulder dystocia increased to 4.5%. When prolongation of the second stage of labor was accompanied by midpelvic delivery and an infant weight of more than 4,000 g, the incidence of dystocia increased to 21%. Benedetti and Gabbe defined the prolonged second stage of labor as one greater than 2 hours in primigravida and greater than 1 hour in multigravida [11].

More than 70% of shoulder dystocia cases occur with infants weighing more than 4,000 g [16]. With macrosomia and/or continued fetal growth beyond term, the trunk, and particularly the chest, grow larger relative to the head. The chest circumference exceeds the head circumference in 80% of cases. The arms also contribute to the greater dimensions of the upper body. Within a barely adequate pelvis, such bulk might easily block fetal rotation from a disadvantageous anteroposterior to the more desirable oblique diameter and thus increase the frequency of the problem.

Discussion

For proper perspective, it is noteworthy that the majority of large infants are delivered without this complication. For example, the Johns Hopkins series [26] included 1,409 infants weighing more than 4,000 g; shoulder dystocia occurred in only 1.7% of cases. The University of Southern California series also demonstrated that shoulder dystocia occurred in only 1.2% of infants weighing more than 4,000 g if prolonged second stage of labor and midpelvic delivery were not complicating factors [11]. These studies are consistent with earlier observations by Bolton [27] of only eight cases of shoulder dystocia among 1,440 infants. However, in infants greater than 4,000 g, the incidence varies from 1.6% to 20.1%.

Any maternal or fetal factor that contributes to an increased incidence of macrosomia will increase the incidence of shoulder dystocia and brachial plexus injury. The larger the baby, the more serious the injury. It is evident that as women continue to develop greater obesity, as well as greater weight gain during the pregnancy, macrosomia has also continued to increase, thus making prevention of shoulder dystocia a more significant issue. Four factors remain as significant contributors to shoulder dystocia: macrosomia, obesity, diabetes, and operative delivery [28]. Harris has stated that "the practitioner can *usually identify* the patient who is a candidate for shoulder dystocia and macrosomia [29]. Unfortunately in 1991, the ACOG attempted to redefine macrosomia from an actual birth weight (4,000 g, or 8 lb 14 oz) to a clinical estimated fetal weight *in utero* of 4,500 g [30]. It is a well-known, proven fact that clinical estimates of fetal weight in large babies will err to the mean and thus underestimate the macrosomic infant. This leads to an unnecessary false sense of security [29].

Shoulder dystocia is not always preventable or predictable; however, in most severe cases, there are often well-defined risk factors or events that could have been identified during the antepartum and intrapartum periods. The care provider must be alert to this problem in those women with significant risk factors [31–36]. A well-prepared obstetrician or midwife can anticipate this problem as a result of routinely identifying those risk factors that predispose to shoulder dystocia. Thus, prevention requires identification of risk factors, which leads to anticipation of the problem [26,31].

Anticipation includes very careful digital evaluation of the bony birth canal, often referred to as clinical pelvimetry. The ACOG has noted that "clinical pelvimetry can be useful to qualitatively identify the general architectural features of the pelvis [2]. " The use of ultrasound to estimate fetal size can be very useful. The ACOG has confirmed the fact that "ultrasonography has been shown to be an extremely valuable tool [5]."

Perspective

The more mature and experienced clinician and reader will quickly observe that some contemporary authors (1993 to present) often misinterpret prior literature date [6]. These misleading by-products need to be kept in mind (i.e., new definitions of midpelvic extractions, macrosomia, and certain mathematical calculations regarding cesarean sections and prevention of injury). Accordingly, one does not have to be a statistician to recognize that the newer definitions and calculations are grossly inaccurate [6,37,38].

The purpose of this book is to bring together the fragmented information, and the diverse literature on this subject, and to present the subject in a logical manner. The material is organized in a simple and useful manner. A critique of various aspects of the problem is presented from the standpoint of current knowledge, statistics, and personal experience.

Prevention of shoulder dystocia will be discussed in the context of the "Three P's"; passenger, passage, and power. Extensive discussion of the identification of risk factors will be based on the preconceptual issues, antepartum factors, intrapartum factors, and the role of ultrasound.

References

1. Creasy R, Resnik R. *Maternal Fetal Medicine*. 5th ed. Philadelphia: Saunders; 2004:677.
2. American College of Obstetricians and Gynecologists. Technical Bulletin No. 218. Dystocia and the augmentation of labor. Washington, DC: ACOG; 1995.
3. Naef R, Martin J. Emergent management of shoulder dystocia. *Obstet Gynecol Clin North Am* 1995;22:247–261.
4. Gonik B, Hollyer V, Allen R. Shoulder dystocia recognition. *Am J Perinatol* 1991;6:31–34.
5. American College of Obstetricians and Gynecologists. Technical Bulletin No. 200. Diabetes and pregnancy. Washington, DC: ACOG; 1994.
6. McLeod A. Editorial comment. *Am J Obstet Gynecol* 1982;144:164.
7. Dignam WJ. Difficulties in delivery, including shoulder dystocia and malpresentation of the fetus. *Clin Obstet Gynecol* 1976;19:3–12.
8. Cunningham F, MacDonald P, Gant N. *Williams Obstetrics*. 18th ed. Norwalk, CT: Appleton-Century-Crofts; 1989.
9. Zuspan F, Quilligan E. *Douglas-Stromme Operative Obstetrics*. 5th ed. Norwalk, CT: Appleton & Lange; 1988.
10. Dignam WJ. Abnormal delivery. In: Schaefer G, Graber EA, eds. *Complications in Obstetric and Gynecologic Surgery*. Hagerstown, MD: Harper & Row; 1981:18–31.
11. Benedetti TJ, Gabbe SG. Shoulder dystocia: A complication of fetal macrosomia and prolonged second stage of labor with midpelvic delivery. *Obstet Gynecol* 1978;52:526–529.
12. Schwartz BC, Dixon DM. Shoulder dystocia. *Obstet Gynecol* 1958;11:468–475.
13. Morris W. Shoulder dystocia. *J Obstet Gynecol Br Commonw* 1955;62:302–306.
14. McCall JO Jr. Shoulder dystocia: A study of after effects. *Am J Obstet Gynecol* 1962;83:1486–1492.
15. Coustan DR, Imarah J. Prophylactic insulin treatment of gestational diabetes reduces the incidence of macrosomia, operative delivery, and birth trauma. *Am J Obstet Gynecol* 1984;150:836–842.

16. Golditch IM, Kirkman K. The large fetus: Management and outcome. *Obstet Gynecol* 1978;52:26–31.
17. Gonik B, Stringer CA, Held B. An alternate maneuver for management of shoulder dystocia. *Am J Obstet Gynecol* 1983;145:882–884.
18. Parks DG, Ziel HK. Macrosomia, a proposed indication for primary cesarean section. *Obstet Gynecol* 1978;52:407–412.
19. Levine MG, Holroyde J, Woods JR, et al. Birth trauma: Incidence and predisposing factors. *Obstet Gynecol* 1984;63::792–797.
20. Gabbe, SG, Mestman JH, Freeman RK, Anderson GV, Lowensohn RI. Management and outcome of class A diabetes mellitus. *Am J Obstet Gynecol* 1977;127:465–469.
21. Van Dorsten J. Shoulder dystocia. Precis: An update in obstetrics & gynecology. *Am Coll Obstet Gynecol.* 1998;6:95–97.
22. Nocon J, Weisbrod L. Shoulder dystocia. In: Goodwin R, ed. *Operative Obstetrics.* Baltimore: Williams & Wilkins; 1995:341.
23. Gonik B, Hollyer V, Allen R. Shoulder dystocia recognition. *Am J Perinatol* 1991;8:31–34.
24. Hopwood HG. Shoulder dystocia: Fifteen years' experience in a community hospital. *Am J Obstet Gynecol* 1982;144:162–166.
25. Sack RA. The large infant: A study of maternal, obstetric, fetal, and newborn characteristics including a long-term pediatric follow-up. *Am J Obstet Gynecol* 1969;104:195–204.
26. Swartz DP. Shoulder girdle dystocia in vertex delivery: Clinical study and review. *Obstet Gynecol* 1960;15:194–206.
27. Bolton RN. Some considerations of excessive fetal development. *Am J Obstet Gynecol* 1959;77:118–121.
28. Lee C. Shoulder dystocia. *Clin Obstet Gynecol* 1987;30:77–82.
29. Harris B. Unexpected mechanical dystocia. In: Fadel H, ed. *Diagnosis and Management of Obstetric Emergencies.* Reading, MA: Addison-Wesley Co.; 1983.
30. American College of Obstetricians and Gynecologists. Technical Bulletin No. 159. Fetal macrosomia. Washington, DC: ACOG; 1991.
31. Ott WJ. The diagnosis of altered fetal growth. *Obstet Gynecol Clin North Am* 1988;15:237–263.
32. Miller JM Jr, Brown HL, Pastorek JG II, Gabert HA. Fetal overgrowth, diabetic versus nondiabetic. *J Ultrasound Med* 1988;7:577–579.
33. Miller JM Jr, Kissling GE, Brown HL, Nagel PM, Korndorffer FA III, Gabert HA. In utero growth of the large for menstrual age fetus. *J Clin Ultrasound* 1989;17:15–17.
34. Landon MB, Mintz MC, Gabbe SG. Sonographic evaluation of fetal abdominal growth: Predictor of the large for gestational age infant in pregnancies complicated by diabetes mellitus. *Am J Obstet Gynecol* 1989;160:115–121.
35. Lindsay MK, Graves W, Klein L. The relationship of one abnormal glucose tolerance test value and pregnancy complications. *Obstet Gynecol* 1989;73:103–106.
36. Cohen W, Acker D, Friedman E. *Management of Labor.* 2nd ed. Rockville, MD: Aspen Publications; 1989:37–42.
37. Gurewitsch E, Johnson E, Hamzehzadeh S, Allen R. Am J Obstet Gynecol 2006;194:486–492.
38. Apuzzio J, Vintzileos A, Iffy L. Shoulder dystocia. In: *Operative Obstetrics.* 3rd ed. London: Taylor & Francis; 2006:253–263.

Part I
Prevention

Chapter 1
Preconceptual Risk Factors

James A. O'Leary

Summary Identification of risk factors and anticipation of shoulder dystocia will help prevent fetal injury.

Keywords: diabetes · macrosomia · obesity

Contents

1.1   Introduction   3
1.2   Maternal Birthweight   4
1.3   Maternal Age   5
1.4   Maternal Height   7
1.5   Obesity   8
1.6   Obesity and Diabetes   11
1.7   Conclusion   11

1.1 Introduction

The simplest and easiest approach to shoulder dystocia is prevention. Thus, obstetricians must have a high level of anticipatory knowledge to avoid this catastrophic event. Such a mindset can only be developed by learning and identifying those risk factors involved in shoulder dystocia. Identification of critical risk factors will lead to anticipation, which in turn will lead to prevention. The risk factors for shoulder dystocia can be divided into preconceptual risk factors, antepartum risk factors, and intrapartum risk factors. This chapter will deal with preconceptual issues.

Risk factors for shoulder dystocia are similar to those for cephalopelvic disproportion [1–14] and can be considered under the triad of the "Three P's": passenger, passage, and power. Preconceptual, or prepregnancy, risk factors relate only to the passage and the patient herself and should be evident to the

J.A. O'Leary
Professor Obstetrics & Gynecology (retired), University of South Florida, Tampa, Florida, USA

J.A. O'Leary (ed.), *Shoulder Dystocia and Birth Injury*,
DOI 10.1007/978-1-59745-473-5_1, © Humana Press, a part of Springer
Science+Business Media, LLC 2009

examiner at the first office visit. Individuals providing obstetric care should have a firm commitment to the recognition of these risk factors and the knowledge and skill to perform clinical pelvimetry. The preconceptual risk factors are an abnormal pelvis, especially the flat or platypelloid pelvis, and those maternal issues that lead to macrosomia.

A strong index of suspicion for a difficult delivery and birth injury is an ongoing responsibility for providers of obstetric care. The optimum time to identify these risk factors is at the first prenatal visit or first gynecologic office visit. Ideally, a woman receiving preconceptual counseling can be alerted to those factors that might be correctable. For example, maternal glucose intolerance will account for 10% of macrosomic infants. Large maternal stature or excessive weight gain in pregnancy will account for slightly more than 50% of macrosomic infants. Thus, women at risk for glucose intolerance or excessive weight gain can be counseled on the need to monitor such events. However, the cause in at least one third of macrosomic infants remains unexplained [15–21].

1.2 Maternal Birthweight

The value of ascertaining maternal birthweight has recently been reconfirmed [22–31]. Klebanoff et al. [22] demonstrated that a mother's birthweight has a strong influence on her child's birthweight. Identifying infants whose macrosomia is due to familial factors is important [23], as this explains some previously "idiopathic" large infants. It may also make it possible to distinguish those infants with benign macrosomia from the subset of infants that are high risk or large for gestational age (LGA). Furthermore, it alerts the obstetrician caring for the small woman who was herself large at birth to the increased possibility of a large infant at delivery. Klebanoff's study was one of the first to examine the effect of a mother's birthweight on her risk of producing a macrosomic infant independent of other known risk factors. It demonstrated that women who were large at birth are at increased risk of giving birth to a large infant. In fact, maternal birthweight is more strongly associated with accelerated fetal growth than is either current maternal height or weight.

This relationship between a mother's own birthweight and the risk of delivering an LGA infant was based on studies in 1,335 women. Compared with women who weighed 8 lb or more at birth, women who weighed 6 to 7.9 lb were only 50% as likely (P = .007), and women who weighed 4 to 5.9 lb were only 15% as likely (P = .002), to give birth to an LGA infant. When this relationship was adjusted for nine other factors known to influence birthweight, including maternal weight and weight gain during pregnancy, maternal birthweight was second only to weight gain during pregnancy in predicting the birth of LGA infants. Maternal birthweight was also accurate in the prediction of macrosomia (birthweight >4,000 g). Therefore, a mother's birthweight should become part of the routine obstetric and gynecologic history.

Table 1.1 Key Preconceptual Historical Risk Factors

1.	Maternal birthweight
2.	Prior shoulder dystocia
3.	Prior macrosomia
4.	Preexisting diabetes
5.	Obesity
6.	Multiparity
7.	Prior gestational diabetes
8.	Advanced maternal age

The risk of macrosomia will increase from 15.1% to 31.5% when more than one risk factor is present. Preconceptual counseling will help to identify eight key potential predictors of a shoulder dystocia (Table 1.1). The more factors present, the greater the risk. As suggested, the presence of these factors is not only additive but also may be synergistic.

1.3 Maternal Age

Since 1980, a rather impressive proportion of American women above the age of 35 years began to have babies, and many of these women were pregnant for the first time [19]. In 1950 was coined the hapless term *elderly primigravida* as a descriptor of obstetric risk. Five decades later, older maternal age is increasingly an issue of perinatal concern. Live births to women aged 30 to 34 years increased from 18.9% of all live births in 1982 to 30.6% in 2002. The relative change in live births to women 35 years or older was even larger, with the proportion of live births to women 35 to 39 years of age increasing from 4.7% in 1982 to 14.1% in 2002 and those among women 40 years of age or older increasing from 0.6% to 2.6%. Similar increases in older maternal age categories have been observed in other industrialized countries [16].

As a net result of these factors, a larger percentage of American women are between the ages of 35 and 50 years. Combined with the trend among many women to delay childbearing due to women's career opportunities, advanced education, infertility, control over fertility, late and second marriages, and financial concerns, the birth rate for the 1990s has shown a dramatic increase for women older than 35 years. The United States Bureau of the Census estimates that because of the higher birth rate of women older than 35 years combined with the decrease in the number of women aged 20 to 29 years, the proportion of babies born to these older women has almost doubled by the end of the 1990s compared with the early 1980s. Specifically, as noted by Eastman [24], the proportion of total births in women over 35 years of age has increased from 5% in 1982 to 8.6% in the year 2000. Thus, the impact of older maternal age on pregnancy becomes increasingly important.

Maternal age as a risk factor in pregnancy has a long history, but maternal age as a risk factor for shoulder dystocia has not received great emphasis. The significance of increasing age here is its relationship to increasing birthweight, diabetes, and obesity. In the mnemonic that helps to predict macrosomia, "A DOPE," "A" refers to maternal age, which is associated with increased fetal birthweight as maternal age advances. The mature gravida over age 30 is at much greater risk for macrosomia and therefore shoulder dystocia. She is also at increased risk for obesity, diabetes, and excessive weight gain, as well as postdatism or a postterm gestation.

The definition of advanced maternal age in the obstetric literature is varied. Most authors have designated a lower limit of 35 years, others, 40 years, and a few have even indicated that 45 years represents advanced maternal age. Regardless of the specific age definition, pregnancies in women of advanced maternal age are considered by many to be high risk.

Generally, the incidence of most chronic illnesses increases as a function of age; it is not surprising, therefore, that medical complications are encountered more frequently in women who are older than 35 years. It follows logically that the severity and associated complications of many of these conditions increase, as does their duration, and thus it is likely that older pregnant women will have more advanced forms of chronic disorders. Perhaps the best example is diabetes, the incidence of which increases with age, and most type II, or non–insulin-dependent, diabetics are age 40 or older.

Using a computerized database from a perinatal network, 511 pregnancies in women whose age was 40 years or older at delivery were studied by Spellacy [20]. The oldest woman was aged 52 years. This group represented 1.2% of the 41,335 women delivering. Their pregnancy outcomes were compared with those of 26,759 women whose ages at delivery were 20 to 30 years. The older women were of greater parity and had higher weights. There was also an increased frequency of hypertension, diabetes mellitus, and placenta previa in the older women [24].

Spellacy showed [20] that the older women experienced an increase in infant macrosomia, male sex, stillbirths, and low Apgar scores. They also had a higher incidence of cesarean section and fewer forceps deliveries. The older women whose individual weights were less than 67.5 kg at delivery did not show any difference in hypertension, fetal macrosomia, fetal death rates, or low infant Apgar scores.

The results of the Spellacy study [20] confirm many earlier reported observations. The frequency of pregnancy in older women (>40 years) in this study was 1.2%, which is similar to that reported by others. The older women were of higher weight and had an increased frequency of both hypertension and diabetes mellitus. These factors most probably contributed to the increased frequency of cesarean section in older women.

The impact of maternal age is also noted in infant outcomes. Thus, older women have heavier infants with significant increases in macrosomia, low Apgar scores, and fetal deaths. When maternal obesity is removed as a factor, there are no differences in maternal hypertension, macrosomia, fetal deaths, and Apgar scores. Older women more frequently have male infants, shoulder dystocia, and brachial plexus injuries. Although advanced maternal age may have an adverse effect on pregnancy and delivery, the major impact seems to be related to the effect of increased weight and parity rather than to age itself.

As studies have shown, mature gravidas, age 30 years and over, can be expected to be heavier and have more macrosomic infants, with a concomitant risk for shoulder dystocia. The risk for macrosomia with increasing maternal age is as follows:

Maternal Age (y)	Incidence of Macrosomia (%)
10–19	4
20–29	8
20–29	8
30–39	12

It is difficult to separate maternal gestational diabetes, obesity, and antenatal weight gain from the age factor. The clinician must be aware that older mothers are at risk for increased fetal weight. This awareness should trigger more thorough nutritional counseling, fastidious measurement of fetal growth, liberal use of ultrasound, careful checking for maternal glucose intolerance, and strict control of antenatal weight gain.

The overwhelming majority of studies in the obstetric literature describe a significantly higher rate of cesarean births in older women. Kirz et al. [15] noted an increased use of cesarean delivery for the older age group. No one specific indication for cesarean birth showed an increase in the pregnancies of women over 34 years of age. It may be that the increase is cesarean births for older women is a self-fulfilling prophecy. Because the pregnancies have been considered high risk, the physician may use a lower threshold for terminating the labor process. Pregnant women of advanced maternal age received epidural anesthesia significantly more often than did younger parturients. This may be a contributing factor to the higher rate of forceps and vacuum deliveries for the older age group and to the incidence of shoulder dystocia and birth injury.

1.4 Maternal Height

It is a well-known fact that short obstetric patients have more difficult and prolonged labor. The risks of shoulder dystocia and cesarean section are higher among short women, particularly those with large fetuses, than among tall women.

In a study of 7,543 low-risk women, short stature (less than 5 feet 2 inches) was associated with nearly a doubling in the risk of cesarean section among women delivering their first child (odds ratio 1.72) as well as multiparous women (odds ratio 2.09). Tall stature (more than 5 feet 5 inches) halved the risk in first deliveries (odds ratio 0.42). Tallness had no impact on subsequent births, whose risk of cesarean section (odds ratio 1.01) was about the same as that of average-height women (5 feet 2 inches to 5 feet 4 inches).

On the basis of these results, "physicians should consider the timely and judicious use of cesarean section in short women." Short women also had nearly twice the risk of shoulder dystocia (odds ratio 1.8) compared with that of tall women (odds ratio 0.58).

Absolute weight gain, regardless of height, also had an impact. The authors determined that when weight gain was over 35 lb, there appeared to be an increase in the risk of adverse outcomes. Height however, did not modify the effect of weight gain on outcomes [25].

1.5 Obesity

Maternal obesity is a very serious obstetric risk factor. In a discussion of shoulder dystocia or macrosomia, it must be given strong emphasis. It may have greater importance than does diabetes mellitus. Over the past 15 years, Americans have significantly increased their annual consumption of food from as much as 600 lb per year to more than 700 lb per year, and thus obesity is on the increase.

The literature supports a relationship between obesity and coexisting medical illnesses such as diabetes and hypertension. Perinatal adverse outcomes include an increased incidence of stillbirth and congenital anomalies. There is also an established relationship between maternal obesity and fetal macrosomia [26]. Since 1991, there has been a 50% to 70% increase in the rate of obesity in adults of reproductive age [2].

There is strong evidence for the relationship between macrosomia and shoulder dystocia; current case-control studies have demonstrated a higher prevalence of obesity in pregnancies affected by shoulder dystocia than in the corresponding control group [26].

In this large, prospectively collected cohort, it was found that obese and morbidly obese patients were at increased risk for gestational diabetes. The incidence of gestational diabetes in both obese (6.3%) and morbidly obese (9.5%) patients was increased compared with the control group (2.3%). These findings are consistent with previous studies. Creasy and Resnick [27] reported the incidence of gestational diabetes to be 24.5% for patients with a body mass index (BMI) greater than 40 compared with 2.2% for patients with a BMI of 20 to 24.9 (P < .0001). These authors reported an incidence of gestational diabetes of 14.2% for patients with a BMI greater than 35 compared with 4.3% for patients with a BMI of 19 to 27 (P < .01). for nulliparous patients, the cesarean delivery rate was 20.7% for the control group, 33.8% for obese, and 47.4% for morbidly obese patients [28].

The relationship between maternal size and fetal size is interesting. These findings confirm this association. These authors [28] found that both obese and morbidly obese patients have a significantly increased risk for birthweight greater than 4,500 g compared with controls. These findings are important to remember when clinically estimating fetal weight in the labor room. The clinician should know that a large fetus is more common in the obese and morbidly obese population.

Obese patients may have difficulty completing the second stage of labor secondary to soft tissue dystocia, and operative vaginal delivery may be used to expedite delivery in such a situation. After controlling for birthweight, the current study found that morbidly obese patients were more likely to have an operative vaginal delivery than were patients with a BMI less than 30. However, once again the odds ratio was less than 2.0 [28].

The effect of obesity alone was investigated by Garbaciak et al. [29] among 16,858 women who delivered their infants within a 12-month period. Complete analysis was possible for 9,667 patients, who were divided into four weight categories and separated into two groups, those with and those without complications. Perinatal mortality, infant size, and the primary cesarean delivery rate were calculated for each group. Among 2,597 women with prenatal complications, there was a significant increase in perinatal mortality ($P < .001$), primary cesarean delivery ($P < .02$), and mean infant birth weight ($P < .01$) in the obese and the morbidly obese gravid women. Obesity alone did not appear to affect the perinatal mortality rate, but it increased the likelihood of cesarean delivery in the morbidly obese patient, shoulder dystocia, and brachial plexus palsy.

In addition to careful measurement of fetal growth and fundal height measurements, the liberal use of ultrasound measurements in obese women is clearly indicated. The early identification of risk factors will permit early therapy, which should include careful dietary counseling, repeated blood sugar measurements, and weight restriction. Anticipation of the need for abdominal delivery should be noted early. Liberal use of labor induction may be helpful, as well as ultrasound measurements of fetal size at term. The recognition of a macrosomic child in the obese mother requires diligent search for any additional risk factors for shoulder dystocia, if vaginal delivery is considered. Cesarean section is indicated if these factors exist. Inability to evaluate the pelvis in such circumstances may justify imaging pelvimetry and/or consultation. The presence of macrosomia of 4,500 g alone is justification for cesarean section in nonobese women. The presence of macrosomia of 4,000 to 4,500 g may in itself be sufficient to warrant abdominal delivery when other risk factors, especially a platypelloid (flat) pelvis, diabetes, and/or obesity, are present.

Johnson and coauthors [30] recently reviewed the complications of pregnancy in 588 obese women who weighed at least 113.6 kg (250 lb) during pregnancy and in a matched control group of women who weighed less than 90.0 kg (200 lb) during pregnancy. The investigators noted that the incidence of pregnancy complicated by obesity more than doubled during the 20-year time interval of the study. The rates of diabetes and hypertension were significantly higher in the obese group (9.9% and 27.6%, respectively) than in the control group (2.2% and 3.1%, respectively). Therapeutic induction of labor was more common for the obese patients (23.5%) than in the control group (2.2%). The rate of failure of attempted inductions was significantly greater in the obese group (1%) than in the control group (1.5%). The indications for induction in the obese group included postdatism, hypertension, preeclampsia, diabetes, and premature rupture of the membranes without effective labor.

Shoulder dystocia occurred approximately twice as often in the morbidly obese patient without prenatal complications (1.78%) when compared with the normal-weight patient (0.81%) [30]. More recent data suggest that a significant increase in cesarean deliveries is present as a function of maternal obesity. If obese gravid women are at increased risk for prenatal complications, this increase in primary cesarean deliveries could be expected. However, between each weight category in those patients without prenatal complications, a significant increase in the number of cesarean sections was present for those patients who were morbidly obese.

Previous reports have concluded that fetal weight is directly proportional to maternal size. Emerson [31] reported that more than 50% of overweight women had babies who weighed over 8 lb (3,630 g). Eastman and Jackson [24] have shown a straight-line correlation between weight of the newborn infant and maternal weight gain in pregnancy of more than 10 lb. They also showed a direct correlation between prepregnant maternal weight and eventual infant birthweight. They believed that these two factors acted independently and additively in determining the baby's weight and concluded that mothers who are heavier prior to conception will deliver heavier babies. Others have not only reported a significant increase in macrosomic babies in obese populations but have also noted a significant lengthening of the gestational period [20–23].

These data reveal a significant difference in mean infant birthweight among obese patients both with and without prenatal complications. As the weight of the mother increases, so does the weight of the newborn infant. Analyzing the correlation of fetal weight with maternal weight revealed that only 24% and 27% of the increase in fetal weight in women with and without prenatal complications, respectively, could be attributed to maternal weight alone. This tendency for increased birthweight as maternal weight increased was also present in those women who had prenatal complications.

Gross et al. [4] recently reported a higher incidence of macrosomic babies in their population of obese women. If this increase of macrosomia is present, it could serve as an explanation for the increase in primary cesarean sections, although this was not found in the study of Gross et al. This difference between studies may be due to the different way obesity was defined in their study and in the aforementioned British study [3] and the fact that Gross et al. did not differentiate obese women from morbidly obese women.

The best way to prevent the problems associated with morbidly obese and obese gravid women would be to eliminate the prepregnant obese state. Because this is not realistically possible, it is necessary for those attending such patients to be aware of the specific complications that can occur. This author recommends that all obese and morbidly obese gravid women have a glucose screening test for diabetes at their initial prenatal visit, and that it be repeated at the beginning of the third trimester, if the previous screen was normal. It seems prudent to avoid vaginal delivery in the morbidly obese patient who is at risk for any type of dystocia that is not easily correctable.

1.6 Obesity and Diabetes

The problems of maternal obesity are difficult to separate from gestational diabetes or overt diabetes; however, Johnson and colleagues [30] reported that in pregnant women weighing more than 250 lb, the incidence of shoulder dystocia was 5.1% compared with 0.6% for control women who weighed less than 200 lb. Spellacy and co-workers [20] reported that for women weighing more than 90 kg, infant birthweight distribution was as follows: 8.2% weighed 2,500 to 3,499 g, 33% weighed 4,500 to 4,999 g, and 50% weighed more than 5,000 g. Shoulder dystocia was identified in 0.3% of the 2,500 to 3,499 g infants, 7.3% of the 4,500 to 4,999 g infants, and 14.6% of the larger infants. Parks and Ziel [32] reported that when maternal prepregnancy or early pregnancy weight was above 90 kg, 5.5% of infants weighed more than 4,500 g compared with 1.9% in a control group. Shoulder dystocia was identified in 13.6% of infants who weighed more than 4,500 g compared with 1.7% in the control group.

The association of macrosomia with mild diabetes mellitus is well established and in the studies discussed above was a significant contributing factor in shoulder dystocia and brachial plexus injury [27].

1.7 Conclusion

Maternal age over 30 years, maternal obesity and height, as well as high maternal birthweight are significant risk factors for macrosomia, and thus the risk of shoulder dystocia is increased in this population. Identification of an abnormal pelvis in these women is critically important.

References

1. Calandra C, Abell D, Beischer N. 1981 Maternal obesity in pregnancy. *Obstet Gynecol* 1981;57:8–14
2. Carpenter M, Coustan D. Criteria for screening tests for gestational diabetes. *Am J Obstet Gynecol* 1982;144:768–772.

3. Edwards L, Dickes W, Alton I, et al. Pregnancy in the massively obese: Course, outcome, and obesity prognosis of the infant. *Am J Obstet Gynecol* 1978;131:479–483.
4. Gross T, Sokol R, King K. Obesity in pregnancy: Risks and outcome. *Obstet Gynecol* 1980;56:446–551.
5. Kerr M. The problem of the overweight patient in pregnancy. *Br J Obstet Gynaecol* 1962;69:988–994.
6. Maeder E, Barno A, Mecklenburg F. Obesity: A maternal high-risk factor. *Obstet Gynecol* 1975;45:669–674.
7. Naeye R. Weight gain and the outcome of pregnancy. *Am J Obstet Gynecol* 1979;135:3–7.
8. Tracy T, Miller G. Obstetric problems of the massively obese. *Obstet Gynecol* 1969;33:204–209.
9. Jovanovic L, Peterson C. Screening for gestational diabetes. *Diabetes* 1985;34:21–26.
10. Leikin E, Jenkins J, Pomerantz G, Klein L. Abnormal glucose screening tests in pregnancy: A risk factor for fetal macrosomia. *Obstet Gynecol* 1987;69:570–74.
11. Gabbe S, Mestman J, Freeman R, Anderson G, Lowensohn R. Management and outcome of class A diabetes mellitus. *Am J Obstet Gynecol* 1977;127:465–469.
12. Grimes D, Gross G. Pregnancy outcomes in black women aged 35 and older. *Obstet Gynecol* 1981;58:614–618.
13. Hansen J. Older maternal age and pregnancy outcome: A review of the literature. *Obstet Gynecol Surv* 1986;41:726–731.
14. Kajanoja P, Widholm O. Pregnancy and delivery in women aged 40 and over. *Obstet Gynecol* 1978;51:47–53.
15. Kirz D, Dorchester W, Freeman R. Advanced maternal age: The mature gravida. *Am J Obstet Gynecol* 1985;152:7–11.
16. Lehman D, Chism J. Pregnancy outcome in medically complicated and uncomplicated patients aged 40 years or older. *Am J Obstet Gynecol* 1987;157:738–744.
17. Martel M, Wacholder S, Lippman A, Brohan J, Hamilton E. Maternal age and primary cesarean section rates: A multivariate analysis. *Am J Obstet Gynecol* 1987;156:305–310.
18. Mestman J. Outcome of diabetes screening in pregnancy and perinatal morbidity in infants of mothers with mild impairment in glucose tolerance. *Diabetes Care* 1980;3:447–451.
19. Modanlcu H, Dorchester W, Thorosian A, Freeman R. Macrosomia—maternal, fetal and neonatal implications. *Obstet Gynecol* 1980;55:420–426.
20. Spellacy W, Miller M, Winegar A, Peterson P. Macrosomia—maternal characteristics and infant complications. *Obstet Gynecol* 1985;66:158–162.
21. Yasin S, Beydoun S. Pregnancy outcome at greater than or equal to 20-weeks gestation in women in their 40s. A case control study. *J Reprod Med* 1988;33:209–212.
22. Klebanoff M, Mills J, Berendes H. Mothers birth weight as a predictor of macrosomia. *Am J Obstet Gynecol* 1985;153:253–258.
23. Coustan D, Widness J, Carpenter M, Rotondo L, Pratt D, Oh W. Should the fifty gram, one hour plasma glucose screening test for gestational diabetes be administered in the fasting or fed state? *Am J Obstet Gynecol* 1986;154:1031–1035.
24. Eastman N, Jackson E. Weight relations in pregnancy. *Obstet Gynecol Survey* 1968;23:1003–1024.
25 Gurewitsch E, Johnson E, Hamzehzadeh S, Allen R. *Am J Obstet Gynecol* 2006;194:486–492.
26. Robinson H, Tkatch S, Mayes A, Bott N, Okun N. Is maternal obesity a predictor of shoulder dystocia? *Am J Obstet Gynecol* 2003;101:24–27.
27. Creasy R, Resnik R. *Maternal-Fetal Medicine*. Fifth ed. Philadelphia: Saunders; 2004:1035.
28. Weiss, J, Malone F, Emig D, et al. Obesity, obstetric complications and cesarean delivery rate—a population-based screening study. *Am J Obstet Gynecol* 2004;190:1091–1097.
29. Garbaciak J, Richter M, Miller S, Barton J. Maternal weight and pregnancy complications. *Am J Obstet Gynecol* 1985;152:238–242.

30. Johnson S, Kolberg B, Varner M. Maternal obesity and pregnancy. *Surg Gynecol Obstet* 1987;164:431–435.
31. Emerson R. Obesity and its association with the complications of pregnancy. *Br Med J* 1962;2:515–519.
32. Parks D, Ziel H. Macrosomia, a proposed indication for primary cesarean section. *Obstet Gynecol* 1978;52:407–412.

Chapter 2
Antepartum Risk Factors

James A. O'Leary

Summary Identification of risk factors allows anticipation of shoulder dystocia and prevention of brachial plexus palsy. Obesity, diabetes, and increased fundal height are the most important risk factors.

Keywords: brachial plexus palsy · diabetes · macrosomia · shoulder dystocia risk factors

Contents

2.1   Introduction   15
2.2   Gestational Diabetes and Borderline Diabetes   16
2.3   Overt Diabetes   20
2.4   Postdate Pregnancy   23
2.5   Obesity   26
2.6   Excessive Weight Gain   27
2.7   Fundal Height   29
2.8   Conclusion   29

2.1 Introduction

The majority of physicians believe that there is a constellation of antepartum and intrapartum clinical features that indicate a predisposition to shoulder dystocia. By recognizing these warning signs, the alert practitioner should be able to avert or manage a shoulder dystocia successfully in *most* circumstances [1].

The major risk factors for shoulder dystocia (Table 2.1), especially those that lead to fetal injury, are included in the mnemonic "A DOPE": age, diabetes (including prediabetes), obesity, postdatism, and excessive weight gain [2–18].

Other risk factors frequently mentioned, such as maternal birthweight, prior shoulder dystocia, multiparity, and a history of birth injury and/or stillbirth,

J.A. O'Leary
Professor Obstetrics & Gynecology (retired), University of South Florida, Tampa, Florida, USA

J.A. O'Leary (ed.), *Shoulder Dystocia and Birth Injury*,
DOI 10.1007/978-1-59745-473-5_2, © Humana Press, a part of Springer Science+Business Media, LLC 2009

Table 2.1 Antepartum Risk Factors

Glucose intolerance or excess
Excessive weight gain
Macrosomia
Short stature
Abnormal pelvic shape
Abnormal pelvic size
Postdatism

must be incorporated into the clinical assessment of obstetric patients, during both the pregnancy and the intrapartum period [18–32].

A 1995 report of 16,471 births defined the key risk factors predictive of shoulder dystocia to be a birthweight in excess of 3,600 g, diabetes, lower social class, Indian origin, obesity, four prior births, and Pitocin (oxytocin, Parke-Davis, Indiana, USA) [19].

2.2 Gestational Diabetes and Borderline Diabetes

Pregnancy-induced glucose intolerance includes gestational diabetes and cases with one abnormal value or two borderline values on a 3-hour glucose tolerance test (GTT); it represents a significant risk factor for macrosomia and shoulder dystocia [20–25]. Gestational diabetes is carbohydrate intolerance induced by pregnancy. This definition excludes the possibility that glucose intolerance may have antedated pregnancy. Use of the diagnostic term *gestational diabetes* communicates the need for high-risk surveillance to third-party payers or others responsible for the financing of health care delivery and to convince women of the need for further testing postpartum. Gestational diabetes is a heterogeneous disorder with varied worldwide prevalence. Indeed, in a 10-year survey [21], the reported prevalence of gestational diabetes varied from 0.15% to 12.3%.

It is well-known that women with fasting hyperglycemia are at greater risk for fetal death and that this danger is not apparent for those with postprandial hyperglycemia only [26]. Today, the perinatal focal point is avoidance of difficult delivery due to macrosomia and of concomitant neonatal morbidity from birth trauma and shoulder dystocia with elevated fasting glucose.

2.2.1 Identification

The obvious advantage of identifying gestational diabetes is increased awareness of potential shoulder dystocia [22–29]. Bochner and colleagues [30] reported the outcomes of 201 gestational diabetics whose fasting and postprandial glucose values were normalized with diet. Fetal abdominal circumference was measured ultrasonically between 30 and 33 weeks. For infants with values over the 90th percentile, 40% weighed more than 4,000 g at delivery, and there was an increased incidence of cesarean section for failure to progress, shoulder dystocia, and birth trauma. Conversely, if the size of the circumference was below the 90th percentile, these complications were not increased compared with the normal population. The predictive value of abdominal circumference measurements greater than the 90th percentile was 56%, thus supporting the role of ultrasound.

It is emphasized that the pregnant woman with a normal fasting glucose level but an abnormal GTT early in pregnancy may develop overt diabetes late in pregnancy and be at increased risk for significant macrosomia. The incidence is estimated to be about 15%, and thus fasting glucose levels should be checked periodically.

All pregnant women should be screened for glucose intolerance in the second trimester. Patients at high risk should receive a repeat screen or its equivalent in the third trimester. The nonfasting 50 g glucose screen should be used. Values above 135 to 140 mg% are considered abnormal. At least 5% to 10% of the gestational diabetics and insulin-dependent patients will have infants who develop macrosomia. The presence of glucose excess, especially if the abnormal value is the fasting blood sugar, will greatly increase risk for shoulder dystocia, especially if any prepregnancy risk factors are present. In O'Shaughnessy's series, approximately 50% of the diabetic pregnancies resulted in large for gestational age (LGA) infants [31].

The diagnosis of gestational diabetes is based on criteria originally proposed by O'Sullivan and Mahan [32], which include at least two abnormal values on a 3-hour oral GTT. The increased incidence of maternal and fetal complications among patients with gestational diabetes is now well established.

Of the 2,276 patients studied by Leikin et al. [20] who underwent screening for gestational diabetes mellitus, 81.5% had normal glucose screening tests after a 50 g carbohydrate load (serum glucose <135 mg/dL). Of the 15.7% who had abnormal glucose screening tests and went on to complete 3-hour GTT, 48.7% were shown to be nondiabetic when further tested with a 3-hour GTT. The 176 women with abnormal glucose screens but normal GTTs were compared with the 1,854 who had normal screening values. The frequency of infants weighing more than 4,000 g was 11.9% in the study group and 6.4% in the control group (P = .0086). When the data were corrected for other macrosomia risk factors (advanced age, multiparity, obesity, white race, and prolonged gestation), there was still a significantly higher frequency of macrosomia in the study group; this demonstrates that patients with minor abnormalities of carbohydrate metabolism during pregnancy are at risk for delivering a macrosomic infant. These results are similar to those of Frisoli et al. [28], who reported macrosomia in 6 infants of a group of 22 mothers who had an abnormal glucose screening but normal findings on GTT between the 30th and 34th weeks of gestation.

In the study of Al-Shawaf et al. [33] of 218 pregnant women with abnormal glucose tolerance, 81.2% had impaired glucose tolerance and 18.8% had gestational diabetes. Gestational diabetic women were of higher parity, more obese, required insulin therapy more often, had more babies weighing more than 4,000 g, and had higher fasting plasma glucose than women with impaired glucose tolerance. Women with gestational impaired glucose tolerance were older, more obese, of higher parity, and had heavier babies than did pregnant women with a normal screening plasma glucose.

It behooves all care providers to consider every obese patient as high risk for shoulder dystocia. The combination of obesity and diabetes makes these patients very high risk for shoulder dystocia, and thus the threshold for cesarean section should be reduced. Langer studied this association in 4,001 patients. He concluded that achievement of targeted levels of glycemic control was associated with enhanced outcome only in women treated with insulin [34]!

2.2.2 One Abnormal Value

All studies suggest that patients with minor abnormalities of carbohydrate metabolism during pregnancy are at risk for delivering a macrosomic infant [35]. Pregnant patients of the type identified in these studies benefit from dietary control and more intensive evaluation of their fasting and postprandial glucose levels. It is necessary to determine whether such measures would prevent the increased incidence of macrosomia in this population and thus limit the potential morbidity of mothers and their infants.

In a report by Lindsay et al. [36], the presence of either a single abnormality on the oral GTT or an abnormal glucose screen was associated with an increased risk of pregnancy complications. It was clear from those data that a single oral GTT abnormality alone could identify such complications. They screened 4,618 pregnant women for gestational diabetes between the 24th and 28th weeks of gestation. Eighty-seven percent had normal results; of the 13% with abnormal screening tests, 139 had one abnormal value on the subsequent 3-hour oral GTT. These women were then compared with 725 randomly selected patients with a normal screening test. The incidence of macrosomia (birthweight >4,000 g) was significantly greater in the study group (18.0%) than in the control group (6.6%), a relationship that persisted after controlling for confounding risk factors by logistic regression modeling. The results prove that patients with one abnormal value on an oral GTT during pregnancy are at risk for delivering macrosomic infants.

Women with one abnormal value on the 3-hour GTT have been found to be at increase risk for fetal macrosomia. If repeated, one third will have gestational diabetes [37].

Gestational diabetes is associated with fetal macrosomia, cesarean delivery, preeclampsia, neonatal hypoglycemia, and perinatal death. In the United States, the most widely accepted screening and diagnosing scheme for gestational diabetes is the National Diabetes Data Group stepwise algorithm, in which a 50-g, 1-hour glucose challenge test (GCT) is administered universally at

24 to 28 gestational weeks, followed by a 100-g, 3-hour GTT in GCT positive patients. A patient is diagnosed with gestational diabetes if two or more of four values are elevated on the GTT. This scheme has false-negative and false-positive rates; the sensitivity and specificity of the GCT are 27% and 89%, respectively. Based on a gestational diabetes prevalence of 5%, the positive and negative predictive values of the GCT are 1% and 95%, respectively; depending on the presence or absence of clinical risk factors, the GCT has a positive predictive value of 12% to 40%. Although an exact estimate of the negative predictive value for the GCT-GTT scheme is difficult to establish, it seems that a significant proportion of GTT-negative patients will develop fetal macrosomia or be identified as diabetic at a later time, especially those with risk factors. The National Diabetes Data Group screening algorithm, has shown that nondiabetic "glucose intolerant" patients identified by the WHO diagnostic criteria are at increased risk for shoulder dystocia, cesarean delivery, and fetal macrosomia [37].

Minor degrees of carbohydrate intolerance during pregnancy have been reported to be associated with an increased risk of macrosomia. Witter and Niebyl [38] evaluated whether the glucose screen is useful in predicting macrosomia in patients who are not gestational diabetics. They agreed that minor abnormalities of carbohydrate metabolism in pregnancy are a risk factor for delivery of a macrosomic infant. Recently Langer et al. [34] observed that women with a positive 1-hour glucocola and normal GTT were at increased risk for cesarean section and shoulder dystocia. The study group had a significantly higher cesarean delivery rate (31.1% vs. 21.1%, P = .043) and shoulder dystocia incidence (9.7% vs. 2.3%, P = .007). The risk for shoulder dystocia was independent of prepregnancy body mass and weight gain during pregnancy.

2.2.3 Abnormal Screen, Normal 3-Hour GTT

It has been reported previously that pregnant women with abnormal 1-hour glucose screens but normal oral GTTs were more likely to deliver a macrosomic infant than were women whose glucose screens were normal. An abnormal glucose screen was defined as greater than 135 mg/dL in one study and as more than 150 mg/dL in the other study [39]. We can confirm these findings. Further, even those women whose glucose screens are more than 135 mg/dL with normal GTTs deliver macrosomic infants more often than do those whose glucose screens are less than 130 mg/dL. This confirms that minor abnormalities in carbohydrate metabolism are a risk factor for delivery of a macrosomic infant. A negative screen does not signal a lesser risk of macrosomia and should not be considered reassuring in women with risk factors.

In summary, a minor abnormality of carbohydrate metabolism in pregnancy is a risk factor for delivering a macrosomic infant. However, the 50-g, 1-hour oral glucose screen at 28 weeks is not a useful screening test for ruling out macrosomia in the pregnant patient with a normal GTT.

2.3 Overt Diabetes

It is unquestioned that overt diabetes has a significant impact on pregnancy outcome. The infant and mother can experience very serious complications. The likelihood of successful outcomes for the infant and the diabetic mother are related to the degree of diabetes control.

The definition of infants of diabetic mothers (IDMs) as either macrosomic or not may be misleading, because it implies a bimodal distribution of birthweights. The distribution of birthweights of IDMs actually is unimodal and is shifted significantly to the right of the reference range, suggesting that irrespective of actual birthweight, IDMs exceed their genetic potential for growth. However, *macrosomia* is a useful term because it defines a group of infants who are at an increased risk for peripartum and, potentially, long-term complications.

Although it is a routine procedure in teaching institutions, the need to screen all pregnant women by a glucose-loading test late in the second trimester of the pregnancy is still not done by some care providers. As a result, a disturbingly high proportion of shoulder dystocia – related fetal injuries can be traced back to undiagnosed, uncontrolled, or inadequately controlled maternal diabetes. There seems to be no justification, therefore, to replace routine testing of gravidas' glucose tolerance by some complex formula [39].

The association between maternal diabetes mellitus and the LGA infant is universally accepted. Fetal overgrowth is the hallmark of a pregnancy complicated by poorly controlled maternal diabetes when the mother has no vascular disease. The large size of the fetus increases the morbidity and mortality risk for both fetus and mother. In 10 published studies, infants weighing 4,500 g or more had higher perinatal and neonatal morbidity and mortality rates [39]. In a study of 801 pregnancies that resulted in deliveries of infants weighing 4,100 g or more, the perinatal morbidity rate was 11.4%. The perinatal mortality rate for a group of 287 newborns who weighed 4,500 g or more at delivery was 18.9 per 1,000, twice the rate of 7 per 1,000 in the control group of 21,678 normal-weight newborn infants. Ten percent of babies born weighing more than 4,500 g required admission to the neonatal intensive care unit compared with 3% of normal-weight newborns [40]. In another study of macrosomic infants, there was a 24-fold increase in the rate of shoulder dystocia and approximately a 150% excess of perinatal death and birth injuries in the 4,500- to 4,999-g weight group compared with infants whose birth weights were 2,500 to 3,499 g [40].

2.3.1 Incidence

The incidence of shoulder dystocia in nondiabetic gravidas vaginally delivering an infant weighing 4,000 to 4,499 g or more than 4,500 g is 10.0% and 22.6%, respectively. In all weight categories, diabetics experienced more shoulder dystocia than nondiabetics. Among them, 31% of vaginally delivered neonates weighing more than 4,000 g experienced shoulder dystocia. Nevertheless, the risk factors of diabetes plus a large fetus (>4,000 g) could predict 73% of shoulder dystocia among diabetics, while a large fetus alone flagged 52% of shoulder dystocia in nondiabetics. Cesarean section is recommended as the delivery method for diabetic gravidas in whom estimated fetal weight is more than 4,000 g. We advise cesarean section for diabetic gravidas who are carrying fetuses estimated to be more than 3,000 g and who experience an abnormal labor.

The group at highest risk for infants with shoulder dystocia are diabetics, including gestational diabetics. They have a 5% risk of traumatic delivery. These infants are husky and fat when compared with other infants of the same weight and age. For this reason, the incidence of shoulder dystocia is greatly increased among diabetic patients with large infants.

For those caring for pregnant diabetics, there is growing concern about the potential birth trauma associated with vaginal delivery. Diabetics tend to have much larger babies on average than nondiabetics and, weight for weight, fetuses of diabetic mothers tend to develop shoulder dystocia more often than do comparable infants of normal women. Therefore, increasingly performing a cesarean section when the ultrasonographic estimate of fetal weight is more than 4,000 g is logical. Although it may be considered too aggressive in some circles, it really cannot be criticized because it does prevent a potentially serious problem, which in diabetic cases can be expected to arise often enough to justify the approach. This author advocates it as well, preferring 4,000 g as the cutoff weight. This also was recommended almost 30 years ago in the 1978 American College of Obstetricians and Gynecologists (ACOG) Technical Bulletin Number 48 [41].

2.3.2 Treatment

A 1995 research report demonstrated that elective cesarean section for infants in excess of 4,000 g would prevent 44% of shoulder dystocias, increase the cesarean section rate by 2%, and halve the perinatal mortality with shoulder dystocia. Elective cesarean section for ultrasonic-proven macrosomia will reduce shoulder dystocia in diabetic women. Similar reductions from 10.2% to 1.4% have confirmed this study [42].

Fetal macrosomia is partially preventable by aggressive control of maternal hyperglycemia with strict diet and insulin therapy. Coustan and Imarah [43] treated gestational diabetics with diet and insulin (starting at 20 U NPH and 10 U regular daily) and halved the rates of macrosomia and operative delivery to 7% and 16%, respectively. The incidence of birth trauma and shoulder dystocia was decreased from 20% to 5%. The 1989 edition of *Danforth's Obstetrics* [29] states that macrosomia can be avoided by closely controlling glucose levels, can be predicted by ultrasound, and, if present, cesarean delivery is warranted.

It has long been debated whether prophylactic insulin will decrease complications related to macrosomia. Coustan and Imarah [43] concluded from a nonrandomized study that routine insulin treatment given to women with gestational diabetes decreased the incidence of macrosomia, midforceps and cesarean deliveries, and birth trauma from shoulder dystocia. Persson and Weldner [44] randomized insulin treatment and diet in 202 women with gestational diabetes and reported no differences in mean birthweight, number of macrosomic infants, or neonatal hypoglycemia [21]. Finally, Leikin and co-workers [20] reported that women with gestational diabetes and fasting euglycemia, when treated by diet alone, had the same incidence of macrosomia as a group of women at high risk for diabetes but who had postprandial euglycemia. In this study, women with fasting hyperglycemia were given NPH insulin in addition to diet therapy, and macrosomia developed only in those who were obese. Importantly, half of these women with gestational diabetes and postprandial hyperglycemia were morbidly obese.

Diabetic macrosomia leads to an increased rate of operative deliveries, perinatal asphyxia, and traumatic skeletal and nerve injuries. As a result of, the disproportionate overgrowth of insulin-sensitive organs, and the greater body size compared with head measurement, macrosomic fetuses of diabetic mothers are at greater risk of birth trauma. In addition, these infants have the potential risk of late diabetes-related sequelae.

When a vaginal delivery of a macrosomic fetus is attempted, there is a higher rate of protracted labor, especially in primigravidas, and the use of oxytocin is more common. Because the progress of labor is more dependent on the size of the fetal head and the maternal pelvis than on the size of the fetal body, not all mothers who deliver macrosomic babies have protracted labor, and the large size of the fetus frequently is missed, or recognition occurs too late. The diabetic mother whose fetus's head-body ratio is disproportionate can have an apparently normal labor curve before presenting the obstetrician with an impacted shoulder at delivery. The shoulder, shoulder-head, and chest-head circumferences are significantly higher among infants with birthweights of 4,000 g or more who had shoulder dystocia than among similar-weight babies delivered without such trauma, even when infants of diabetic mothers were excluded [15]. The incidence of this complication in deliveries of diabetic mothers was 50%, 23%, and 9% for infants weighing 4,500 g or more, 4,000 to 4,499 g, and 3,500 to 3,999 grams, respectively, compared with 23%, 10%, and 2% for deliveries of nondiabetic mothers. Shoulder dystocia has been described in 45% of IDMs weighing more than 4,000 g. The significant increase in the rate of shoulder dystocia is associated with complications such as fetal asphyxia, meconium aspiration, and birth trauma. Head trauma can range in severity from a minor injury to intracranial hemorrhages. These fetuses have a higher rate of broken clavicles and humeri, peripheral nerve injuries of the cervical or brachial plexus, and/or facial palsies. These injuries may be permanent, as in

Erb-Duchenne palsy, or even life threatening in cases of unilateral phrenic nerve paralysis [17,18].

Recommendations for management are divided into two categories: (1) the prevention of diabetes-related macrosomia and (2) the improvement of fetal outcome when macrosomia is present.

Evidence exists that tight glycemic control during a diabetic pregnancy decreases the risk of fetal macrosomia, neonatal hypoglycemia, and the rate of infant mortality [45]. There was a decrease in the rate of macrosomia (from 30.9% to 17.7%) and other diabetes-related morbidity when active screening for diabetes and a rigid control of maternal blood sugar were used [45]. In another study, women whose diabetes was well controlled did not have LGA infants. The factors leading to fetal macrosomia in both diabetic and nondiabetic pregnancies suggest that achieving tight diabetic control does not eliminate entirely the problem of fetal macrosomic. However, good glycemic control will reduce the rate of macrosomia in infants of diabetic mothers [45].

2.4 Postdate Pregnancy

Prolonged pregnancy contributes to excessive fetal size; macrosomia is rare at 37 weeks gestation and is increasingly common thereafter, with the highest rate at 41 weeks gestation and over. However, if there is evidence of accelerated fetal growth near term, many investigators believe that induction of labor before macrosomia is indicated. Fetal size assessment by ultrasound at 36 to 38 weeks gestation would permit induction of labor of LGA fetuses before their size becomes excessive, and it may make the obstetrician aware of possible complications that may arise during delivery.

Prolonged pregnancy should be prevented in women with diabetes and in those with risk factors for macrosomia. Therefore, when fetal macrosomia is suspected in a postdate mother, labor progress should be followed closely, and instrumental delivery should be avoided. If excessive fetal size is recognized before the onset of labor, the high neonatal morbidity will be reduced by elective cesarean section. However, most investigators agree that by obtaining an ultrasound estimation of fetal weight, close to term, the obstetrician would be able to make decisions regarding the safest mode of delivery before the onset of labor.

Postdatism, or the postterm pregnancy, is an important risk factor for shoulder dystocia, and with obesity and diabetes comprises an ominous triad. The current epidemic of obstetric obesity behooves modern-day care providers to reduce the number of large infants. Postdate pregnancy is frequently encountered and often has a poor outcome. Fetal weight exceeding 4,000 g is almost twice as frequent at week 42 as at 40 weeks. A study of 519 pregnancies beyond 41 weeks disclosed that 23% of newborn weighed more than 4,000 g and 4% more than 4,500 g. The fetal risk further increases because the rate of growth of the fetal body exceeds that of the head at and beyond term gestation. A difference of 1.6 cm or more between the chest and head circumferences and a ≥4.8 cm discrepancy between those of the shoulders and the head identify a kind of fetal macrosomia that is highly conducive to shoulder dystocia at birth. A discrepancy of ≥1.4 cm or more between the diameters of the fetal trunk and the head (biparietal diameter) has been found to be more predictive of a fetal weight exceeding 4,000 g than the actual demonstration of such fetal weight by the customary techniques [39]. Inducing labor in these women would have significantly reduced the number of injured infants.

Boyd et al. [46] reported a 21% incidence of macrosomia with infants delivered at 42 weeks compared with 12% at 40 weeks, and suggested induction of labor as a means to prevent shoulder dystocia. In the study by Spellacy et al. [47], the frequency of postdatism was 10.2% among infants with mild macrosomia and 14.8% among those with more severe macrosomia. When multiple risk factors were present along with postdatism, the fetal risks increased even further. Other prenatal risks influence the frequency of shoulder dystocia: short stature, abnormal pelvic morphology (especially the flat pelvis), and reduced pelvic size. Each of these are of greater significance in the postdate pregnancy when accompanied by predisposing prepregnancy and other prenatal risk factors, thus supporting the concept on earlier delivery.

Using a regional network database of 60,456 births, Horger et al. [53] compared 3,457 postdate (≥42 weeks) infants with a control group of 8,135 infants born at 40 weeks gestation. Both patient groups included only uncomplicated pregnancies. Although the differences were small, women who delivered postdate infants had a lower parity and higher weight at delivery. The postdate infants were heavier, more likely to be delivered by forceps or cesarean section, and more likely to experience shoulder dystocia. The higher perinatal morbidity in postdate infants suggests that careful attention should be paid to this high-risk factor especially in regard to shoulder dystocia and its prevention by earlier delivery.

Garbaciak et al. [54] studied a total of 317 consecutive patients with accurately dated pregnancies who were seen because of fetal surveillance at more than 41 weeks gestation and in whom there was an estimation of the fetal weight based on femur length and abdominal circumference at the initial visit. The incidence of macrosomia at 41 weeks gestation was 25.5%. There was a higher incidence of cesarean section because of arrest and protraction disorders in the postdate pregnancies in which the infant was macrosomic (22%) versus those in which the infant was not macrosomic (10%, P < .01). In a control group of 100 consecutive women delivered between 38 and 40 weeks gestation, the incidence of macrosomia was 4%, significantly lower than the rate in the postdate patients (P < .01). Thus, earlier delivery would have had improved infant outcome.

Because fetal body size continues to grow faster than fetal head size, the risk of shoulder dystocia increases with gestational age, especially after 40 weeks. Of all shoulder dystocias, 40% occur in births of pregnancies attaining 41 weeks and 60% after 41 weeks. The risk of shoulder dystocia for postterm infants is four times that for term infants. In births of 43 weeks gestation or greater, the risk for shoulder dystocia is 6%, and the risk of cesarean section increases. Birth trauma with vaginal delivery and meconium aspiration with cesarean section are the main risk of postdate infants. Induction after 39 weeks is indicated if the cervix is favorable and will be beneficial if the infant is approaching macrosomia. This will reduce the incidence of serious shoulder dystocia.

A recent report shows that the risk to the fetus of continuing the pregnancy beyond 41 weeks gestation is far greater than originally appreciated [47]. Recent data also prove that the risk of cesarean delivery after the routine induction of labor at term is lower than previously reported, possibly due to the availability of newer cervical ripening agents [47].

The largest of these trials was the Canadian Multicenter Postterm Pregnancy Trial (CMPPT), which randomized 3,407 low-risk women with uncomplicated singleton pregnancies at or after 41 weeks gestation to induction of labor within 4 days of randomization or expectant management to 44 weeks [47]. These authors concluded that the incidence of adverse perinatal outcomes in low-risk but not high-risk pregnancies at or after 41 weeks gestation is very low. These conclusions are further reinforced by a recent meta-analysis of randomized controlled trials reported in the Cochrane Library [48]. The Cochrane report also suggests that the routine induction of labor at or after 41 weeks is associated with a reduction in perinatal mortality, with no increases in the rate of instrumental delivery, use of analgesia, or cesarean delivery regardless of parity, cervical effacement, and induction method [48].

The difference between the earlier studies, which showed an increase in the cesarean delivery rate with routine induction of labor [17,18], and the more recent studies [13–15] may be attributed to the availability and routine use of cervical ripening agents. Indeed, the introduction of preinduction cervical maturation has lowered the rate of failed and serial inductions, reduced fetal and maternal morbidity, shortened hospital stays, lowered medical costs, and possibly decreased the rate of cesarean delivery [48].

To summarize, several recent studies demonstrate that the risk to the fetus and to the mother of continuing pregnancy beyond 41 weeks gestation are far greater than originally appreciated. The risks of routine labor induction, primarily failed induction leading to cesarean delivery, also are lower than previously thought [48]. For these reasons, induction of labor should be routine at an earlier gestational age than is currently the norm—specifically, at 39 to 41 weeks gestation. The greater the number of risk factors for shoulder dystocia, the earlier the induction should be scheduled.

A key clinical skill for all obstetricians and midwives who manage postdate pregnancies and macrosomia is the ability to accurately evaluate the cervix and determine its favorability. When inducing for macrosomia, carefully performed clinical pelvimetry and ultrasound are essential tools. So often, care providers neglect these critically important steps, or perform them in a perfunctory manner. When practicing induction of labor in high-risk pregnancies, it is important to exclude contraindications to vaginal delivery especially cephalo-pelvic disproportion.

2.5 Obesity

Pregnancy outcome is compromised regardless of the level of maternal obesity [40].

Unfortunately for the obstetrician, obesity and adult-onset diabetes fre-quently coexist. Maternal obesity has an independent effect on fetal macro-somia and has a strong diabetes-independent influence on fetal growth.

Obese and morbidly obese individuals are at significant risk for macrosomia, shoulder dystocia, hypertensive disease, preeclampsia, diabetes mellitus, and urinary tract infections. The reader is referred to Chapter 1 for an in-depth review. The incidence of obesity varies among women of various racial and socioeconomic groups. African Americans and Hispanics are at increased risk for being obese, with the rate for African-American women approaching 45% [2,13]. In addition, women who are obese tend to be older and multiparous [45].

The analysis of Tallarigo et al. [23] associates maternal obesity with a significant increase in antenatal complications and an increased incidence in perinatal mortality. It was interesting to note that there was an increase in shoulder dystocia and cord accidents in obese and morbidly obese patients who did not have prenatal complications. In the morbidly obese patients without prenatal complications, there was also a significant increase in meconium staining and late decelerations of the fetal heart rate. These observations may account for the increased incidence of primary cesarean delivery in the morbidly obese patient without prenatal complications.

It is a widespread misconception that the increased rate of postoperative complications in obese women warrants preferential delivery of morbidly obese gravidas by the vaginal route. In fact, there are data to indicate that the incidence of shoulder dystocia among grossly obese women may be almost 10-fold higher than in the general population [15]. Therefore, morbid obesity is a consideration for, rather than against, abdominal delivery.

Maternal obesity is known to have serious obstetric complications. The literature supports a relationship between obesity and coexisting medical ill-nesses such as diabetes and hypertension [10]. Perinatal adverse outcomes include an increased incidence of stillbirth and congenital anomalies. There is also an established relationship between maternal obesity and fetal macrosomia [49]. There is strong evidence for the relationship between macrosomia and shoulder dystocia; the current evidence for an independent relationship between maternal obesity and shoulder dystocia is strong. Case-control studies have demonstrated a higher prevalence of obesity in pregnancies affected by shoulder dystocia than in the corresponding control groups. Since 1991, there has been a 50% to 70% increase in the rate of obesity in adults of reproductive age [3]. In the general population, obesity has long-term health implications such as uterine cancer, diabetes mellitus, and heart disease [3]. The current obstetric literature demonstrates that obesity does impact perinatal outcomes [30].

Common descriptions of obesity include absolute body weight (pounds or kilograms), body mass index (BMI; weight in kilograms divided by height in meters squared), and percentage of ideal body weight [4]. In 1990, the Institute of Medicine (IOM) published definitions of weight categories using BMI as the units of measurement [5]. The following criteria were used for the weight-for-height categories: underweight, BMI less than 19.8; normal weight, BMI 19.8 to 26.0; overweight, BMI greater than 26.0 to 29.0; and obese, BMI greater than 29.0. However, the IOM subcommittee noted that any cutoff was arbitrary "since none of the weight-for-height classification schemes has been validated against pregnancy outcome [28]."

The relationship between maternal size and fetal size is interesting. It has been reported that both obese and morbidly obese patients have a significantly increased risk for birth weight greater than 4,500 g compared with controls [30]. These findings are important to remember when clinically estimating fetal weight in the labor room. The clinician should know that a large fetus is not necessarily more common in the obese and morbidly obese population, but a macrosomic fetus is.

Obese patients may have difficulty completing the second stage of labor secondary to soft tissue dystocia, and operative vaginal delivery may be used to expedite delivery in such a situation. After controlling for birthweight, morbidly obese patients are more likely to have an operative vaginal delivery than are patients with a BMI less than 30.

For nulliparous patients, the cesarean delivery rate was 20.7% for the control group, 33.8% for obese, and 47.4% for morbidly obese patients [45]. Obesity is an independent risk factor for adverse obstetric outcome and is significantly associated with an increased cesarean delivery rate and birth injury.

2.6 Excessive Weight Gain

Maternal weight gain ranks high as a significant risk factor for macrosomia. Boyd et al. [46] found that a weight gain of 20 kg would be additive with the risk factors of obesity and being 7 days postdate. The risk of excessive weight gain has been detailed by Dor et al. [50] but questioned by Parks and Ziel [51]. It can be assumed that the excess glucose intake exposes the infant to a greater growth stimulus and adds greater risk if prepregnancy abnormalities have been noted. Excessive weight gain causes the incidence of macrosomia to increase from 1.4% to 15.2%.

Seidman et al. [2] studied the association between maternal weight gain during pregnancy and the infant's birthweight in 14,121 term singleton births. The parturients were stratified into four body-mass categories, three age groups, four parity groups, and three levels of educational attainment. A separate multiple regression analysis was performed for each category to control for the confounding effect of gestational age, maternal social class, ethnicity, cigarette consumption, marital status, age, parity, education, and weight/ height ratio. A significant positive influence of prenatal weight gain on birthweight was found for all subgroups. The effect varied depending on maternal prepregnancy body mass, age, parity, and the level of formal education.

A significant positive linear relationship is found between maternal weight gain and birthweight for all levels of prepregnancy body mass, age, parity, and education. These results confirm earlier reports [4,6,52,53] that birthweight increases as prepregnancy body mass increases. The effect of maternal weight gain on birthweight decreases with increases in body mass indices. However, weight gain is significantly associated with birthweight even among very obese women. It seems that for the obese mother, the impact of her weight gain on the birthweight of her infant is diminished. Thus, the lower weight gain observed for overweight women may be appropriate, and such limited weight gains may even reduce the rate of macrosomia [54] and aid in subsequent weight loss [55].

Birthweight correlates positively with maternal age and is more dependent on maternal weight gain as maternal age increases. Weight gain is found to have the smallest effect on birthweight for the teenage group. Parity is found to exert an independent and additive effect with weight gain on birthweight, after controlling for the important confounding effects of maternal age and prepregnancy body mass. The problem of maternal weight gain and birthweight is significantly increased for women with more years of schooling. This association may reflect better nutrition [14,20] and prenatal care [21] among better educated women.

The advice mothers receive has been shown to have a significant effect on final weight gain [16,55]. Appropriate weight-gain advice by prenatal care providers, in conjunction with better maternal compliance, could have a positive effect on birth outcomes. Better understanding of the influence of maternal factors such as age, parity, education, and prepregnancy body mass on weight gain may strengthen the credibility and perhaps the influence of dietary advice to pregnant women. Previous studies have shown that a mother's optimal weight gain in pregnancy depends on her body build. Underweight women need to gain more than do overweight women. This author suggests that recommendations for a minimal weight gain in pregnancy be determined for the individual woman after considering not only her weight for height but also her age and parity. Nonobese primigravidas and teenage women should gain more weight than should older and multiparous women.

A Mayo Clinic research study has concluded that although no single maternal variable is a consistent predictor of macrosomia, maternal BMI, Leopold estimated fetal weight, and intrapartum fundal height appear to be the best predictors [34].

2.7 Fundal Height

Mothers experiencing higher symphysis-fundus measurements at term have a much higher incidence of shoulder dystocia. Fundal height is an easy screening method for everyone to follow uterine growth. It gives us a suspicion of macrosomia (absolute birthweight) and identifies mothers needing ultrasound exams. In these patients, the use of ultrasound has been shown to be the best method to predict fetal weight [51] and document excessive fetal growth weights.

2.8 Conclusion

Because of fetal complications, it is important to identify the women at risk for having a macrosomic infant so that the delivery method can be evaluated. Women delivering macrosomic infants tend to be older and to have an increased parity. More characteristically, they have one of three problems: obesity, diabetes mellitus, and postmaturity. Macrosomia would be expected in obese and diabetic pregnant women because the principal substrate for fetal growth is glucose, which is elevated in these two conditions.

With this information, the obstetrician can better detect and plan for the management of macrosomia. Ultrasound scans can now approximate fetal weight. Therefore, it would seem prudent to scan all women in labor who are obese, have diabetes mellitus, who are postterm, or who have gained excessive weight to determine an estimated fetal weight. Because there is an error of about 10% in this estimate, it seems reasonable to deliver by cesarean section all low-risk infants whose estimated weight is more than 4,500 g and all high-risk infants whose estimated weight is more than 4,000 g and thus avoid fetal trauma. This plan could reduce perinatal injuries for macrosomic infants without greatly increasing the number of cesarean deliveries.

Obesity is a high-risk factor and deserves great respect on the part of clinicians and greater emphasis in our teaching program. The same emphasis must be placed on the presence of borderline carbohydrate intolerance postdatism, maternal weight gain, and maternal birthweight.

References

1. Phalen J, Strong T. Shoulder dystocia. *Female Patient* 1988;13:73–80.
2. Seidman D, Ever-Hadani P, Gale R. The effect of maternal weight gain in pregnancy on birth weight. *Obstet Gynecol* 1989;74:240–247.
3. Gormican A, Valentine J, Satter E. Relationships of maternal weight gain, prepregnancy weight, and infant birthweight. *J Am Diet Assoc* 1980;77:662–667
4. Harrison G, Udall J, Morrow G. Maternal obesity, weight gain in pregnancy, and infant birth weight. *Am J Obstet Gynecol* 1980;136:411–412.

5. Kliegman R, Gross T. Perinatal problems of the obese mother and her infant. *Obstet Gynecol* 1985;66:299–303.
6. Seidman D, Slater P, Ever-Hadani P, Gale R. Accuracy of mother's recall of birthweight and gestational age. *Br J Obstet Gynaecol* 1987;94:731–735.
7. Naeye R. Weight gain and the outcome of pregnancy. *Am J Obstet Gynecol* 1979;135:3–9.
8. Palmer J, Jennings G, Massey L. Development of an assessment form: Attitude toward weight gain during pregnancy. *J Am Diet Assoc* 1985;85:946–949.
9. Shepard M, Hellenbrand K, Bracken M. Proportional weight gain and complications of pregnancy, labor, and delivery in healthy women of normal prepregnant stature. *Am J Obstet Gynecol* 1986;1555:947–954.
10. Rush D, Davis H, Susser M. Antecedents of low birthweight in Harlem, New York City. *Int J Epidemiol* 1972;1:375–387.
11. Dohrmenn K, Lederman S. Weight gain in pregnancy. *J Obstet Gynaecol Neonatal Nurs* 1986;15:446–453.
12. Taffel S, Keppel K. Advise about weight gain during pregnancy and actual weight gain. *Am J Public Health* 1986;76:1396–1399.
13. Jacobson H. Current concepts in nutrition: Diet in pregnancy. *N Engl J Med* 1977;297:1051–1053.
14. Kleinman J, Madans J. The effects of maternal smoking, physical stature and educational attainment on the incidence of low birth weight. *Am J Epidemiol* 1985;121:843–855.
15. Elliott J, Garite T, Freeman R, McQuown D, Patel J. Ultrasonic prediction of fetal macrosomia in diabetic patients. *Obstet Gynecol* 1982;60:159–162.
16. Golditch I, Kirkman K. The large fetus: Management and outcome. *Obstet Gynecol* 1978;52:26–30.
17. Modanlou HD, Dorchester WL, Thorosian A, Freeman RK. Macrosomia-maternal, fetal, and neonatal implications. *Obstet Gynecol* 1980;55:420–424.
18. Sack PA. The large infant: A study of maternal, obstetric, fetal, and newborn characteristics including a long-term pediatric follow-up. *Am J Obstet Gynecol* 1969;104:195–204.
19. Yeo G, Lim Y, Yeong C, Tan T. An analysis of risk factors for the prediction of shoulder dystocia in 16,471 consecutive births. *Ann Acad Med Singapore* 1995;24:836–840.
20. Leikin EL, Jenkins JH, Pomerantz GA, Klein L. Abnormal glucose screening tests in pregnancy: A risk factor for fetal macrosomia. *OB Gynecol* 1987;69:570–576.
21. Pritchard JA, MacDonald PC, Gant NF, eds. *Williams Obstetrics*. 17th ed. Norwalk, CT: Appleton-Century-Crofts; 1985:668.
22. Sox HC. Probability theory in the use of diagnostic tests. *Ann Intern Med* 1986;104:60–66.
23. Tallarigo L, Giampietro O, Penno G, Miccoli R, Gregori G, Navalesi R. Relation of glucose tolerance to complications of pregnancy in non-diabetic women. *N Engl J Med* 1986;315:989–993.
24. Watson WJ. Serial changes in the 50-g oral glucose test in pregnancy: Implications for screening. *Obstet Gynecol* 1989;74:40–46.
25. Carpenter MW, Coustan DR. Criteria for screening tests for gestational diabetes. *Am J Obstet Gynecol* 1982;144:768–772.
26. Gabbe SG, Mestman JH, Freeman RK, Anderson GV, Lowensohn RI. Management and outcome of class A diabetes mellitus. *Am J Obstet Gynecol* 1977;127:465–469.
27. Mestman JH. Outcome of diabetes screening in pregnancy and perinatal morbidity in infants of mothers with mild impairment in glucose tolerance. *Diabetes Care* 1980;3:447–451.
28. Frisoli G, Naranjo L, Shehah N. Glycohemoglobins in normal and diabetic pregnancies. *Am J Perinatol* 1985;2:183–185.
29. Scott J, DiSara P, Hammond C, Spellacy W. *Danforth's Obstetrics*. 6th ed. Philadelphia: JB Lippincott; 1990.
30. Bochner CJ, Medearis AL, Williams J III, Castro L, Hobel CJ, Wade ME. Early third-trimester ultrasound screening in gestational diabetes to determine the risk of macrosomia and labor dystocia at term. *Am J Obstet Gynecol* 1987;157:703–708.

31. O'Shaughnessy R, Russ J, Zuspan FP. Glycosylated hemoglobins and diabetes mellitus in pregnancy. *Am J Obstet Gynecol* 1979;135:783–789.
32. O'Sullivan J, Mahan CM. Criteria for the oral glucose tolerance test in pregnancy. *Diabetes* 1964;13:278–280.
33. Al-Shawaf T, Moghraby S, Akiel A. Does impaired glucose tolerance imply a risk in pregnancy? *Br J Obstet Gynaecol* 1988;10:236–241.
34. Langer O, Yogev Y, Xenakis E, Brustman L. Overweight and obese in gestational diabetes: The impact on pregnancy outcome. *Am J Obstet Gynecol* 2005;192:1768–1776.
35. Stamilio D, Olsen T, Ratcliffe S, Schder H, Macones G. False positive 1-hour glucose challenge test and adverse perinatal outcomes. *Obstet Gynecol* 1989;103:148–156.
36. Lindsay MK, Graves W, Klein L. The relationship of one abnormal glucose tolerance test value and pregnancy complications. *Obstet Gynecol* 1989;73:103–105.
37. American College of Obstetricians and Gynecologists. Technical Bulletin #200. Washington, DC: ACOG; 1994.
38. Witter FR, Niebyl JR. Abnormal glucose screening in pregnancy in patients with normal oral glucose tolerance tests as a screening test for fetal macrosomia. *Int J Gynecol Obstet* 1988;27:181–184.
39. Carpenter M. Rationale and performance of tests for gestational diabetes. *Clin Obstet Gynecol* 1991;34:544–557.
40. Neiger R. Fetal macrosomia in the diabetic patient. *Clin Obstet Gynecol* 1992;35:138–150.
41. American College of Obstetricians and Gynecologists. Technical Bulletin #48. Washington, DC: ACOG; 1978.
42. Conway D, Langer O. Elective delivery of infants with macrosomia in diabetic women. *Am J Obstet Gynecol* 1998;178:922–925.
43. Coustan D, Imarah J. Prophylactic insulin treatment of gestational diabetes reduces the incidence of macrosomia, operative delivery, and birth trauma. *Am J Obstet Gynecol* 1984;150:836–842.
44. Persson PH, Weldner BM. Reliability of ultrasound fetometry in estimating gestational age in the second trimester. *Acta Obstet Gynecol Scand* 1986;65:481–483.
45. Weiss J, Malone F, Emig D, et al. Obesity, obstetric complications and cesarean delivery rate-a population-based screening study. *Am J Obstet Gynecol* 2004;190:1091–1097.
46. Boyd ME, Usher RH, McLean, FH. Fetal macrosomia: Prediction, risks, proposed management. *Obstet Gynecol* 1983;61:715–720.
47. Spellacy WN, Miller SJ, Winegar A. Pregnancy after 40 years of age. .*Obstet Gynecol* 1986;68:452–457.
48. Norwitz E. Postdate pregnancy 2000; September. OBG Management; 68–72.
49. Pondaag W, Thomas R. Natural history of obstetric brachial plexus palsy: A systemic review. *Develop Med Child Neural* 2004;46:138–144.
50. Dor N, Mosberg H, Stern W, Jagani N, Schulman H. Complications in fetal macrosomia. *N Y State J Med* 1984;84:302–309.
51. Parks DG, Ziel HK. Macrosomia, a proposed indication for primary cesarean section. *Obstet Gynecol* 1978;52:407–412.
52. Miller JM Jr, Brown HL, Pastorek JG II, Gabert HA. Fetal overgrowth diabetic versus nondiabetic. *J Ultrasound Med* 1988;7:577–579.
53. Horger EO, Smythe AR. Pregnancy in women over forty. *Obstet Gynecol* 1977;49:257–262.
54. Garbaciak J, Richter M, Miller S, Barton J. Maternal weight and pregnancy complications. *Am J Obstet Gynecol* 191185;152:238–242.
55. Adams MM, Oakley GP, Marks JS. Maternal age and births in the 1980s. *JAMA* 1982;247:493–497.

Chapter 3
Role of Ultrasound in Shoulder Dystocia

James A. O'Leary

Summary Early recognition of maternal risk factors combined with early ultrasound are key to recognition of large infants. Using multiple ultrasound parameters, greater accuracy is achieved.

Keywords: asymmetrical large infants · macrosomia

Contents

3.1	Introduction	33
3.2	Early Macrosomia Detection	35
3.3	Estimation of Fetal Weight	36
3.4	Head Measurements	36
3.5	Abdominal Measurements	37
3.6	Diabetes and Ultrasound Measurements	39
3.7	Obesity and Ultrasound Measurements	40
3.8	Serial Measurements	41
3.9	Computed Tomography	41
3.10	Growth Rates	42
3.11	Soft Tissue Thickness	42
3.12	Shoulder Ratios	43
3.13	Conclusion	43

3.1 Introduction

Ultrasonography has been shown to be an *extremely valuable tool* in evaluating fetal growth and estimating fetal weight (see ACOG Tech. Bull. no. 200, 1994). It continues to be the mainstay for assessing risk of labor induction in diabetic pregnancies [1].

Competent clinical examination, physical exam, and estimated fetal weight "should enable experienced examiners to arrive at fairly accurate conclusions" [2].

J.A. O'Leary
Professor Obstetrics & Gynecology (retired), University of South Florida, Tampa, Florida, USA

J.A. O'Leary (ed.), *Shoulder Dystocia and Birth Injury*,
DOI 10.1007/978-1-59745-473-5_3, © Humana Press, a part of Springer
Science+Business Media, LLC 2009

"Sonographic cephalometry often enhances appreciably the confidence of the estimate" [2, 3]. More recently, Dor et al. [4] have demonstrated that ultrasound exams are more accurate than the physical exam.

Ultrasound is an extremely valuable tool in evaluating fetal growth, estimating fetal weight, and determining hydramnios and malformations [5]. The use of ultrasound to estimate fetal weight has been greatly improved (thus supplanting clinical estimation almost universally in America) and is playing a pivotal role in obstetric management. Most importantly, fetal weight estimates provide the basis for recognition of abnormal fetal growth. The combination of fetal physical variables makes estimated weights substantially more accurate [1]. It is noteworthy that macrosomic infants (4,000 g) almost invariably exhibit abnormal fat deposition in the check pad and paraspinal area [1].

The prenatal recognition of altered fetal growth is an important goal for every obstetrician [6–15]. This early determination of excessive growth affords the clinician the opportunity to treat the problem and prevent adverse outcomes. The recognition of risk factors for macrosomia, combined with careful serial physical measurements of fundal height, serial estimates of fetal weight by palpation, and serial ultrasound determinations, will greatly simplify the diagnosis of macrosomia [16–24]. Appropriate consultation should help to clarify the more difficult clinical cases.

The recognition of risk factors for excess growth dictates early ultrasound dating of the pregnancies and serial ultrasound examinations in the second and third trimesters [25–27]. Failure to identify these factors eliminates the best chance for early diagnosis and treatment. To improve perinatal care, the evolution and the extent or severity of macrosomia should be determined and quantified as early as possible and prior to term or attainment of maximal size and weight. Clinically, it is more useful to recognize that fetal weight above the 90th percentile for gestational age is a more meaningful definition of macrosomia than is absolute birthweight [28–36]. Indications for ultrasound are given in Table 3.1

Table 3.1 Indications for Serial Ultrasound Exams

Prior macrosomia
Obesity
Glucose intolerance
Excessive weight gain
Prior birth injury
Pregnancy of 41 weeks or more
Maternal weight:height ratio elevated
Polyhydramnios
Maternal perception
Fundal height increase

3.2 Early Macrosomia Detection

Very recently, Manogura [37] reported on the early detection of excessive fetal growth in 70 women who developed gestational diabetes. She observed that early suggestion of accelerated fetal growth offers a window of opportunity to optimize glycemic management of the mother and potentially prevent macrosomic stillbirth and perinatal morbidity. The women underwent serial assessments, including standardized ultrasound exams for nuchal translucency screening (11 to 14 weeks gestation), detailed evaluation of anatomy (18 to 20 weeks gestation), and formal fetal echocardiogram (22 to 24 weeks gestation and then every 4 weeks thereafter).

The Gardosi method was used to predict individual fetal growth potentials based on fetal gender and the mother's height, weight, parity, ethnic, and other characteristics. Estimated fetal weights from imaging were converted to percentiles, with large for gestational age (LGA) defined as above the 90th percentile. Early differences were seen between the 27 LGA infants and infants born at normal weights. By 24 weeks gestation, LGA infants had a median estimated fetal weight in the 54th percentile, significantly higher than the 48th percentile for normal-weight neonates. At 24 weeks, an estimated weight that was above the 58th percentile predicted an LGA baby with a sensitivity of 30% and a specificity of 84%.

If this trend continued at 28 weeks, then the odds of having an LGA baby were four times higher. At 28 weeks, future LGA babies were at a median 72 nd percentile of estimated fetal weight compared with the 51st percentile for normal-weight infants. An estimated fetal weight of greater than the 58th percentile at 28 weeks increased the sensitivity of predicting macrosomia to 63%, with a specificity of 87%.

"The potential to interrupt this progression by intensive midtrimester glycemic management deserves further study," the investigator concluded.

Elevated estimated fetal weight percentiles on ultrasound did not predict adverse perinatal outcomes such as shoulder dystocia, cesarean delivery, or neonatal complications.

The experience of most authors [38–47] parallels that of Hadlock [8], who contends that LGA fetuses are a nonhomogeneous population with two main forms of macrosomia. The first is symmetric macrosomia in which accelerated growth of all fetal parameters (i.e., fetal weight, length, head circumference, and abdominal circumference) exceed the 90th percentile for gestational age. Generally, this form of *constitutional macrosomia* is more commonly noted in patients with large stature and tends to recur in subsequent pregnancies. On the other hand, asymmetric macrosomia occurs in diabetic patients. In these asymmetric LGA fetuses, the head and femur measurements vary in size and length but fall below the 90th percentile rank. Fetal abdominal circumference and thigh diameter, however, both reflect soft tissue mass and may be significantly larger than normal [48–51].

Although several formulas are now available for sonographic estimation of fetal weight, to date only two noteworthy studies have carefully evaluated the accuracy of fetal weight estimation for the detection of macrosomia. Presumably, this is because of the possible errors associated with such estimates, which range from ±16% to ±20%. Clearly, such a range of estimates would result in a number of false-negative and false-positive results [13]. Korndorffer [18] studied the applicability of fetal weight estimation formulas, which were tested in 64 fetuses of diabetic mothers. The standard deviation of differences was 322 g and the multiplier was 0.781. Korndorffer concluded that the variation in standard deviations of mean differences required caution by the obstetrician and advised use of clinical judgment and percentile ranks of fetal sonar parameters in addition to weight estimates when planning delivery of suspected macrosomic fetuses.

3.3 Estimation of Fetal Weight

The philosophy that sonographic assessment of fetal weight at term is unacceptably unreliable is not shared by many prominent experts [52]. Langer and associates calculated that, using an estimated fetal weight threshold of 4,250 g as an indication for abdominal delivery for diabetic women, 76% of diabetes-related brachial plexus injuries could be prevented [53]. It is interesting that with due recognition of its limitations, sonographic estimation of the fetal weight has been relied upon in many clinical situations, ranging from the determination of the expected date of confinement to detection of fetal growth and the diagnosis of discordance between twins.

Ott and Doyle [10] reported their experience using the weight estimation equation of Shepard [28] in 595 patients undergoing real-time ultrasound examination within 72 hours of delivery. The prevalence of LGA features in this population was 12%. Overall, LGA infants were detected for a sensitivity of 73.5%. There were a number of false-positive results, as the predictive value of a positive test was only 63.2%. However, this method was 95% specific, and a normal estimated fetal weight was predictive of a normally grown infant in 96% of cases.

Although estimation of weight appears to be simple, clinicians should be cautioned that the formulas are associated with a 95% confidence range of 15% to 22%. Using a figure of 15%, the predicted weight would have to exceed 4,700 g for all fetuses to truly weigh in excess of 4,000 g. Similarly, to eliminate false-negative results, an estimated weight below 3,600 g would be required.

3.4 Head Measurements

Crane et al. [13] evaluated multiple biparietal diameter measurements in 74 patients in an attempt to diagnose those fetuses destined to be large at birth. Using two or more biparietal diameter values two standard deviations above the mean, they were able to correctly identify 25 of 26 LGA fetuses. Remarkably, all 48 normally grown infants were found to have normal biparietal diameters *in utero*. In the study by Tamura et al. [12] of diabetic women, only 9 of 67 fetuses were found to have a biparietal diameter greater than the 90th percentile. Similarly, the researchers serially studied diabetic women during the third trimester and found normal head circumference growth in the LGA group [12]. Wladimiroff et al. [14] have also noted that only 7% of LGA infants will have a biparietal diameter above the 90th percentile. The normal progression of fetal head growth in diabetic pregnancies was described by Ogata et al. [15] who confirmed that, in contrast with the fetal liver, the fetal brain is not sensitive to the growth-promoting effects of insulin.

3.5 Abdominal Measurements

"Sonographic measurements of the fetal abdominal circumference have proved to be *most helpful* in predicting fetal macrosomia. Using serial sonographic examinations, accelerated abdominal growth can be identified by 32 weeks gestation. Measuring subcutaneous fat in the fetus is sensitive for detecting macrosomia in diabetic mothers" [5]. Recent studies of an abdominal circumference of 35 cm identified more than 90% of macrosomic patients who were at risk for shoulder dystocia [54].

A recent prospective study of 332 women having an ultrasound estimated fetal weight of more than 3,400 g within 14 days of delivery has been shown to be a valuable tool in predicting asymmetric growth [5]. The authors developed an index for asymmetry by subtracting the biparietal diameter (BPD) from the abdominal diameter (AD). A distribution curve was generated to determine the optimal cutoff for shoulder dystocia prediction. The mean asymmetry index was significantly higher in the shoulder dystocia group (P = .0002). Above the cutoff was 25% for unselected cases and 38.5% for diabetics. The authors concluded that an asymmetry (AD minus BPD $\geq$ 2.6 cm) significantly increased the risk of shoulder dystocia. This finding was true in both diabetic and non-diabetic populations [55].

Wladimiroff and colleagues [14] were among the first to address ultrasound diagnosis of the LGA infant when they described ultrasonographically detected growth characteristics in 30 LGA infants, including 11 infants of diabetic women [21]. These authors noted that head-to-chest ratios fell below the 5th percentile in 53% of the LGA group compared with 2% of normal infants. In this study, fetal chest measurements were obtained caudal to the cardiac pulsations and actually represented an upper abdominal measurement. Elliott et al. [16] analyzed biparietal diameter and chest diameter measurements in 70 diabetic women undergoing ultrasound examination within 30 weeks of delivery. A macrosomia index was calculated for each fetus by subtracting the biparietal diameter from the chest diameter. These authors found 20 of 23 (87%) infants weighing in excess of 4,000 g had a macrosomia index of 1.4 cm or greater. Whereas this approach seems quite sensitive, it is associated with a high false-positive rate, as only 61% of those screened positive were truly macrosomic at birth. Elliott et al. [16] emphasized that the macrosomia index may be most helpful in recognizing infants at risk for birth trauma.

More recent studies [56–71] demonstrate that abdominal measurements are probably the most reliable sonographic parameter for the detection of macrosomia *in utero*. However, much of the available data again come from studies of pregnancies complicated by diabetes mellitus.

Gilby studied 1,996 women at 36-plus weeks with an ultrasound examination within 1 week of delivery and found fetal abdominal cirumference (AC) was useful in predicting macrosomia. AC predicted infants >4,500 g better than those >4,000 g. Almost all macrosomic infants >4,500 g had an AC of ≥35 cm (68 of 69, or 99%), but many nonmacrosomic infants were also in this group (683). AC of ≥38 cm occurred in 99 infants, and 37 of 69 (53.6%) weighing >4,500 g were identified. Most infants (78%) with AC ≥38 cm weighed >4,000 g. Gilby et al. [72] concluded that fetal AC was very helpful in identifying potential macrosomic infants. If AC was =35 cm, the risk of infant birthewight >4,500 g was =1%. if AC was ≥38 cm, the risk was 37%(37 of 99), and>50% of these infants were identified (37 of 69, or 53.6%).

It appears that serial ultrasonography can establish the onset of accelerated abdominal growth in diabetic pregnancies. Ogata and colleagues [15] provided the first description of serial ultrasonographic assessment for the evaluation of fetal macrosomia. These authors performed several measurements of abdominal circumference in 23 diabetic women during the third trimester. In 10 fetuses who proved to be macrosomic at birth, accelerated abdominal growth was detectable by 28 to 32 weeks gestation. They confirmed these findings in a study of diabetic women examined on at least three occasions during the third trimester. Growth curves for femur length and head circumference were similar for both appropriate for gestational age (AGA) and LGA fetuses.

Hadlock et al. [66] evaluated another method to identify the macrosomic fetus *in utero*. Applying the femur length to abdominal circumference ratio, these authors studied 156 fetuses within 1 week of delivery. Using a cutoff ratio of less than 20.5% representing the 10th percentile, they were able to detect only 63% of their LGA population. Mintz and Landon [6] used a femur length to abdominal circumference ratio of less than 21% as the cutoff and could only identify 58% of LGA infants of diabetic mothers. These disappointing results have been confirmed by Benson et al. [34] who studied 157 fetuses of diabetic mothers and noted a 64% sensitivity and only a 36% predictive value with a femur length to abdominal circumference ratio of less than 20%. Similarly, in a larger study of 210 nondiabetic women, Miller et al. [35] reported that a femur length to abdominal circumference ratio of less than 21% was able to identify only 21 of 88 (24%) LGA fetuses.

3.6 Diabetes and Ultrasound Measurements

Bochner [27] and colleagues conducted a study to determine whether an early third trimester fetal abdominal circumference measurement can be used in gestational diabetes patients to predict macrosomia and labor dystocia at term. The predictive accuracy of a 30- to 33-week abdominal circumference measurement was tested, using the 90th percentile as the discriminant point. The study consisted of 201 euglycemic patients with gestational diabetes who maintained weekly fasting glucose levels less than 100 mg/dL with dietary management alone. The predictive accuracy of 30- to 33-week fetal abdominal circumference measurement was 96.4% for ruling out macrosomia and 56.3% for predicting macrosomia. Patients with fetal abdominal circumference measurements greater than the 90th percentile at 30 to 33 weeks had a significantly increased incidence of cesarean section for failure to progress, shoulder dystocia, and birth trauma, whereas patients with abdominal circumference measurements less than or equal to the 90th percentile were at no greater risk than the general population. These results suggest that the latter patients are not at increased risk for macrosomia, cesarean section, or birth trauma at term, as long as their weekly glucose testing remains within normal limits. Thus, efforts to decrease the incidence of macrosomia and its attendant risks should focus on those gestational diabetic patients whose fetal abdominal circumference is greater than the 90th percentile at 30 to 33 weeks.

The Bracero et al. [19] study suggests that the LGA fetuses of diabetic gravid patients seem to have disproportionately accelerated abdominal growth when compared with LGA and AGA fetuses of nondiabetic gravid patients and AGA fetuses of diabetic gravid patients. Furthermore, an abdominal diameter to femur length ratio greater than 1.385 and an abdominal diameter to biparietal diameter ratio greater than 1.065 have a high predictive value for detecting fetuses of diabetic gravid patients destined to develop macrosomia. On the other hand, these ratios cannot differentiate genetically predisposed LGA fetuses from AGA fetuses. The salient feature in LGA fetuses of diabetic gravid patients is accelerated abdominal growth; thus, serial measurements of the fetal abdomen should predict LGA infants [19]. Reliance on serial abdominal measurements alone requires exact knowledge of gestational age. The use of ratios could thus detect accelerated abdominal growth in patients with uncertain dates.

The detection of evolving diabetic macrosomia by serial ultrasound measurements of the fetal biparietal diameter and abdominal circumference is very important. In 23 insulin diabetics [11] (classes A to C), the biparietal diameter values of all fetuses fell within the normal range. However, abdominal circumference values for only 13 of 23 fetuses fell within the normal range of measurements for fetuses of nondiabetic pregnancies. In the other 10 fetuses, abdominal circumference values exceeded the upper limits of normal for nondiabetic pregnancies between 28 and 32 weeks gestation; these infants were all macrosomic at birth, and their subcutaneous fat estimated by skinfold thickness was significantly increased.

These observations indicate that ultrasound may identify disparate growth rates of various fetal structures in the latter part of pregnancy. Sokol et al. were able to improve the accuracy [73] of identifying the macrosomic fetus compared with reliance on the equation by Hadlock et al. [17]. A fetus was found to be at significantly increased risk for birth weight >4,000 g when the estimated fetal weight based on abdominal circumference is larger than that based on either head circumference or femur length or when there is a large within-subject variance in estimated fetal weight based on abdominal circumference, femur length, and head circumference. They also found that there were significantly different groups of patients whose estimated fetal weights require different equations for better estimates. Even given ultrasonographic measurements, taking into account maternal height, weight, and presence of diabetes mellitus can improve macrosomia detection. Although these findings remain to be optimized and validated, the approach used here appears to yield better predictions than the current "one function fits all" approach.

Elliott and associates [16] detected macrosomia in a diabetic population by determining the difference between the fetal trunk diameter and the biparietal diameter. Using 1.4 cm as the threshold between macrosomia (defined in their study as a birthweight greater than 4,000 g) and nonmacrosomia, they were able to detect 87% of such fetuses. Their false-positive rate, however, was 39%.

In 147 fetuses of diabetic mothers, Tamura and associates [12] compared biparietal diameter, head circumference, and abdominal circumference percentile ranks to birthweight percentiles in the latter part of pregnancy. Estimates of fetal weight by the method of Shepard et al. [28] were also calculated from these data and compared with actual birthweight percentile values. They noted (1) abdominal circumference values greater than the 90th percentile correctly predicted macrosomia (defined as a birthweight greater than the 90th percentile for age) in 78% of cases, and (2) biparietal diameter and head circumference percentiles were significantly less predictive of macrosomia. By comparison, estimated fetal weights greater than the 90th percentile correctly predicted macrosomia in 74% of cases.

When both the abdominal circumference and the estimated fetal weight exceeded the 90th percentile, however, macrosomia was correctly diagnosed in 88% of cases. Vaginal delivery was attempted in 109 of 147 diabetic gravidas. The percentage of cesarean delivery for disproportion in fetuses predicted to be macrosomic was 28.3%. On the other hand, the percentage of cesarean section in fetuses predicted not to be macrosomic was less than 0.7%, a statistically significant difference ($\chi^2 = P > .05$).

3.7 Obesity and Ultrasound Measurements

Weiss et al. have attempted to determine in 207 women if maternal obesity has an adverse impact on the prenatal ultrasound prediction of neonatal macrosomia in the diabetic population [74]. The incidence of fetal macrosomia increased significantly in the obese population when compared with the normal population (30% vs. 15%, P = .05). The ability of ultrasonography to accurately predict neonatal macrosomia did not vary significantly with increasing maternal body mass index. They concluded that ultrasound prediction of macrosomia is not affected by obesity. The increased positive predictive value in the obese population is likely a reflection of the increased incidence of macrosomia in this subgroup of patients [74].

3.8 Serial Measurements

Serial ultrasound examinations were performed by Landon et al. [21] during the third trimester in 79 pregnant women with diabetes to establish the onset of accelerated fetal growth. At least three ultrasound examinations were performed, with a minimum scan interval of 2 weeks. Growth curves constructed for femur length and head circumference were similar for 48 AGA fetuses and 31 LGA fetuses. The mean changes in femur length and head circumference (expressed as centimeter per week during the early and late third trimester) did not differ statistically between these two groups. Abdominal circumference growth was clearly accelerated at 32 weeks gestation in the LGA group compared with the AGA group. A change in abdominal circumference of 1.2 cm per week over the period of 32 to 39 weeks gestation has been determined to be an optimal cutoff for detecting excessive fetal growth (sensitivity 84%, specificity 85%). A change in abdominal circumference of 1.2 cm per week was present in 4 of 4 LGA fetuses (>4,000 g), in 17 of 21 (81%) fetuses with birthweights 4,000 to 4,499 g, and in 5 of 6 (83%) whose weight exceeded 4,500 g. It appears that improved detection of the LGA fetus in diabetic pregnancies can be accomplished by the use of serial ultrasonography during the third trimester [21].

3.9 Computed Tomography

Kitzmiller [22] conducted a feasibility study of the use of computed tomography to measure the width of the fetal shoulder diameter, abdominal circumference, and femur length of each fetus. Neither the patient nor the physician staff managing the labor and delivery were aware of the ultrasound results. Complete records of 43 patients were available for analysis. Nine (21%) patients were delivered by cesarean section for cephalopelvic disproportion. Five (12%) women had cesarean section for other indications. Of the 29 patients who delivered vaginally, 8 (21%) infants had shoulder dystocia. The mean birthweight in the shoulder dystocia group was 4,805 g. The mean birthweight in the non–shoulder dystocia group was 3,670 g (P < .01). The mean difference between abdominal diameter and biparietal diameter was significantly greater in the dystocia group (2.1 ± 0.6 cm) than in the group without dystocia (1.4 ± 0.8 cm)

(P < .05). All of the shoulder dystocia cases had abdominal diameter minus biparietal diameter differences of 1.5 cm or greater, and none of the cases with abdominal diameter minus biparietal diameter differences less than 1.5 cm had shoulder dystocia. Using abdominal diameter minus biparietal diameter difference ≥1.5 cm for the prediction of shoulder dystocia with vaginal delivery, sensitivity equals 100%, and specificity equals 53%. The results of this study prove that fetal ultrasound measurement should be performed when there is a clinical risk for macrosomia. If the abdominal diameter minus biparietal diameter difference is ≥1.5 cm, primary cesarean section should be considered.

3.10 Growth Rates

The purpose of the investigation by Songster and Golde [75] was to avoid macrosomia by predicting birthweight. Retrospective calculations from a previously collected database of sonograms performed on third-trimester fetuses indicated that a mean growth rate of 180 g per week occurred during this period. In the current study, ultrasound examinations were performed prospectively on 20 diabetic gravidas 1 to 6 weeks prior to delivery. Scans were performed using real-time linear array equipment, and standard views of the fetal biparietal diameter and the fetal abdomen were obtained. Fetal weight was calculated by the method of Shepard et al. [28], and daily fetal growth was projected at a rate of 180 g per week. Patients were evaluated weekly for delivery in accordance with their medical and obstetric condition and the birthweight prediction of their fetus. Neonatal birthweight was compared with this predicted value. The average calculated weight was 3,487 ± 326 g compared with the mean actual birthweight of 3,514 ± 405 g. The mean absolute difference between predicted and measured birthweight was 269.2 ± 190 g. This error is similar to the observed standard deviation of 106 g/kg associated with predictions using Shepard's weight formula. The average interval from scan to delivery was 3.9 weeks.

The largest infant weighed 4,180 g and the smallest weighed 2,840 g. None of the 20 infants suffered birth trauma, and all infants were discharged in good condition. The authors [28] conclude that the prediction of birthweight based on preterm ultrasound measurements is a helpful method for anticipating fetal macrosomia and preventing birth trauma.

3.11 Soft Tissue Thickness

The goal of the study by Winn and associates [76] was to evaluate the utility of measuring the nonmuscular soft tissue thickness of the fetal arm in the prenatal diagnosis of fetal macrosomia. The study showed patients had uncomplicated, singleton pregnancies with gestational ages of at least 37 weeks and estimated fetal weight of 3,500 g. The ultrasound examinations were done within 7 days of delivery. The tissue thickness was measured on a cross section at the midregion of the fetal humerus. The estimated fetal weight by biparietal diameter and abdominal circumference was calculated from Shepard's formula [28] provided the cephalic index was normal. The estimated fetal weight by abdominal circumference and femur length was obtained from the table of Hadlock et al. [66] Results were based on a study population of 44 patients. The means and standard deviations of shoulder thickness and birthweights were 6.0 ± 1.0 mm and $3,947 \pm 611$ g, respectively. When the measurement was between 5 and 7 mm, the estimated fetal weight by abdominal circumference and femur length was within 5% of the birthweight in 72% (26 of 36) of the cases. There was one case with a thickness of 4.0 mm in which the birthweight was underestimated by more than 5%. When the measurement was greater than 7.0 mm, the birthweight was underestimated in 71% (5 of 7) of the cases. This report concluded that the accuracy of predicting the birthweights of macrosomic neonates can be improved by using the measurement of the nonmuscular soft tissue thickness of the fetal arm. It is hoped that this easily obtained fetal parameter will facilitate the clinical management of pregnancies with macrosomic fetuses.

3.12 Shoulder Ratios

Modanlou et al. [9] showed that neonates experiencing shoulder dystocia had significantly greater shoulder-to-head and chest-to-head proportions than either macrosomic neonates delivered by cesarean section for failed progress in labor or macrosomic neonates delivered without shoulder dystocia. Moreover, neonates of diabetic mothers also showed significantly greater shoulder-to-head and chest-to-head size differences than did neonates of nondiabetic mothers of comparable weight. These authors recommended that a chest minus head circumference difference of 1.6 cm or a shoulder minus head circumference difference of 4.8 cm as demonstrated by ultrasound be considered the anthropometric proportions indicating the possibility of shoulder dystocia. If disproportion is detected prenatally in LGA infants or in a diabetic pregnancy, cesarean delivery would be recommended to avoid birth injury [9].

3.13 Conclusion

Many parameters have been devised to diagnose large infants; however, no single test establishes a perfect diagnosis of macrosomia, and multiple parameters must be monitored. All studies should include evaluation of the amniotic fluid volume, biparietal diameter, femur length, abdominal circumference, and estimated fetal weight. In high-risk cases (unexplained polyhydramnios, history of macrosomia, obesity, excessive weight gain, diabetes mellitus), additional measurements such as the head circumference to abdominal circumference ratio and the femur length to abdominal circumference ratio also must be evaluated. Similarly, evaluation of suspected excessive fetal growth requires careful evaluation of serial abdominal circumference measurements at 2- to 3-week intervals using all of the above techniques. Careful ultrasonic monitoring of fetuses with suspected or documented macrosomia should decrease much of the morbidity and mortality associated with shoulder dystocia [76].

We can conclude that the clinical tools currently available will allow us in many circumstances to estimate the fetal weight accurately enough to justify undertaking cesarean section as a major surgical intervention to prevent labor and thereby avoid shoulder dystocia. We have to accept some shortcomings related to the limited state of the art, but when coupled with other clinical issues, a decision frequently can be made.

References

1. Manning F. General principles and applications of ultrasound. Creasy R, Resnik R, eds. Maternal-Fetal Medicine. Fourth ed. Philadelphia: W.B. Saunders; 2004:315–356.
2. Pritchard J, MacDonald P, eds. Techniques to evaluate fetal health. Williams Obstetrics (chapter 15). 15th ed. New York: Appleton-Century-Crofts; 1966:329–367.
3. Pritchard J, MacDonald P, eds. Techniques to evaluate fetal health. Williams Obstetrics (chapter 15). 17th ed. New York: Appleton-Century-Crofts; 1985:668.
4. Dor P, Weiner H, Sofrin O, et al. Clinical and sonographic fetal weight estimates. *J Reprod Med* 2000;45:390–394.
5. Chervenak F, Gabbe S. Obstetric ultrasound. Gabbe S, Niebyl J, Simpson J, eds. *Obstetrics*. Fourth ed. New York: Churchill Livingston; 2002:251–311.
6. Mintz MC, Landon MB. Sonographic diagnosis of fetal growth disorders. *Clin Obstet Gynecol* 1988;31:44–53.
7. Campbell S, Wilkin D. Ultrasonic measurement of fetal abdominal circumference in the estimation of fetal weight. *Br J Obstet Gynaecol* 1975;82:689–696.
8. Hadlock FP. Evaluation of fetal weight estimation procedures. :Deter J, Harrist S, Birnholz R, Hadlock J, eds. *Quantitative Obstetrical Ultrasonography*. New York: John Wiley & Sons; 1986;113–118.
9. Modanlou HD, Komatsu G, Dorchester W, Freeman RK, Bosu SK. Large for gestational age neonates: Anthropometric reasons for shoulder dystocia. *Obstet Gynecol* 1982;60:417–421.
10. Ott WJ, Doyle S. Ultrasonic diagnosis of altered fetal growth by use of a normal ultrasonic fetal weight curve. *Obstet Gynecol* 1984;63:201–208.
11. Tamura RK, Sabbagha RE, Depp R, Dooley SL, Socol ML. Diabetic macrosomia: Accuracy of third trimester ultrasound. *Obstet Gynecol* 1986;67:828–831.
12. Tamura RK, Sabbagha RE, Dooley SL, Vaisrub N, Socol ML, Depp R. Realtime ultrasound examinations of weight in fetuses of diabetic gravid women. *Am J Obstet Gynecol* 1985;153:57–61.
13. Crane JP, Kopta MM, Welt SI. Abnormal fetal growth patterns: Ultrasonic diagnosis and management. *Obstet Gynecol* 1977;50:205–209.
14. Wladimiroff JW, Bloemsa CA, Wallenburg HCS. Ultrasonic diagnosis of the large for dates infant. *Obstet Gynecol* 1978;52:285–289.
15. Ogata ES, Sabbagha R, Metzger BE, Phelps RL, Depp R, Freinkel N. Serial ultrasonography to assess evolving fetal macrosomia: Studies in 23 pregnant diabetic women. *JAMA* 1980;243:2405–2408.

16. Elliott JP, Garite TJ, Freeman RK, McQuown DS, Patel JM. Ultrasonic prediction of fetal macrosomia in diabetic patients. *Obstet Gynecol* 1982;60:159–161.
17. Hadlock FP, Harrist RB, Fearneyhough TC, Deter RL, Park SK, Rossavik IK. Use of femur length/abdominal circumference ratio in detecting the macrosomic fetus. *Radiology* 1985;154:503–508.
18. Korndorffer FA, Kissling GE, Brown HL, Gabert HA. Recognition of the overgrown fetus in utero ponderal indices. *Am J Perinatol* 1987;4:86–89.
19. Bracero LA, Baxi LV, Rey HR, Yeh MN. Use of ultrasound in anternatal diagnosis of large for gestational age infants in diabetic gravid patients. *Am J Obstet Gynecol* 1985;152:43–48.
20. Murata Y, Martin CB. Growth of the biparietal diameter of the fetal head in diabetic pregnancy. *Am J Obstet Gynecol* 1973;115:252–255.
21. Landon MB, Mintz MC, Gabbe SG. Sonographic evaluation of fetal abdominal growth: Predictor of the large for gestational age infant in pregnancies complicated by diabetes mellitus. *Am J Obstet Gynecol* 1989;160:115–121.
22. Kitzmiller JL. Macrosomia in infants of diabetic mothers: Characteristics, causes, prevention. Jovanovic L, Peterson CM, Fuhrman K, eds. *Diabetes and Pregnancy, Teratology, Toxicity, and Treatment*. New York: Praeger; 1986:121.
23. Ott WJ. The diagnosis of altered fetal growth. *Obstet Gynecol Clin North Am* 1988;15:237–263.
24. Miller JM Jr, Brown HL, Khawli OF, Pastorek JG II, Gabert HA. Ultrasonographic identification of the macrosomic fetus. *J Ultrasound Med* 1988;7:577–579.
25. Miller JM Jr, Brown HL, Khawli OF, Pastorek JG II, Gabert HA. Ultrasonographic identification of the macrosomic fetus. *Am J Obstet Gynecol* 1988;159:1110–1114.
26. Dorman KJ, Hansmann M, Redford DH, et al. Fetal weight estimation by realtime ultrasound measurement of biparietal and transverse trunk diameter. *Am J Obstet Gynecol* 1982;142:652–655.
27. Bochner CJ, Medearis AL, Williams J III, Castro L, Hobel CJ, Wade ME. Early third-trimester ultrasound screening in gestational diabetes to determine the risk of macrosomia and labor dystocia at term. *Am J Obstet Gynecol* 1987;157:703–708.
28. Shepard MJ, Richards VA, Berkowitz RL. An evaluation of two equations for predicting fetal weights by ultrasound. *Obstet Gynecol* 1982;142:47–51.
29. Deter RL, Harrist RB, Hadlock FP, Carpenter RJ. Fetal head and abdominal circumference: A critical re-evaluation of the relationship to menstrual age. *J Clin Ultrasound* 1982;10:365–369.
30. Williams RL, Creasy RK, Cunningham GC, Hawes WE. Fetal growth and perinatal viability in California. *Obstet Gynecol* 1982;59:624–628.
31. Platt LD, Devore G, Golde S et al. The use of femoral soft tissue diameters in the prediction of macrosomic babies. *Official Proceedings, AIUM Annual Meeting Denver* 1982:97.
32. Miller JM, Korndorffer FA, Gabert HA. Fetal weight estimates in late pregnancy with emphasis on macrosomia. *J Clin Ultrasound* 1986;14:437–441.
33. Deter RL, Rossavik IK. A simplified method for determining individual growth curve standards. *Obstet Gynecol* 1987;70:801–807.
34. Benson CB, Doubilet PM, Saltzman DH, et al. Femur length/abdominal circumference ratio: Poor predictor of macrosomic fetuses in diabetic mothers. *J Ultrasound Med* 1986;5:141–144.
35. Miller JM Jr, Kissling GA, Brown HL, Gabert HA. stimated fetal weight: Applicability to small and large for gestational age fetus. *J Clin Ultrasound* 1988;16:95–98.
36. Spinnato JA, Allen RD, Mendenhall HW. Birthweight prediction from remote ultrasound examination. *Obstet Gynecol* 1988;71:893–897.

37. Manogura A. Early fetal growth rate helps predict macrosomia. *OB-GYN News* 2007;42:6,2–3.
38. Thurnau GR, Tamura RK, Sabbaha R, et al. A simple estimated fetal weight equation based on real time ultrasound measurements of fetuses less than thirty-four weeks' gestation. *Am J Obstet Gynecol* 1983;145:557–561.
39. Vintzileos AM, Campbell WA, Rodis JF, et al. Fetal weight estimation formulas with head, abdominal femur, and thigh circumference measurements. *Am J Obstet Gynecol* 1987;157:410–414.
40. Benson CB, Doubilet PM, Saltzman DH. Sonographic determination of fetal weights in diabetic pregnancies. *Am J Obstet Gynecol* 1987;156:441–447.
41. Boyd ME, Usher RH, McLean FH, Kramer MS. Obstetrics consequences of postmaturity. *Am J Obstet Gynecol* 1988;158:334–338.
42. Jimenez JM, Tyson JE, Reisch JS. Clinical measures of gestational age in normal pregnancies. *Obstet Gynecol* 1983;61:438–441.
43. Devore G, Berkowitz RL. The use of portable realtime ultrasound in the assessment of fetal weight during labor in the high risk patient. *Clin Obstet Gynecol* 1982;25:203–208.
44. Patterson RM. Estimation of fetal weight during labor. *Obstet Gynecol* 1985;65:330–334.
45. Timor-Tritsch IE, Itskovich J, Brandes JM. Estimation of fetal weight by realtime sonography. *Obstet Gynecol* 1981;57:653–658.
46. Warsof SL, Wolf P, Coulehan J, Queenan JT. Comparison of fetal weight estimation formulas with and without head measurements. *Obstet Gynecol* 1986;67:569–574.
47. Watson WJ, Soisson AP, Harlass FE. Estimated weight of the term fetus. Accuracy of ultrasound vs clinical examination. *J Reprod Med* 1988;33:369–373.
48. Yarkoni S, Reece EA, Wan M, et al. Intrapartum fetal weight estimat5ion: A comparison of three formulae. *J Ultrasound Med* 1986;5:707–711.
49. Gabbe SG, Mestman JH, Freeman RK, et al. Management and outcome of class A diabetes mellitus. *Am J Obstet Gynecol* 1977;127:465–469.
50. Warsof SL, Gohari P, Berkowitz RL, Hobbins JC. The estimation of fetal weight by computer assisted analysis. *Am J Obstet Gynecol* 1977;128:881–886.
51. Hadlock FP, Harrist RB, Sharman RS, Deter RL, Park SK. Estimation of fetal weight with the use of head, body and femur measurements: A prospective study. *Am J Obstet Gynecol* 1985;151:333–338.
52. Apuzzio J, Vintzileos A, Iffy L. Operative Obstetrics. Third ed. London: Taylor & Francis 2006;256.
53. Langer O, Berkus MD, Huff RW, Samueloff A. Shoulder dystocia: Should the fetus weighing >/- 4000 grams be delivered by cesarean section? *Am J Obstet Gynecol* 1991;165:831–837.
54. Jazayeri A, Heffron J, Phillips R, Spellacy W. Macrosomia prediction using ultrasound fetal abdominal circumference of 35 centimeters or more. *Obstet Gynecol* 1999;93:523–526.
55. Miller R, Johnson B, Devine P. Sonographic "fetal asymmetry" predicts shoulder dystocia. *Am J Obstet Gynecol* 2007;189:545.
56. O'Sullivan JB, Mahan CM. Criteria for oral glucose tolerance test in pregnancy. *Diabetes* 1964;13:278–282.
57. Doubilet PM, Greenes RA. Improved prediction of gestational age from fetal head measurements. *Am J Radiol* 1984;142:797–801.
58. Brenner WE, Edelman DA, Hendricks CH. A standard of fetal growth for the United States of America. *Am J Obstet Gynecol* 1976;126:555–559.
59. Acker DB, Sachs BP, Friedman EA. Risk factors for shoulder dystocia. *Obstet Gynecol* 1985;66:762–767.
60. Mintz MC, Landon MB, Gabbe SG, et al. Shoulder soft tissue width as a predictor of macrosomia in diabetic pregnancies. *Am J Perinatol* 1989;6:240–243.

61. Ianniruberto A, Gibbons JM. Predicting fetal weight by ultrasound B scan cephalometry: An improved technique with disappointing results. *Obstet Gynecol* 1971;37:689–693.

62. Campbell WA, Vintzileos AM, Neckles S, et al. Use of the femur length to estimate fetal weight in premature infants: Preliminary results. *J Ultrasound Med* 1985;4:583–588.

63. Vintzileos AM, Neckles S. Campbell WA, et al. Ultrasound fetal thigh calf circumferences and gestational age independent fetal ratios in normal pregnancy. *J Ultrasound Med* 1985;4:287–291.

64. Dubowitz LMS, Dubowitz O, Goldberg C. Clinical assessment of gestational age in the newborn infant. *J Pediatr* 1970;77:1–7.

65. O'Brien GD, Queenan JT. Growth of the ultrasound fetal femur length during normal pregnancy. Part I. *Am J Obstet Gynecol* 1981;141:833–838.

66. Hadlock FP, Kent WR, Lloyd JL, et al. An evaluation of two methods for measuring fetal head and body circumference. *J Ultrasound Med* 1982;1:359–364.

67. Hill LM, Breckle R, Wolfgram KR, et al. Evaluation of three methods for estimating fetal weight. *J Clin Ultrasound* 1986;14:171–174.

68. Deter RL, Hadlock FP, Harrist RB, Carpenter RJ. Evaluation of three methods for obtaining fetal weight estimates using dynamic image ultrasound. *J Clin Ultrasound* 1981;9:421–426.

69. Hohler CW, Kreinick CJ, Warford SHS, et al. A new method for prediction of fetal weight from ultrasound measurement of fetal abdominal circumference, thigh circumference and femur length. *J Ultrasound Med* 1983; Suppl 2:107–110.

70. McLean F, Usher R. Measurements of liveborn fetal malnutrition infants compared with similar gestation and with similar birthweight normal controls. *Biol Neonate* 1970;16:215–219.

71. Williams J III, Kirz DS, Worthen NJ, Oakes GK. Ultrasound prediction of shoulder dystocia. *Soc Perinatol Obstet* 1985;11:27.

72. Gilby I, Williams M, Spellacy W. Fetal abdominal circumference measurements of 35 and 38 cm as predictors of macrosomia. *J Reprod Med* 2000;45:936–938.

73. Sokol R, Fchik L, Dombrowski M, Zadar I. Correctly identifying the macrosomic fetus. *Am J Obstet Gynecol* 2000;182:1489–1495.

74. Weiss J, Shevell T, Cleary J, Malone F, Divine P. Macrosomia at birth: the accuracy of prenatal ultrasound diagnosis in the obese diabetic population. *Obstet Gynecol* 2002;99:193.

75. Songster G, Golde S. The prediction of fetal weight at term by preterm ultrasound. *Soc Perinatol Obstet* 1986;141:157.

76. Winn H, Holcomb W, Mazor M, et al. The utility of nonmuscular soft tissue thickness in the diagnosis of fetal macrosomia. *Procedeings Soc Perinatol Obstet* 1989;286.

Chapter 4
Intrapartum Risk Factors

James A. O'Leary

Summary Maternal weight, estimated fetal weight, fundal height, abnormal labor patterns, and need for operative delivery identify a group of women at great risk for shoulder dystocia.

Keywords: abnormal labor · fundal height · macrosomia · operative delivery · oxytocin

Contents

4.1 Introduction 49
4.2 The Initial Exam 50
4.3 Labor: The End Point 51
4.4 Prior History 51
4.5 Risk Factors 52
4.6 Oxytocin 52
4.7 Midpelvic Delivery 53
4.8 Teaching Tools 55
4.9 Conclusion 57

4.1 Introduction

Most authors contend that there is a constellation of clinical features that indicate a predisposition to shoulder dystocia and that by recognizing these warning signs, the alert practitioner should be able to avert or manage a shoulder dystocia successfully [1].

No single maternal variable is a consistent predictor of delivering a macrosomic infant; maternal body mass index, Leopold estimated fetal weight, and intrapartum fundal height are the best predictors [2].

J.A. O'Leary
Professor Obstetrics & Gynecology (retired), University of South Florida, Tampa, Florida, USA

J.A. O'Leary (ed.), *Shoulder Dystocia and Birth Injury*,
DOI 10.1007/978-1-59745-473-5_4, © Humana Press, a part of Springer
Science+Business Media, LLC 2009

Using a statistical model, it is possible to identify adverse combinations of factors that are associated with shoulder dystocia and neonatal injury along with a relatively low false-positive rate. The best model included birthweight in combination with maternal height and weight as well as gestational age and parity. A score above 0.5 detected 50.7% of the shoulder dystocia cases with brachial plexus injury along with a false-positive rate of 2.7% [3].

The intrapartum prevention of shoulder dystocia begins with a review of potential prepregnancy and antepartum risk factors. The possibility of a shoulder dystocia should be assessed first from the standpoint of how likely it is to occur. Second, if the probability of dystocia is high, a determination should be made as to the degree of difficulty (severe, moderate, or mild) that is likely to occur. For example, if there is a likelihood of difficulty, when there is a flat or platypelloid pelvis, cesarean section would be indicated.

4.2 The Initial Exam

The initial intrapartum physical assessment may be helpful, especially if there is a high index of suspicion for shoulder dystocia. However, the best we can do with our hands placed on the abdomen is to approximate the 10% to 15% error of ultrasound. When we measure uterine size by caliper or tape measure, that is, the vertical height of the fundus above the pubic symphysis (fundal height), we can add a greater degree of objectivity.

A recent study was undertaken to determine whether there is any difference in the rate of error of estimated fetal weight (EFW) in cases of shoulder dystocia compared with controls [4]. Women whose delivery was complicated by shoulder dystocia were studied and compared with a control group matched for parity, race, labor type (spontaneous or induced), and birthweight. During the 5-year study period, there were 206 cases of shoulder dystocia that met all study criteria. There was no difference in the number of patients that had EFW underestimation error 20% or greater (shoulder dystocia 9.8% vs. control 12.8%; $P = .38$). There was also no difference in the number of patients that had EFW underestimation error 20% or greater between shoulder dystocia with and without injury (injury 8.3% vs. no injury 7.1%; $P = .79$). The authors concluded that EFW underestimation error in cases of shoulder dystocia is an infrequent event and does not occur more often than in deliveries without shoulder dystocia.

In patients with high risk for shoulder dystocia, a proper, careful, and meticulous assessment of fetal weight is a major obligation of the care provider at the time of hospital admission. The obstetrician must exert a concerted effort to diagnose macrosomia prior to attempting delivery. The obstetrician must make things happen (an active role) rather than watch what happens (a passive role) or, even worse, wonder what is happening (no role).

Benedetti and Gabbe [5] stated that optimum management of shoulder dystocia involves anticipation and prevention. It seems clear that when the obstetrician is confronted with a pregnancy complicated by the previously mentioned factors, cesarean section is the safest, most prudent mode of delivery.

4.3 Labor: The End Point

Using labor as an end point for cesarean section has definite risks in a woman with multiple predisposing factors [5–19]. Labor may be too fast, too slow, or, as in most cases, normal. Labor abnormalities can help identify women at risk for shoulder dystocia. Dor et al. [16] reported a 46% incidence of failure to progress in a group of macrosomic infants, and Mondanlou et al. [20] described a 63.3% incidence of cephalopelvic disproportion and a 21.1% incidence of failure to progress in a similar group of patients. The value of a prolonged second stage as a marker for shoulder dystocia has been clearly defined by Benedetti and Gabbe [5]. In their study, an abnormal second stage with macrosomia was associated with an increase in the incidence of shoulder dystocia from 1.2% to 23%. A significant reduction in a broad variety of conditions and circumstances conductive to arrest of the shoulders at birth have been identified.

Inadequacy of the pelvis can make vaginal delivery difficult or impossible. Reduction of the anteroposterior diameter (platypelloid pelvis) is particularly important. However, excessive size of the fetus may preclude its passage even through a pelvis that is adequate by definition. Fetopelvic disproportion may be caused by the fact that, under certain circumstances, the width of the shoulders exceeds the greatest diameter of the head. This situation may lead to arrest of the shoulders in the process of delivery.

Small maternal stature is often associated with diminished pelvic dimensions. By predisposing to increased fetal size, excessive weight gain during pregnancy is conducive to the inability of the shoulders to pass through the birth canal. Although relatively seldom mentioned in the literature, the mother's own birthweight is a useful predictor of that of her child and, thus, of the risk of arrest of the shoulders at delivery [21].

4.4 Prior History

Previous delivery of a large child is a risk factor for shoulder dystocia rather than reassurance about the woman's ability of giving birth to another big baby uneventfully. High recurrence rates have been reported after a preceding shoulder dystocia [5]. Family history of diabetes is a predisposing factor for gestational diabetes and, thus, another unfavorable prognostic factor.

It is widespread misconception that the increased rate of postoperative complications in obese women warrants preferential delivery of morbidly obese gravidas by the vaginal route. In fact, there is data to prove that the incidence of shoulder dystocia among grossly obese women may be almost

10-fold higher than that in the general population [21]. Therefore, morbid obesity is a consideration for, rather than against, abdominal delivery.

Although it is a routine procedure in most teaching institutions, the need to screen all pregnant women by a glucose-loading test late in the second trimester of the pregnancy is still not uniformly done. As a result, a disturbingly high proportion of shoulder dystocia–related fetal injuries can be traced back to undiagnosed, uncontrolled, or inadequately controlled maternal diabetes. There seems to be little justification, therefore, to replace routine testing of gravidas' glucose tolerance by some complex formula and calculate diabetic predisposition based on maternal age, race, body mass index, family history, and previous pregnancy outcome [21]. Absence of screening for glucose intolerance makes the patient at greater risk for shoulder dystocia.

Minor degrees of glucose intolerance that do not fulfill the criteria for gestational diabetes still predispose to fetal macrosomia and its consequences. Contrariwise, excessive fetal weight gain can be avoided in the majority of diabetic patients by strict diet and, if necessary, by the use of insulin [21].

4.5 Risk Factors

It has been suggested that maternal weight gain exceeding 35 lb (15.6 kg) may increase the risk of large for gestational age fetal status by as much as 10-fold [21]. According to most authorities, prolongation of the pregnancy beyond the expected date of confinement increases the fetal risk exponentially, as fetal weight exceeding 4,000 g is almost twice as frequent at week 42 of the gestation as at week 40 [21]. The fetal risk further increases because the rate of growth of the fetal body exceeds that of the head at and beyond term gestation. A difference of 1.6 cm or more between the chest and head circumferences and a ≥ 4.8 cm discrepancy between those of the shoulders and the head identify a kind of fetal macrosomia that is highly conducive to shoulder dystocia at birth. A discrepancy of ≥ 1.4 cm or more between the diameters of the fetal trunk and the head (biparietal diameter) has been found more predictive of a fetal weight exceeding 4,000 g than the actual demonstration of such fetal weight by the customary techniques [21].

Protraction or arrest disorder during the first stage can be found in its background with relative frequency. Even more important is a prolonged second stage or one associated with protraction or arrest disorder [21].

4.6 Oxytocin

Uterine stimulation with oxytocin is a suspected predisposing factor. However, because its use is frequently prompted by the occurrence of protraction or arrest disorder, its role is difficult to determine with certainty. The same applies to conduction anesthesia, the administration of which frequently leads to the use

Table 4.1 Intrapartum Risk Factors

Prolonged second stage
Protracted descent
Arrest of descent
Failure of descent
Macrosomia
Abnormal first stage
Molding
Need for midpelvic delivery

of oxytocin [21]. There is a close relationship between the delivery of the fetus by forceps or vacuum extractor and arrest of the shoulders at birth.

Hypotonic uterine inertia or dysfunction may at times represent a protective mechanism, for women with a large baby, a small pelvis, or disproportion. Therefore, prior to commencing oxytocin stimulation, clinical evaluation of the underlying cause is a minimum standard of care. Arrest and protraction disorders are known to be associated with an increased incidence of shoulder dystocia [1,22,23].

When abnormalities of labor occur, they are unfortunately a late phenomenon. Arrest of descent, failure of descent, protracted descent, or a prolonged second stage occur at a time when all parties involved would like to conclude the process. Fatigue, frustration, and physician ego can also be compounding variables. Intrapartum risk factors are summarized in Table 4.1

It has been shown [1] that the labor pattern gives some warning of shoulder dystocia and that if the obstetrician were thus alerted, he or she could do a cesarean section instead of permitting vaginal delivery or vacuum extractor. Certain labor abnormalities may be predictive of cephalopelvic disproportion, particularly protracted descent and arrest patterns of labor, and these patterns in turn are somewhat more common in association with shoulder dystocia [5]. However, there is no specific abnormality in the first stage of labor that reliably predicts shoulder dystocia often enough to be clinically useful. Is there any labor abnormality in the second stage that may be predictive? When Acker et al. [11] studied this question, they confirmed that an increased frequency of protraction and arrest disorders are accompanied by dystocia; however, they also found exceedingly rapid or precipitate labors followed by shoulder dystocia as well. The mechanism by which shoulder dystocia occurs among precipitate labors is unclear, but we can conjecture that it may be related to the fact that there is insufficient time in the course of fetal descent for the fetal shoulders to accommodate their dimensions to the architecture of the maternal pelvis.

4.7 Midpelvic Delivery

There is a close relationship between the delivery of the fetus by forceps or vacuum extractor and arrest of the shoulders at birth [21].

Since an important early paper specifically referred to "midpelvic extraction," contemporary papers frequently imply that only the by-now largely abandoned midforceps and midvacuum extraction operations are predisposing. In fact, at the time of the publication of the quoted paper, the term *midpelvic extraction* incorporated those procedures that, on the basis of a recent reclassification [21], are now referred to as low-forceps and low-vacuum extractions. Similar confusion has derived from the redefinition of the term *macrosomia*, indicating a birth weight of 4,500 g versus the traditional definition of 4,000 g. Papers published after this reclassification usually interpreted the term as a body weight exceeding 4,500 g. Actually, writers who referred to *macrosomia* prior to 1992 implied a weight exceeding 4,000 g. These misleading by-products of well-intentioned innovations need to be kept in mind. Contemporary authors often misinterpret old literature data [21], especially those serving as defense expert witnesses.

There is universal agreement that the use of extraction instruments increases the risk of shoulder dystocia. However, opinions vary with regard to the magnitude of the increase of the risk from as little as 1.4-fold [20] to as much as 10- to 17-fold. The wide difference among various estimates may be due to the fact that they are often used in cases of protracted or arrested second-stage complications that are conducive themselves to arrest of the shoulders at birth. Whereas the use of any kind of extraction instrument predisposes to shoulder dystocia, sequential application of vacuum extractor and forceps, in any order, increases the risk exponentially. Because they are conducive to protracted labor and malrotation, deflexion and asynclitism of the fetal head have similar effects [21].

Midpelvic delivery in women with abnormal descent curves and prolonged second stage and the tragic outcomes have been well defined [5]. The triad of meconium, molding, and macrosomia is a definite warning in these clinical situations. Epidural and saddle-block anesthesias have also been incriminated as disposing to shoulder dystocia [5,12]. Maternal glucose intolerance and macrosomia in conjunction with an abnormal labor is more than sufficient reason to perform a cesarean section. Seigworth [24] reported that 77% of infants with a shoulder dystocia weighed more than 4,000 g and that 49% were delivered with the use of midforceps. Benedetti and Gabbe [5] showed that a higher percentage of infants more than 4,000 g were delivered with the vacuum extractor than with midforceps. They proposed that the difference between the two methods was that the vacuum extractor could deliver a larger infant than could forceps.

It is widely recognized in clinical practice that prolonged second-stage labors are closely correlated with shoulder dystocia [25,26,27,28]. Moreover, cases in which a prolonged second stage is terminated by forceps delivery, particularly midforceps, are also associated with subsequent shoulder dystocia [29–36]. Many such forceps deliveries are deemed necessary for such indications as arrest of descent, transverse arrest, or maternal exhaustion. If done after cephalopelvic disproportion has been ruled out, they perhaps can be considered appropriate. If the forceps procedure is indicated and shoulder dystocia follows in these cases, the obstetrician should not be faulted for the complication, even though it occurred as a result of the operative delivery.

4.8 Teaching Tools

A recent edition of *Williams Obstetrics* [16] contains a number of broad statements pertinent to the recognition of shoulder dystocia. The text states that a reliable prediction of shoulder dystocia is impossible. However, McLeod [31] notes that most serious cases can be predicted. The Williams Obstetricstext states that a predictable diagnosis of macrosomia is extremely difficult but advises the clinician that identification of risk factors might enable him or her to more accurately predict problem cases.

An obstetrician's decision to deliver a macrosomic infant vaginally must be dependent on not only the adequacy of the pelvis and the ability to exclude the platypelloid type clinically or radiologically [32] but also several other factors as well [28–39]. Pertinent data may be divided into antepartum and intrapartum factors. We decided to evaluate these factors with regard to outcome. Specifically, we wanted to know whether it was possible to determine early in labor whether we could identify those women at risk for shoulder dystocia. Analysis of our experience led us to develop a scoring index that will indicate to the care provider those patients at great risk.

The scoring method and antepartum risk factors are listed in Table 4.2 After completion of the antepartum score, all women with low and intermediate scores were evaluated by an intrapartum score Table.4.3 These two simple scoring systems numerically evaluate the pertinent factors in determining whether to allow the vaginal delivery of an infant when shoulder dystocia is a concern. Retrospective analysis revealed that complications of labor and delivery occurred with much greater frequency in those patients who had an intrapartum score of 3 or less. In addition, infants with low scores delivered vaginally were frequently severely depressed, necessitating endotracheal resuscitation. Four injuries occurred in this low-score group. All were directly related to the difficulty in extracting the shoulders.

Table 4.2 Antepartum Shoulder Dystocia Score:A Teaching Tool

Factor	0	1	2
Estimated fetal weight (lb)	9 ½	8 ½–9 ½	8 ½
Maternal weight gain (lb)	>35	25–35	25
Maternal weight (lb)	>180	150–180	150
Glucose intolerance	Yes	Suspect	No
Gestational age (wk)	>42	41–42	<41

A combined score of 0 to 3 represents great risk, 4 to 7 intermediate risk, and 8 to 10 negligible risk.

Table 4.3 Intrapartum Shoulder Dystocia Score: A Teaching Tool

Factor	0	1	2
Second stage	Prolonged	Borderline	Normal
Birthweight (lb)	>9 ½	8 ½–9 ½	8 ½
Forceps	Mid	Low-mid	Low
First stage	Arrest	Protraction	None
Antepartum score	1–4	5–7	8–10

A combined score of 0 to 3 represents great risk, 4 to 7 intermediate risk, and 8 to 10 negligible risk.

In the 137 deliveries with high scores, only one infant required resuscitation; this followed precipitate labor of 40 minutes. No fetal mortality and no injuries were encountered in the high-score group. If cesarean section had been performed in all 43 patients with low scores, the fetal outcome would have been far better, although some cesarean sections would have been performed unnecessarily. Because the unequivocal diagnosis of any shoulder dystocia labor comes at a time when there is no turning back, fetal morbidity and mortality will be reduced only if disproportion is recognized prior to the onset of delivery.

We have shown that by the use of a scoring index as a teaching tool, potentially difficult deliveries may be recognized early in labor, indeed, on admission, provided there has been some prior active labor. It would appear that all cases of overt fetopelvic disproportion and, more importantly, most cases of subclinical disproportion will be manifested by a low score (0 to 3). An intermediate score of 4 to 7 may be indicative of a problem. Further evaluation by radiologic means may be helpful. There should be no difficulty with shoulder dystocia delivery when the score is high. In fact, where abnormal labor exists, oxytocic stimulation may be used to advantage. This score represents an index of sound clinical judgment. It has been devised not to replace an obstetrician's acumen but to facilitate the evaluation of risk factors involved in the decision to allow a patient to continue in labor or to be delivered by cesarean section. As a teaching tool, it has proved helpful.

This author submits that the key to the proper analysis and solution of the controversy about predicting shoulder dystocia resides in the recognition and acceptance of a reliable method to assess the patients' condition early in the course of her pregnancy and labor so that a proper course can be followed. Intimately and inextricably involved with such an assessment is the inherent capability of the method to assist the clinician in determining which labors can be stimulated safely and judiciously with oxytocin.

A retrospective analysis demonstrated that there was a threefold increase in the need for resuscitation of babies born to patients with low scores. The fetal injury with scores of 0 to 3 was 17% compared with 3% for scores of 4 or greater.

Although these are preliminary observations, we propose that to achieve better results with shoulder dystocia, clinicians carefully evaluate the various components of the shoulder dystocia scores. We submit that the use of the scores will afford the clinician a good method by which to choose dysfunctional labors that can be safely stimulated with oxytocin. The educational value for younger physicians using the scores has been obvious to those involved in teaching the house staff.

4.9 Conclusion

All of the risk factors for macrosomia must be reconsidered at the beginning of labor, and the severity of each factor must be considered. As the number and severity of risk factors increases, so does the likelihood of a shoulder dystocia; for example, a maternal weight of 250 lb is certainly of greater significance than that of 180 lb. The same is true for maternal weight gain, maternal age, and gestational age.

Careful clinical pelvimetry and meticulous ultrasound examination is mandatory. If doubt remains regarding fetopelvic relationships, consultation and/ or pelvimetry can be used to resolve the diagnostic dilemma. The old adage "if in doubt get more data" is certainly applicable to intrapartum assessments.

References

1. Phelan J, Strong T. Shoulder dystocia. *Female Patient* 1988;13:73–76.
2. Brost B, Calhoun B, Misko C. Evaluation of clinical risk factors for delivering a macrosomic infant. *Am J Obstet Gynecol* 2003;S121:#209.
3. Dyachenko A, Ciampi A, Fahey J, Mighty H, Oppenheimier L, Hamilton E. Prediction of risk for shoulder dystocia with neonatal injury. *Am J Obstet Gynecol* 2006;195:1544–1549.
4. Mehta S, Blackwell S, Hendler R, et al. Accuracy of estimated fetal weight in shoulder dystocia and neonatal birth injury. *Am J Obstet Gynecol* 2005;192:1877–1881.
5. Benedetti T, Gabbe S. Shoulder dystocia: A complication of fetal macrosomia and prolonged second stage of labor with midpelvic delivery. *Obstet Gynecol* 1978;52:526–531.
6. Cruikshank D, White C. Obstetric malpresentations: Twenty years' experience. *Am J Obstet Gynecol* 1973;116:1097–1104.
7. Golditch I, Kirkman K. The large fetus: Management and outcome. *Obstet Gynecol* 1978;52:26–30.
8. Modanlou H, Dorchester W, Thorosian A, Freeman R. Macrosomia—maternal, fetal, and neonatal implications. *Obstet Gynecol* 1980;55:420–424.
9. Sack R. The large infant: A study of maternal, obstetric, fetal, and newborn characteristics including a long-term pediatric follow-up. *Am J Obstet Gynecol* 1969;104:195–204.
10. Dignam W. Abnormal delivery. Schaefer G, Graber E, eds. *Complications in Obstetric and Gynecologic Surgery*. Hagerstown, MD: Harper & Row; 1981:18–31.
11. Acker D, Sach B, Friedman E. Risk factors for shoulder dystocia in the average-weight infant. *Obstet Gynecol* 1986;67:614–618.
12. Dignam W. Difficulties in delivery, including shoulder dystocia and malpresentation of the fetus. *Clin Obstet Gynecol* 1976;19:3–12.
13. Gross T, Sokol R, Williams T, et al. Shoulder dystocia: A fetal physician risk. *Am J Obstet Gynecol* 1987;156:1408.
14. Harris B. Shoulder dystocia. *Clin Obstet Gynecol* 1984;27:1–6.

15. O'Connor T, Cavanaugh D, Knuppel R, eds. *Obstetric Emergencies*. Philadelphia: Harper & Row; 1982:243–251.
16. Dor N, Mosherg H, Stern W, Iagami N, Schulman H. Complication in fetal Macrosomia. *J Med* 1984;84:302–309.
17. Seeds J. Malpresentations. In: Gabbe S, Niebyl Jr, Simpson J, eds. *Obstetrics, Normal and Problem Pregnancies*. New York: Churchill-Livingstone; 1986:453.
18. Smeltzer J. Prevention and management of shoulder dystocia. *Clin Obstet Gynecol* 1986;29:2–9.
19. Hopwood H. Shoulder dystocia: Fifteen years' experience in a community hospital. *Am J Obstet Gynecol* 1982;144:162–167.
20. Modanlou H, Komatsu G, Dorchester W, et al. Large for gestational age neonates: Anthropometric reasons for shoulder dystocia. *Obstet Gynecol* 1982;60:417–423.
21. Apuzzio J, Ventzileos A, Iffy L. *Operative Obstetrics*. Third ed. London & New York: Taylor and Francis.
22. Bahar A. Risk factors and fetal outcomes in cases of shoulder dystocia. *Br J Obstet Gynecol* 1996;103:868–872.
23. Bofill J, Rust D, Deiedas M. Shoulder Dystocia and operative vaginal delivery. *J Mat Fetal Med* 1997;6:220–224.
24. Seigworth G. Shoulder dystocia. *Obstet Gynecol* 1966;28:767–771.
25. Hibbard L. Shoulder dystocia. *Obstet Gynecol* 1969;34:424–429.
26. McCall J Jr. Shoulder dystocia. A study of after effects. *Am J Obstet Gynecol* 1962;83:1486–1491.
27. Coustan D, Imarah J. Prophylactic insulin treatment of gestational diabetes reduces the incidence of macrosomia, operative delivery, and birth trauma. *Am J Obstet Gynecol* 1984;150:836–842.
28. Gonik B, Stringer C, Held B. An alternative maneuver for management of shoulder dystocia. *Am J Obstet Gynecol* 1983;145:882–888.
29. Elliott J, Garite T, Freeman R, et al. Ultrasonic prediction of fetal macrosomia in diabetic patients. *Obstet Gynecol* 1982;60:159–165.
30. Ogata E, Sabbagha R, Metzger B, et al. Serial ultrasonography to assess evolving fetal macrosomia. *JAMA* 1989;243:2405–2409.
31. McLeod A. Editorial comment. *Am J Obstet Gynecol* 1982;144:164.
32. Borell U, Fernstrom I. Radiographic studies of the rotation of the foetal shoulders during labor. *Acta Obstet Gynecol Scand* 1958;37:54–61.
33. Chen S, Aisaka K, Mori H, Kigawa T. Effects of sitting position on uterine activity in labor. *Obstet Gynecol* 1987;69:67–73.
34. Chestnut D, Bates J, Choi W. Continuous infusion epidural analgesia with lidocaine: Efficacy and influence during the 2nd stage of labor. *Obstet Gynecol* 1987;69:323–327.
35. Cohen W. Influence of the duration of second stage labor on perinatal outcome and puerperal morbidity. *Obstet Gynecol* 1977;49:266–269.
36. Hellman L, Prystowsky H. The duration of the second stage of labor. *Am J Obstet Gynecol* 1952;63:1223–1233.
37. Katz M, Lunenfeld E, Meizner I, Bashan N, Gross J. The effect of the duration of second state of labor on the acid base state of the fetus. *Br J Obstet Gynaecol* 1987;94:425–430.
38. Svigos J. The macrosomic infant: A high risk complication. *Med J Aust* 1981;1:245–249.
39. O'Brien J, Usher R, Maughan G. Causes of birth asphyxia and trauma. *Can Med Assoc J* 1966;94:1077–1081.

Chapter 5
Pelvimetry

James A. O'Leary

Summary Clinical pelvimetry, a digital exam of the bony landmarks in the pelvis, is critically important to proper labor and delivery management. Abnormal bone structure, size, or shape is conducive to an abnormal labor and/ or shoulder dystocia.

Keywords: dystocia mechanisms · flat pelvis · impaction · pelvimetry · prenatal assessment

Contents

5.1 Introduction 59
5.2 Clinical Pelvimetry 60
5.3 Prenatal Assessment 61
5.4 Mechanism of Labor and Delivery 63
5.5 Shoulder Dystocia Issues 63
5.6 Shoulder Impaction Mechanism 64
5.7 The Labor Exam 66
5.8 Conclusion 67

5.1 Introduction

In many, if not a majority of cases, shoulder dystocia can and should be anticipated [1]. The power, the passenger, the passage is the triad that helps the process. Unaffected by the ebb and flow of modern technology, dimensions of the passage alone remain constant. The introduction of radiographic pelvimetry into clinical practice contributed to the understanding of the fetopelvic relationship during the labor process. Recognition of the fetal risks associated with exposure to irradiation largely removed diagnostic radiographic techniques from contemporary obstetric practice. An untoward effect of this

J.A. O'Leary
Professor Obstetrics & Gynecology (retired), University of South Florida, Tampa, Florida, USA

J.A. O'Leary (ed.), *Shoulder Dystocia and Birth Injury*,
DOI 10.1007/978-1-59745-473-5_5, © Humana Press, a part of Springer
Science+Business Media, LLC 2009

development has been the loss of obstetricians' interest in the physiology of the labor and delivery process. Therefore, it is of utmost importance to understand the function of the pelvis and to commit to memory the types, the dimensions, and prognosis for birth of the four basic pelvic types. There is danger in ignorance as the practitioner will be making decisions regarding route of birth, which can have grave consequences to mother and infant. The increasing use of the vacuum extractor and cesarean operation for delivery of second-stage labor arrest has also contributed to a decreased emphasis on knowledge of pelvic types and their influence on descent and rotation of the fetal head. However, such knowledge will often allow prediction or explanation of abnormal labor, especially in the descent phase. Further evidence of the value of clinical pelvimetry is found in the studies of Caldwell [2–5]. He noted a cesarean section for all infants of 73.3% when the pelvis was considered inadequate and 19.5% when it was described as adequate. Because of the potential hazards associated with x-rays, such radiologic examinations have limited place in modern-day obstetric practice. Computed tomography (CT) scanners can be used to calculate pelvic measurements, with negligible amounts of radiation to mother and fetus, but at great expense. However, the obstetrician and the nurse midwife have at their fingertips an effective and readily available tool with few working parts to break down: clinical pelvimetry. All the clinician needs is a pair of hands and awareness of a few measurements. Therefore, this chapter will focus on the pelvic structures and architecture that have obstetric significance and are predictors of birth outcomes [6].

5.2 Clinical Pelvimetry

Documentation for clinical pelvimetry should be succinct [6] and include the following:

Pubic arch
Angle of symphysis
Notch
Spines
Sidewalls
Coccyx
Diagonal conjugate or measurement for examining finger
Obstetric conjugate if calculable
Bituberous or measurement of outlet

Knowledge of pelvic measurements and a sequential technique for clinical pelvimetry should facilitate the assessment of pelvic capacity and the formulation of a prognosis for vaginal birth. Competent clinical examination will enable experienced examiners to arrive at fairly accurate conclusions [7].

The size of the examiner's hand and the length of the fingers probably have little effect on the accuracy of clinical pelvimetry. Knowledge of pelvic architecture and expertise in recognizing the pelvic landmarks are more important parameters for accuracy than size alone. The practitioner who has small hands must be more inventive in hand placement and must learn to position patients to the best advantage. The practitioner with small hands should remember that when positioning the hand to begin the examination, the middle and index finger should be straight, with the thumb extended at greater than 90°. The ring finger and the pinky should be flexed across the palm, with the first and second joints extended. This position decreases the angulation of the hand between the extended middle finger and the flexed first and second fingers, allowing partial admission of these two fingers posteriorly into the anterior vagina to increase the length of the examining fingers. When positioning the patient, ask her to place her fists under her buttocks; this will bring the pelvis anterior, decreasing the angle between the pelvis and the examining table and thus increasing the efficiency of the small examining hand [6].

Inadequacy of the pelvis can make vaginal delivery difficult or impossible. Reduction of the anteroposterior diameter (platypelloid, or flat, pelvis), is particularly important. However, excessive size of the fetus may preclude its passage even through a pelvis that is adequate by definition.

For some care providers, clinical pelvimetry may be a lost art and skill, but one that can be easily rediscovered. In many instances, it is not done or is only superficially performed. The pelvis represents the missing link in the prevention of shoulder dystocia. Shoulder dystocia will occur 8 to 10 times more frequently in women with a flat, or platypelloid, pelvis. Thus, one must remember that there is no such pelvis as a "proven" pelvis, and that this is especially true of the flat pelvis. The platypelloid (flat) pelvis with its very large subpubic arch should be the easiest to identify by clinical examination and once recognized should alert the clinician to the possibility of a problem with the shoulders and their relationship to the pelvic inlet.

5.3 Prenatal Assessment

Every patient presenting for prenatal care should be evaluated carefully to determine adequacy of the birth canal. Digital evaluation (clinical pelvimetry) is an essential part of the overall physical examination. This easily taught skill is often neglected and requires a one-on-one relationship between teacher and student. Evaluation of the bony pelvis is easily performed immediately after a vaginal delivery. This type of self-education can be effective and should be strongly encouraged.

In general, the size of the pelvis can be determined to be large or ample, small, or borderline. An examination of the essential landmarks and measurements should allow one to make a determination of normality or abnormality, with only a few instances of significant doubt. The inability to determine size or morphology should elevate one's index of suspicion and thus demand a more careful intrapartum assessment or possible consultation. Even with limited experience, one can easily develop a mental image of the birth canal.

Acceptable minimum normal limits are diagonal conjugate, 12.0 cm; sacrosciatic notch, two finger-breadths; sacrum not palpable at the midpelvic level; ischial spines not prominent; side walls not convergent; subpubic arch greater than 80 degrees; intertuberous diameter 9 to 10 cm. Where there is any doubt of the validity of earlier findings, the measurements should be repeated, insofar as possible, late in pregnancy or during labor.

Surviving among the many clinical measurements is the diagonal conjugate. Easily performed and accurately quantifiable, this measurement, suggested by Smellie [8], enables the examiner to determine the possibility of an anteroposterior measurement greater than 11.5 cm, thereby making obstetric conjugate rarely less than 10 cm [9]. The importance of this information was underscored by the study of Joyce et al. [10] in a review of pelvimetry studies [11–17]. These authors noted a cesarean section rate of 60% when the obstetric conjugate was less than 10 cm in vertex presentations, compared with a rate of 34% when the obstetric conjugate was greater than 10 cm.

A careful clinical examination will disclose the essential dimensions and shape of the pelvis. In general, the characteristics of the anterior segment of the inlet will correspond with the anterior portion of the lower pelvis. A subpubic arch with a well-rounded apex and ample space between the ischial tuberosities is associated with a gynecoid anterior segment at the inlet. A subpubic arch with a narrow angle and straight rami, convergent side walls, and prominent spines is associated with a narrowed, android anterior segment of the inlet and cephalopelvic disproportion. A narrow subpubic arch with straight side walls is characteristic of an anthropoid anterior segment at the inlet, and possible disproportion. Finally, a wide subpubic arch with straight or divergent side walls and a wide interspinous diameter will be associated with a flat anterior segment at the inlet and shoulder dystocia! [18]

The posterior segment can best be characterized by palpation of the sacrospinous ligament and the sacrosciatic notch. A narrow notch (associated with a short sacrosciatic ligament of less than two finger-breadths) suggests an android posterior segment. A sacrosciatic ligament length of two to three finger-breadths is suggestive of a gynecoid posterior segment. If the ligament is directed backward and the spines are close together, the posterior segment of the inlet is probably anthropoid. If the ligament is directed laterally and the spines are far apart, the posterior segment of the inlet is likely to be flat [19].

These pelvic configuration assessments can be made at the time of a pelvic examination when the patient is admitted to the labor unit or can be part of the initial prenatal examination. The advantages of performing the assessment when the patient is hospitalized in labor are the increased relevance of the information at that time and the probability that the individual performing the examination will be incorporating the results into a comprehensive assessment of the patient's labor.

5.4 Mechanism of Labor and Delivery

Danforth [20] stated that shoulder dystocia may be anticipated if the baby is large or if the inlet is small. An understanding of the labor mechanism and the mechanisms of shoulder engagement at the inlet is basic to an understanding of shoulder dystocia.

With a gynecoid or android type of pelvis, the fetal head will engage in the transverse position 60% to 70% of the time. The anthropoid pelvis predisposes to engagement in the occiput anterior or posterior position. After the fetal head enters the pelvis in the transverse position, it is carried downward and backward until it impinges on the sacrum low in the midpelvis. It is at this point that internal rotation begins [20].

Anterior rotation of the fetal head is practically complete when the head makes contact with the lower aspects of the pubic rami.

The common occurrence of engagement and descent predominately in the posterior pelvis is usually associated with a normal progress of labor and spontaneous delivery. However, when engagement and descent occur predominately in the forepelvis, there is a higher incidence of abnormal progress of labor and a higher rate of operative delivery. If the fetal head is descending in the posterior pelvis, the cervix will usually be felt posteriorly in the vagina, whereas engagement and descent in the forepelvis must be suspected if the cervix is palpated in a forward position, closer to the symphysis than to the sacrum [19].

5.5 Shoulder Dystocia Issues

Different concepts have been offered regarding the attitude and position of the fetal shoulders at the time of their impaction. Common teaching holds that, with vertex presentation, the fetal head descends in the transverse position, during which the bisacromial diameter parallels the anteroposterior midline of the maternal pelvis. While the fetal head is undergoing flexion, descent, internal rotation, birth by extension, restitution, and external rotation, the shoulders are generally considered to engage and descend in either the anteroposterior or an oblique diameter of the maternal pelvis. When anterior shoulder impaction occurs, the anterior shoulder is overriding the superior aspect of the pubic bone in the midline, is unengaged and lying in an oblique diameter, or is engaged in an oblique diameter and is unable to descend further or to rotate internally [21].

The shoulders of an average fetus, with bisacromial diameter of 12.4 cm, are just small enough to fit comfortably through the widest diameter of the average pelvic inlet. Unusually broad shoulders will fit if there is sufficient room for a degree of adduction and flexion. Most adults can hunch their shoulders to reduce the diameter by a quarter to a third. The more flexible fetus should do as well or better [19].

Frequently in shoulder dystocia, neither shoulder has a chance to adduct and flex. The shoulders are trapped in an extended and abducted position, overriding the brim of the pelvis and immobilized by traction of the soft tissues of the lower birth canal, which clutch the infant's neck like a tight turtleneck sweater. Further traction risks brachial plexus injury.

Some authors [22–24] have considered that when anterior shoulder impaction occurs, the posterior shoulder is held above the level of the sacral promontory (bilateral dystocia). Others maintain that it is compacted firmly and tightly in the hollow of the sacrum (unilateral dystocia). It is possible that both groups are correct and that either situation may prevail. No formal suggestion of this possibility seems to have been declared, however, and no method has been developed by which these possible situations might be differentiated. Consequently, no contrasts have been drawn between existing maneuvers as to which may be the more appropriate in a given situation. For example, perhaps the rotational and posterior arm extraction maneuvers would be more applicable when the posterior shoulder has descended deeply into the maternal pelvis. On the other hand, the maneuver described by O'Leary (cephalic replacement) may intuitively be thought to be more expeditious when the posterior shoulder has remained unengaged [19].

Normally, after the delivery of the head, external rotation or restitution occurs, returning the head to its natural perpendicular relationship to the shoulder girdle. The fetal sagittal suture usually is oblique to the anteroposterior diameter of the outlet, and the shoulders occupy the opposite oblique pelvic diameter. As the shoulders descend in response to maternal pushing, the anterior shoulder emerges from its oblique axis under one of the pubic rami. If, however, the anterior shoulder descends in the anteroposterior diameter of the outlet and the fetus is relatively large for the outlet, impaction behind the symphysis can occur, blocking further descent. Shoulder dystocia also occurs with an extremely rapid delivery of the head, as can occur with vacuum extraction or forceps. It can result also from overzealous external rotation of the fetal vertex by the obstetrician [19].

During the normal mechanism of labor in a gynecoid pelvis, the fetal head engages and descends to the midcavity in a transverse position. As internal rotation and delivery of the fetal head occur, the shoulders engage in the inlet, generally in an oblique diameter (although this is quite variable). As the fetus descends through the birth canal and the head undergoes the cardinal movements, a process of *shoulder molding* probably occurs. This term refers to the gradual way in which the shoulders and trunk accommodate the conformation of the birth canal during descent to ensure proper engagement of the shoulders. The posterior shoulder is then able to negotiate the sacral promontory, and the anterior shoulder slips beneath the symphysis and emerges under the subpubic arch [21].

5.6 Shoulder Impaction Mechanism

Several factors may confound, individually or in combination, the normal shoulder mechanism. These may relate to the fetus, the use of regional anesthesia, the bony pelvis, the rate of descent, or maternal position.

   Unlike the head, the shoulders are mobile structures, both anterior-posteriorly and superior-inferiorly. Shoulder size and mobility are limited solely by the bony attachment to the manubrium by the clavicle and the many attachments of the clavicle, scapula, and humerus in the head, spine, and thorax. These latter attachments are by muscles that can be stretched and by nerve roots that can be avulsed by superior or inferior traction. The manubrium and chest wall are also plastic and compressible, permitting the thorax to be delivered through the pelvis [25].

   The shoulders individually are much smaller than the head, and the manubrium, thorax, and spine are mobile with respect to the head and each other, permitting a multitude of adaptation in the traverse of the pelvis.

   It is not surprising then that the irregular midpelvis and outlet seldom present a problem for the delivery of the shoulders of an infant whose head has been delivered. The sacrosciatic notch and hollow of the sacrum accommodate the posterior shoulder during delivery of the anterior and the obturator foramen, and the outside world can accommodate the anterior shoulder during the descent and delivery of the posterior. Outlet obstruction is solely by soft tissue and can be relieved by an adequate episiotomy [25].

   However, the pelvic inlet presents a different and potentially more serious problem. In most normal infants, the minimum bisacromial dimension is larger than either the suboccipital-bregmatic diameter or the biparietal diameter that must traverse the pelvic inlet. Moreover, the pelvic inlet is a smooth ovoid without irregularities to accommodate the shoulders during delivery of the upper thorax [25].

   If both shoulders traverse the inlet at the same time, or are pushed or pulled there, an "undeliverable" dystocia is potentially created at the pelvic inlet for many term-sized infants. This is especially true when they are in the shorter anterior-posterior diameter with the anterior shoulder lodged at the pubic symphysis and the posterior shoulder wedged into the sacral promontory. There is always substantially more room in an oblique or transverse diameter, but even in these wide diameters, the shoulders of a large fetus may traverse the inlet together. Comprehension of this simple truth, first recognized by Woods, is as important to the obstetrician managing a shoulder dystocia as the realization that corks will not fit into the bottle sideways is to the vintner. In both cases, forcing the impossible will do damage to the passenger or passageway [25].

   Of course, this undeliverable situation does not normally occur. Usually, the more posterior shoulder slips through the inlet obliquely and comes to rest in either the hollow of the sacrum or sacrosciatic notch during the final extension of the head. The more anterior shoulder remains out of the true pelvis or slips obliquely into the obturator foramen after the posterior shoulder enters the pelvis. The anterior shoulder then either enters the inlet or rotates from the foramen spontaneously or when gentle posterior superior pressure is applied to the fetal head and neck [25].

   The first essential maneuver, descent of the posterior shoulder into the pelvis, is entirely unobserved by the obstetrician at a normal delivery.

The second maneuver is often applied as posterior-inferior traction. This usually is of no consequence, because there is usually sufficient room to deliver the posterior shoulder over the sacrum or sacrospinous ligament while the anterior shoulder is being delivered under the symphysis pubis. Traction in the delivery of the anterior shoulder is nonetheless not helpful in normal delivery and a harmful habit when shoulder dystocia is present [25].

The important element of this process is the stepwise, sequential, rather than simultaneous, delivery of the shoulders through the "impossible diameter" of the pelvic inlet. The more posterior shoulder must enter the pelvis first, because it is more distant from the outlet and under traction with respect to the head and neck [25]. The cardinal sign that the first maneuver has not occurred is an apparent tendency for the delivered fetal head to return from where it came ("turtle sign"). This is caused by reverse traction from a posterior-superior shoulder that has not negotiated the pelvic inlet. This situation would usually arise only for infants with a large chest and shoulders, which limit the body and shoulder mobility necessary for this maneuver and decrease the relative room in which to accomplish it [25].

It is essential to recognize that the entry of the posterior shoulder into the pelvis has not occurred, because application of traction at this time has potentially severe adverse consequences in an already difficult situation. The anterior shoulder is wedged into the pubis, further impacting the posterior shoulder. Forces are applied that tend to impede, rather than promote, delivery of the posterior shoulder into the pelvis. Any traction applied further stretches the brachial plexus cervical roots of the posterior arm, and a brachial plexus palsy is the usual result [25].

5.7 The Labor Exam

Pelvic examination should also include confirmation of the presenting part, its station and position; its cephalic degree of flexion, molding, and presence or absence of asynclitism; and dilatation and effacement of the cervix with application of presenting part. Imaging pelvimetry affords relatively precise measurements plus the important determination of pelvic configuration. Although not widely used, it may be obtained at any time during pregnancy. In evaluating the probabilities of vaginal delivery, it is well to remember the essential diameters of the fetal head at term: biparietal, 9.25 cm; suboccipital bregmatic, 9.5 cm; occipitofrontal, 11.75 cm; and occipitomental, 13.5 cm. Although these cannot be determined clinically, the biparietal diameter can be determined quite accurately by expert repeated ultrasonography regardless of cephalic or breech presentation. These means of assessing pelvic capacity to allow passage of the passenger are fundamental for appropriate management [19].

Abdominal examination findings must be considered in the total assessment. Palpation and visualization determine the lie, presentation, and position of the fetus and allow an estimation of its weight. If engagement of the fetal head has not taken place, as determined by the Pawlik grip, estimation of inlet capacity can be determined by a modification of Muller's impression method. Fundal pressure is combined with downward pressure of the fetal head in the axis of the inlet. The extent of its downward displacement through the pelvic inlet can then be determined by vaginal palpation.

Finally, if there is a previous delivery record, it can be helpful in pelvic evaluation if one reviews the length of labor, position of the fetus, use of forceps, the outcome, and the newborn's weight. Favorable past history, however, may be misleading, as each subsequent fetus increases in size. However, a history of prior weights greater than 9 lb significantly increases the risk of shoulder dystocia. Birth intervals of 10 years or greater demand special attention, as in many cases the later infants are significantly larger.

5.8 Conclusion

Anatomic details should be thoroughly known to every practicing attendant. Any insecurity should be corrected by reviewing standard textbooks and studying pelvic models.

Using tests available today, we can predict with increasing accuracy which patient is going to have a large baby. If we were to rely on only one available technology, we would frequently overestimate or underestimate infant weight. Although we can more accurately estimate the infant weight, additional information obtainable in the prenatal course might reliably tell us which cases may warrant an elective cesarean section. Examination of the bony pelvis can be useful, especially if we can identify the flat pelvis or architecture that is so grossly small or deformed as to be obviously inadequate to accommodate an average-to-large infant through the pelvis; the latter is a rare finding these days.

Remember, if the subpubic arch is abnormal, there will always be other abnormalities!.

References

1. McLeod A, Haywood H. Shoulder dystocia: Fifteen years experience in a community hospital. *Am J Obstet Gynecol* 1982;144:162–167.
2. Caldwell WE, Moloy HC. Anatomical variations in the female pelvis and their effect in labor with a suggested classification. *Am J Obstet Gynecol* 1933;26:479–505.
3. Caldwell WE, Moloy HC, D'Esopo DA. Further studies on the pelvic architecture. *Am J Obstet Gynecol* 1934;28:482–500.
4. Caldwell WE, Moloy HC, D'Esopo DA. The more recent conceptions of the pelvic architecture. *Am J Obstet Gynecol* 1940;40:558–565.
5. Caldwell WE, Moloy HC, D'Esopo DA. Studies on pelvic arrests. *Am J Obstet Gynecol* 1938;36:928–961.
6. Diegmann E, Nichols RF. The bony pelvis (chapter 3). *Operative Obstetics* Second ed. New York: McGraw Hill, p23–28.

7. Pritchard J, MacDonald P, Gant NF, eds. *Williams Obstetrics.* 17th ed. Norwalk, CT: Appleton-Century-Crofts; 1985:668.
8. Smellie W. *Smellie's Treatise on the Theory & Practice of Midwifery* (McClintock AH, ed.). London, England: A.H. McClintock; 1877:1.
9. Mengert WF. Estimation of pelvic capacity. *JAMA* 1948;138:169–173.
10. Joyce DN, Giwa-Sagre F, Stevenson GW. Role of pelvimetry in active management of labor. *Br Med J* 1975;4:505–509.
11. Weinberg A. Obstetrical prognosis and treatment on basis of pelvic architecture. *N Y State J Med* 1940;40:1530–1539.
12. Boyd ME, Usher RH, McLean FH. Fetal macrosomia: prediction, risks, proposed management. *Obstet Gynecol* 1983;61:715–722.
13. Dor N, Mosberg H, Stern W, Jagani N, Schulman H. Complications in fetal macrosomia. *N Y State J Med* 1984;84:302–309.
14. Spellacy WN, Miller S, Winegar A, Peterson PQ. Macrosomia–maternal characteristics and infant complications. *Obstet Gynecol* 1985;66:158–163.
15. Acker DB, Sachs BP, Friedman EA. Risk factors for shoulder dystocia. *Obstet Gynecol* 1985;66:762–767.
16. Borell U, Fernstrom I. The movements at the sacro-iliac joints and their importance to changes in the pelvic dimensions during parturition. *Acta Obstet Gynecol Scand* 1957;36:42–57.
17. Borrell U, Fernstrom I. Radiographic studies of the rotation of the fetal shoulders during labor. *Acta Obstet Gynecol Scand* 1958;37:54–61.
18. Floberg J, Belfrage P, Ohlsen H. Influence of pelvic outlet capacity on labor. A prospective pelvimetry study of 1429 unselected primiparas. *Acta Obstet Gynecol Scand* 1987;66:121–126.
19. Gabbe S, Niebyl J, Simpson J. *Obstetrics.* Fourth ed. New York: Churchill Livingstone; 2002:358–362.
20. Danforth DN. A method of forceps rotation in persistent occiput posterior. *Am J Obstet Gynecol* 1953;65:120.
21. Hibbard L. Shoulder dystocia. *Obstet Gynecol* 1969;34:424–429.
22. Russell JCG. Molding of the pelvic outlet. *J Obstet Gynaecol Br Commonw* 1969; 76:817–820.
23. Young J. Relaxation of the pelvic joints in pregnancy: Pelvic arthropathy of pregnancy. *J Obstet Gynaecol Br Commonw* 1940;47:493–524.
24. Gonik B, Allen R, Sorab J. Objective evaluation of the shoulder dystocia phenomenon: Effect of maternal pelvic orientation on force reduction. *Obstet Gynecol* 1989;74:44–48.
25. Smeltzer J. Prevention & management of shoulder dystocia. *Clin Obstet Gynecol* 1986;29:299–308.

Part II
Treatment

Chapter 6
Recognition of Disproportion

James A. O'Leary

Summary Recognition of molding, fundal height measurement, estimated fetal weight, and clinical pelvimetry will lead to the diagnosis of cephalopelvic disproportion.

Keywords: caput · cephalopelvic disproportion · engagement · fundal height · molding

Contents

6.1	Signs and Symptoms..	72
6.2	Engagement	73
6.3	Intrapartum Reevaluation	75
6.4	Caput and Deflexion	76
6.5	Failure to Progress	77
6.6	Cephalopelvic Assessment	77
6.7	Muller-Hillis Maneuver	78
6.8	Fundal Height	79
6.9	Trial of Labor..	80
6.10	Molding	81
6.11	Clinical Pearls...	84
6.12	Active Management of Labor	85
6.13	Conclusion	86

> *Competent clinical examination should enable experienced examiners to arrive at fairly accurate conclusions.*
> —*Williams Obstetrics,15th edition, p. 689*

J.A. O'Leary
Professor Obstetrics & Gynecology (retired), University of South Florida, Tampa, Florida, USA

J.A. O'Leary (ed.), *Shoulder Dystocia and Birth Injury*,
DOI 10.1007/978-1-59745-473-5_6, © Humana Press, a part of Springer
Science+Business Media, LLC 2009

6.1 Signs and Symptoms

The ability to recognize early signs of impending disproportion is essential for those providing obstetric care [1–9]. Absolute indications for cesarean delivery are few and should be predetermined before the onset of labor [8]. Severe pelvic contraction that precludes vaginal delivery is seldom encountered. It may be found in dwarfs and others with congenital or acquired deformities (e.g., kyphoscoliosis and spondylolisthesis). Osteomalacia, which occurs in geographic areas where nutritional rickets exists, may also produce insurmountable pelvic contractions. Surprisingly, although extensive pelvic fractures following automobile or other accidents usually heal with some pelvic distortion, there is usually sufficient accommodation to allow vaginal delivery. Occasionally, however, the resultant contraction is of such magnitude as to prohibit vaginal delivery. Judgmental decision in these cases rests on the clinical assessment of the pelvis [10–14].

All instances of excessive fetal size, that is 10 lb or more (4,550 g), preferably are delivered by cesarean section [15–22]. Exceptions may be made when the pelvis is unusually large. Disproportion may prevent the proper and even fitting of the presenting part into the lower uterine segment and cervix, one of the requisites for effective contractions in labor [23–30]. If the head is held up by bony disproportion, it may fit improperly, resulting in irregular or ineffective uterine contractions [24–25].

An important part of this evaluation process is the careful and thoughtful estimation of fetal size. The most common methods are palpation of the uterus including Leopold's maneuvers, the measurement of the height of the uterus from symphysis pubis to fundus, and ultrasonic scanning/measuring. Normally, the uterine fundus grows in a linear fashion from week to week from approximately 24 to 38 weeks of gestation, with fundal height in centimeters approximately equal to the gestational age in weeks [31]. Thus, consistent fundal growth provides some indirect information regarding fetal size, particularly when the growth exceeds 40 cm. Unfortunately, such estimates are bedeviled by differences in operator competence, technique, and maternal habitus. The accuracy of weight predictions based on combined examinations is very helpful. Abdominal palpation by Leopold's maneuvers provides the clinician with helpful information regarding fetal size but generates more accurate information concerning fetal lie and presentation. These traditional measures have been largely improved upon in current practice by the use of ultrasonography.

Asynclitism can be found frequently with cephalopelvic disproportion. Instead of converting itself, the asynclitism may become permanent during the balance of the labor if a large enough caput succedaneum develops to hold the head in that position [32, 33]. In this situation, uterine inertia is the result. Some cases can be handled by oxytocin stimulation, but if true cephalopelvic disproportion is the cause, it must be recognized at the earliest opportunity and cesarean section performed at once.

A developing caput succedaneum on the fetal head can be an indication of the strength of contractions and the degree of disproportion [26]. The station of the head is also a helpful sign, as a well-flexed occiput anterior position, with the head at the level of the ischial spines, indicates that the largest diameter of the fetal head has already entered the inlet. If the head is not at station zero, fundal or suprapubic pressure should be exerted in a downward direction in an attempt to determine whether the head will enter the pelvic inlet. A history of previous deliveries may be a reliable guide, but a baby only slightly larger than those previously delivered may not be capable of passing through the pelvis. If progress is unsatisfactory and evaluation determines this is due to disproportion, cesarean section delivery gives a lower perinatal mortality than a difficult operative vaginal delivery. Maternal morbidity is also lower.

There is little to be gained by allowing a patient to labor without normal descent for more than 2 hours in the second stage; indeed, there may be great hazard [23]. When the head fails to engage after 1 hour in the second stage because of inlet contraction, cesarean section should be performed. In most cases, the problem can be solved before 1 hour has passed. Shoulder dystocia occurs when the baby's shoulders are too large to enter the inlet or when they present in an unfavorable diameter [33]. The bisacromial diameter is the long diameter and, when space is at a premium, this longest diameter must adapt to the long diameter of the inlet. As a rule, the shoulders present to the inlet with the bisacromial diameter either in the anteroposterior diameter of the pelvis or in one of the oblique diameters. If the shoulders are large, and the anteroposterior diameter of the pelvis is relatively short, the anterior shoulder overhangs the symphysis and fails to engage. The problem is relatively unusual in the anthropoid pelvis, in which the anteroposterior is long; it is more common in the flat pelvis. Shoulder dystocia should be anticipated if the baby is large or if the inlet is small.

Fetal position must be determined accurately because occiput posterior positions or deflexed attitudes may impede an otherwise normal labor by virtue of larger presenting diameters [23]. Furthermore, the best clinical evidence of a tight fit is the effect on the fetal cranium, where molding (overlapping the cranial bones with distortion of the fetal skull) and marked formation of caput succedaneum can be noted.

6.2 Engagement

The determination of engagement is of major significance. Engagement is said to have occurred when the biparietal diameter of the fetal skull has passed the level of the pelvic bony inlet. It has been well established that an unengaged vertex at the time of the onset of labor bodes poorly for pelvic delivery in a nullipara. Multiparous women, however, frequently present in labor with unengaged fetal heads; no prognostic significance may necessarily be attributed to this.

The presence or absence of compensatory space can be established both anteriorly and posteriorly by digital examination in the presence of the fetal skull [23]. Generally, this should agree with the prenatal assessment of the pelvic architecture. Most important, however, is the presence or absence of fetal head fixation within the pelvis and the presence of thrust on the presenting part during a contraction.

In the evaluation of disproportion, it is recognized that there are many variables concerned in addition to the pelvis and the head. These are especially the character of the contraction, the axis of drive, the state of the membranes, the amount of molding, and the degree of flexion of the head [23–25]. Moreover, the size of the head in relation to the size of the pelvis is important. If the head is small enough, it can, of course, descend in any diameter without being influenced in the slightest by relative narrowing or widening at various levels in the pelvis. But when the head is large enough that all of the pelvic space must be used, there is at each level generally only one pelvic diameter through which the biparietal diameter should pass. A knowledge of this optimal diameter, which presupposes a working knowledge of clinical pelvimetry principles, is a prerequisite to safe delivery, for without knowing the pelvic variations or the effects of the pelvic features on the mechanisms of labor, it is impossible to approach this appraisal. In our teaching, we insist that the details of the four parent pelvic types be learned. With this as a basis, and recognizing that mixed pelves are the rule rather than the exception, two dicta have been helpful in the appraisal and prediction of disproportion [8,23,24]. These are

1. The biparietal diameter is the narrowest diameter of the fetal head and should therefore be directed through the narrowest diameter of the pelvis at any given level.
2. The occiput tends to rotate to the widest or most ample portion of the pelvis at any given level.

Using these dicta, an attempt is made to outline the specific effect of each of the major pelvic features on labor mechanisms in the following manner.

If all the space is to be used, the position of the head at the time of engagement is determined by the shape of the inlet. In the flat pelvis, with anteroposterior narrowing, the biparietal diameter adjusts itself to the narrowed anteroposterior section, and engagement in the transverse position is the rule [23]. In the anthropoid pelvis [27], with typically narrowed forepelvis and ample posterior segment, engagement in the posterior position is to be expected. In the android pelvis, with narrow forepelvis and short posterior segment, the occiput is expected to rotate away from either of these areas and to engage in the transverse position. Transverse engagement also occurs in 70% of gynecoid pelves, as the anteroposterior diameter is slightly shorter than the widest transverse diameter [25].

6.3 Intrapartum Reevaluation

As has been mentioned, pelvic examinations done late in pregnancy, and especially during labor, tend to yield considerably more information than do those done earlier [23]. The maternal soft tissues are much more elastic and less resistant. The patient tends to be more cooperative and relaxed, especially between uterine contractions. This is, therefore, an especially good time to evaluate fetopelvic relationships in detail.

Every patient in labor should be studied carefully to ascertain whether there is disproportion between the fetal head and the pelvis [21]. Up to this point in pregnancy, pelvic evacuation reflects the examiner's subjective perception of the pelvis with reference to a fetal head envisioned to be of average size. Now, for the first time, an ideal reference structure is available for determining pelvic adequacy, namely, the very fetal head that must traverse the birth canal. For the most part, the same dimensions and characteristics of the pelvic architecture are studied as in the earlier examination. However, these can now be gauged more meaningfully against the dimensions of the presenting fetal head. Special attention, of course, should be paid to those patients previously considered to have a guarded prognosis because of constricted pelvic capacity [33].

Friedman et al. [34] note that the history of prior labors may or may not be useful, and that the patient who has had previous dysfunctional labor may have a normal pelvis that will present no special difficulties in the current labor. More likely, however, one who has had a long and hard precedent labor, a difficult forceps delivery, or a baby with evidence of birth injury may be at considerably increased risk [22]. This is particularly true if the fetus is now larger than any delivered before. Such patients are candidates for disproportion and should be watched closely.

Of equal importance to Friedman [29] are patients who have had a prior uncomplicated labor and delivery and who, because of such good obstetric performance, tend to be supervised less carefully in subsequent labors. Their management is often delegated to the least experienced member of the obstetric team. This is a common practice, contributing to delays in recognizing labor problems and in effecting appropriate action. Excessive delays are the unfortunate results of erroneously held impressions that once a patient has had a vaginal delivery, she will follow suit in subsequent pregnancies. Although cephalopelvic disproportion is uncommon in multiparas, it occurs with sufficient frequency to warrant constant vigilance.

Friedman states that the nullipara who enters labor at term with an unengaged fetal head is suspect for inlet dystocia. About 5% of nulliparas present in this manner at the onset of labor. Cesarean section can be anticipated under these circumstances in almost one third of the patients as a consequence of associated cephalopelvic disproportion.

All aspects of the evaluation described for antepartum clinical screening should be repeated in detail for the parturient. Much new information can thus be acquired to aid in her assessment. For example, factors relating to presentation and position of the fetus are obviously important, along with an evacuation of the degree of ossification and the configuration of the fetal head. One can gain an impression of the firmness of the bones, the sharpness of the parietal contours, the size of the fontanelles, the extent to which the cranial plates overlap during uterine contractions, and the width of the cranial dome [22]. These items tend to be of only limited usefulness, however, unless they are shown to be extreme variations from the norm. When extremes are encountered, they serve as important signals that a serious dystocic problem probably exists.

6.4 Caput and Deflexion

Excessive caput formation is usually associated with molding [22]. These findings are useful especially when they are shown to be significant variations from the norm. When extremes are encountered, they serve as important signals that a serious dystocic problem probably exists.

Excessive caput formation is usually associated with molding [22]. The presence of either may delude the casual observer. It is now recognized that most labors associated with cephalopelvic disproportion are characteristically dysfunctional. Most often, there are one or more arrest patterns, namely, secondary arrest of dilatation, prolonged deceleration phase, arrest of descent, or failure of descent. When these disorders are encountered in the course of a labor, cephalopelvic disproportion must be considered and definitively ruled out. It has been shown by Friedman [26] that the combination of documented disproportion and one of these arrest patterns demands cesarean section without further trial of labor. Obviously, the documentation necessary should be obtained in as objective a manner as possible, and the limitations of subjective digital evaluations must be recognized.

Evaluation of fetal cranial flexion is an important issue that is peculiarly absent from the discussion of disproportion or instrumental delivery in many standard texts [35]. In a normally sized term infant, with the chin flexed on the chest, the suboccipitobregmatic diameter is presented to the pelvic inlet (approximately 9.5 cm). This is the smallest presenting diameter of a term-size fetus. As the fetal head progressively deflexes from this position, ever larger diameters are presented to the birth canal. In brow presentation, the occipito-mental diameter (approximately 12.5 cm) presents. Marked cranial deflection often accompanies absolute disproportion and is an important sign for clinicians. Lesser degrees of deflection are common, especially in posterior and transverse presentations. Many cranial deflections correct spontaneously as labor progresses [35]. For brow and face presentations, clinical associations for deflection also include anencephaly (face) and other fetal anomalies, true disproportion high maternal parity, prematurity, and premature membrane rupture. Brow, but not face, presentations virtually always result in obstructed labor unless the baby is very small or the maternal pelvis is unusually large [31].

6.5 Failure to Progress

Several terms are used to describe patterns of inadequate labor progress or dystocia. The most common are cephalopelvic disproportion (CPD) and failure to progress (FTP) [31]. Classically, dystocia is described as resulting either from true or relative disparity between the capacity of the maternal pelvis and the fetal head, due to bony architecture, soft tissue resistance (including the cervix), fetal malpresentation, or a combination of these conditions [31]. After engagement, dystocia usually arises from some combination of inadequate uterine powers and ineffectual maternal bearing-down efforts accompanied by fetal malpositioning and varying degrees of maternal soft tissue and cervical resistance. However, as discussed in more detail below, the greatest cause for failure of vaginal delivery in many labors is inadequate uterine activity [31].

In clinical management, the issues to be considered include (a) excluding true disproportion, (b) establishing the fetal presentation, and (c) determining if adequate uterine activity is present. At times, the initial examination will promptly direct management. As an example, some malpresentations are undeliverable vaginally, face, if mentum posterior, or fixed transverse lie, which should lead to a prompt cesarean delivery. The relative fetopelvic relationship is another important issue. Disproportion is a statement concerning the size of the fetal presenting part in comparison with the amount of space available in the bony pelvis. Classically, disproportion is stated as either absolute or relative [35]. In absolute disproportion, the fetal head cannot transit the maternal pelvis as it is simply too large or the pelvis is too small. Failure of descent and/or dilatation is inevitable. This is an uncommon diagnosis. In the much more frequent condition of relative disproportion, there exists sufficient room to safely deliver the child by the use of obstetric maneuvers, despite the failure of the natural forces. These maneuvers are either pelvic traction, instrumental delivery (by forceps or vacuum extractor), or uterine propulsion via oxytocin administration [31].

6.6 Cephalopelvic Assessment

Once it is recognized that the patient in labor is at risk for cephalopelvic disproportion, there must be careful reevaluation. Two essential features of such reevaluation include a dynamic form of assessment to determine the "thrust" of the fetal head in the birth canal and, rarely, radiographic cephalopelvimetry to compare more objectively pelvic capacity with fetal head volume. The physician tries to determine by as direct a method as possible if the fetal head is likely to pass through the pelvis. When the patient is in active labor, the fetal head tends to be closely applied to the pelvic inlet (and midpelvis, if more deeply engaged), making evaluation of the cephalopelvic relationships especially meaningful.

Abdominal examination is too often ignored in this regard. It can be important for ascertaining whether the plane of the biparietal diameter of the fetal head has actually passed through the inlet. Using the symphysis pubis as a landmark, one can determine the level of the fetal head in reference to the pelvic inlet. This method is not as accurate as vaginal assessment of the station of the forward leading edge of the fetal presenting part with reference to the plane of the ischial spines. Nevertheless, it is recommended as an adjunct for ensuring that perceived descent is true descent and not merely a reflection of the molding of the fetal cranium.

Additional relevant information can be obtained by palpating the fetal head with the fingers of one hand placed intravaginally and those of the other suprapubically. With the head forced down into the inlet by a uterine contraction, the anterior parietal boss projects onto the posterior surface of the pubis. Any overriding here suggests inlet disproportion. If the fetus is presenting in an occiput posterior position, the forehead will be prominent anteriorly over the symphysis.

6.7 Muller-Hillis Maneuver

A most important dynamic test of the pelvic capacity to accommodate the fetal head is the Muller-Hillis maneuver [35]. In this procedure, an assistant forces the head down into the inlet. With fingers inside the vagina, the physician determines how far into the pelvis the fetal head will advance. Hillis [35] simplified the maneuver by evaluating the fetal descent while applying uterine fundal pressure with one hand placed on top of the uterus and the other intravaginally. Optimal results are obtained by using this maneuver during a uterine contraction. This approach is more reliable after the cervix is well dilated, because the maternal soft parts, if resistant, may prevent the head from engaging under the limited amount of downward pressure that one can exert safely.

The Muller-Hillis maneuver is a simple clinical examination that judges descent of the fetal head with fundal or suprapubic pressure. In conducting this examination, the cervix should be dilated to 4 to 5 cm. Fundal or suprapubic pressure is applied at the height of the spontaneous or induced contraction during a vaginal examination. The clinician notes the descent, flexion, and rotation of the presenting part. Acceptable descent with this maneuver is one station (or 1 cm). This examination may make the patient uncomfortable unless she has already received an epidural analgesia/anesthesia, and she should be forewarned [31].

Although the Muller-Hillis maneuver is useful, the clinical importance of this information should not be overstated. If a contraction combined with abdominal pressure results in additional descent of the presenting part, it simply suggests that there is additional space available in the pelvis. If the application of fundal pressure fails to result in additional descent or rotation, it is more likely, but not absolutely certain, that disproportion exists. At best, the Muller-Hillis maneuver is an estimation of pelvic adequacy. The test is meaningless unless interpreted with the additional information derived from observation of the progress of labor and other estimation of pelvic capacity [31]. For example, if the presenting pattern fails to descend spontaneously or with the Muller-Hillis maneuver and marked cranial molding is present, you probably have CPD! Also, abdominal palpation may indicate a high presenting part, suggesting a face or brow presentation, or may note the head overriding the pubic symphysis leading to additional procedures such as real-time ultrasonography and pelvic examination to confirm malpresentation and/or fetal anomaly [31].

Observing the thrust of the fetal head during a uterine contraction while simultaneously applying pressure to the uterine fundus immediately tells the observer whether the head is tightly fixed in the pelvis or is capable of additional caudal movement. It will give the clinician a good appreciation of whether additional space is available for descent. If the fetal head appears to flex and rotate in the manner we recognize to be best suited for the pelvis, it is reasonably certain that effective contractions will eventually succeed in furthering descent and, barring other difficulties, ultimately permit vaginal delivery.

6.8 Fundal Height

According to *Williams Obstetrics*, competent clinical examination should enable examiners to arrive at fairly accurate fetal weight conclusions [36]. Mothers experiencing higher symphysis to fundus measurements at term have a much higher incidence of shoulder dystocia [37]. This is an easy screening method for everyone to follow uterine growth [38]. It provides a suspicion of macrosomia (absolute birth weight) and identifies mothers needing ultrasound exams. The use of ultrasound has been shown to be the best method to predict fetal weight [39]. Frequent clinical estimations of fetal weight may help to select appropriate candidates for cesarean section delivery without a trial of labor [38].

When a patient is admitted in labor or for induction of labor, the abdominal examination should include the fundal height measurement. At term, you should become concerned about the size of the fetus when the fundal measurement is greater than 36 to 38 cm. As the measurement approaches 40 cm or greater, the risk of having a baby that weighs more than 8 lb becomes more likely, and problems such as cephalopelvic disproportion or shoulder dystocia become increasingly more common [37].

The infant's size may be evaluated and estimated when the maternal height and the fundal measurements are taken into account. A fundal measurement of 36 to 38 cm in an average-sized woman is usually indicative of a moderately sized infant of 7 to 8 lb at term; a fundal measurement of 38 to 40 cm may indicate an infant of about 8 to 9 lb, whereas one of 40 to 42 cm may correlate with an infant weight of about 9 to 10 lb, and one of 42 to 44+ cm may be indicative of an infant weighing about 10 lb or more unless hydramnios or a multiple pregnancy is present. In one study, in patients who had fundal measurements at term that were above the 90th percentile (in which the relationship between the maternal height and the symphysis-fundal height were adjusted), there was a higher incidence of abnormal labor and operative delivery. These patients and fetuses experienced an increased amount of shoulder dystocia, meconium aspiration, birth asphyxia, brachial plexus injuries, and midforceps deliveries [37]. Bernard et al. emphasized the importance of fundal height measurements above 40 cm and recommended cesarean section if a high level of suspicion for macrosomia is reasonable [40].

6.9 Trial of Labor

Trial of labor is a popular practice of contemporary obstetrics. Although it cannot be defined with precise limitations, it is the length of labor during which the clinician becomes convinced that the patient cannot be safely delivered vaginally. Reasonable judgment should permit such a decision to be made within 2 to 3 hours of good labor. Disproportion in all such cases is not absolute, but rather is usually of a minor degree. Good labor causes cephalic molding that is confirmed by examination and ultrasound and provides a reasonable assessment of pelvic capacity by a trial of labor. Molding is usually underappreciated by clinicians. Borderline contractions may occur at the inlet, midpelvis, or outlet, or may involve all levels of the pelvis. Inlet contraction is present when the anteroposterior diameter is 10 cm or the transverse diameter is less than 12 cm. At the midpelvic level, interspinous measurement of 9.5 cm or less is indicative of contraction. This also applies to the transverse diameter of the outlet.

Some degree of disproportion is usually suspected during earlier prenatal examinations. It may be further evident in the nullipara at term when the presenting head is found unengaged above the pelvic brim. This is particularly true of inlet contraction. Failure or protraction of descent during labor, not failure of cervical dilation, is the hallmark of disproportion. Unless soft tissue impediments block the descent, clinical pelvimetry gives a reasonably accurate portrayal of the contraction. Acceptance of trial labor then is made on the basis of borderline contraction confirmed early in labor with the mother and fetus in good condition.

Predicated on these factors, management is directed to augmentation of labor if needed, close observation by fetal monitoring, reassessment at frequent intervals, and operative delivery if required. As long as good quality of labor is maintained, that is, adequate contractions (>60 mm Hg) and progressive cervical dilation, stimulation is unwarranted. If, however, uterine activity is incoordinate or hypotonic, and if there is no significant disproportion, stimulation with oxytocin infusion may be initiated. The objective is to achieve a cervical dilation of more than 1.2 cm per hour in the nullipara and more than 1.5 cm per hour in the multipara. To improve further the quality of labor, if the head is well engaged and there is no danger of cord prolapse, the membranes may be ruptured when the cervix is 5 to 6 cm dilated. Artificial rupture of the membranes serves no purpose other than providing a vehicle to measure intrauterine pressure and direct fetal electrocardiograms. Some patients appear to have improved contractions after amniotomy if the head becomes a good dilating wedge [26,27].

A reasonable trial period (2 hours) should allow the adequacy of the inlet to be tested relatively early in labor. As evidence that the biparietal diameter has passed through the inlet, the presenting part is palpable at the level of the spines. Narrowing or foreshortening of the midpelvis, however, may not be challenged by the advancing head until later in labor. Accordingly, assessment of contraction at this level requires a longer period of labor, at times to complete dilation of the cervix, and repeated aseptic vaginal examination, to ascertain if the biparietal diameter can descend past the prominent ischial spines. If so, at this stage the advancing head fills the hollow of the sacrum, and the presenting bony part is within a finger-breadth of the perineum between contractions. If this low-midstation has been achieved, it may be assumed that delivery can be completed through a comparably narrow outlet [26,27].

After several hours of labor at any level of contraction, there is mounting evidence that passage of the head cannot occur without risk of traumatic operative vaginal delivery, cesarean section is indicated. The perturbations of difficult high or midforceps delivery or a vacuum extraction of a head wedged within an inadequate tight bony birth canal present grave danger of fetal skull and brain injury, neuromuscular injury incident to difficult shoulder delivery, and attendant danger of maternal soft tissue laceration and hemorrhage. If an arrest pattern is diagnosed and signs of disproportion are present, cesarean section again is indicated.

6.10 Molding

Molding will always be the single best clinical evidence of disproportion. Although it is a frequently used term, it is poorly understood, and most clinicians are unable to properly define the various grades of molding.

The classic clinical evidence for true disproportion or CPD is progressive molding of the presenting part without descent of the presenting part. If CPD is present, vaginal delivery is unacceptably dangerous or impossible. True CPD is quite uncommon, and the diagnosis is always suspect without an adequate trial of labor. This can be a surprisingly difficult diagnosis. The clinician's challenge is to make an accurate evaluation of the fetopelvic relationship to identify cases in which some element of disproportion exists and cesarean delivery is indicated versus those in which the dystocia is relative and it is appropriate to consider oxytocin stimulation or operative vaginal delivery [31].

In establishing the correct diagnosis, close analysis of the course of labor using a partogram is helpful. Classic protraction and/or arrest disorders are common with disproportion. In poorly progressing labor, the requirement for oxytocin labor augmentation, even with the resumption of normal progress, is additive with epidural anesthesia and results in a higher incidence of cesarean or instrumental delivery. Not surprisingly, the maternal and fetal risk for mechanical birth injury is higher under these circumstances, and operative vaginal delivery is to be attempted only with great care. Fortunately, most cases of dystocia are due to relative disproportion and respond promptly to oxytocin stimulation, lengthened labor, or simple amniorrhexis with resumption of progress and eventual vaginal delivery [35].

If extensive cranial molding is present, it is difficult for the clinician to determine whether the mass of the head is descending or if simply molding and edema account for the movement of the cranial mass deeper into the maternal pelves. In this setting, station cannot be accurately judged based solely on palpation of the leading edge of the presenting part, and other clinical findings become important [31].

If the labor trial is to be used in the diagnosis of cephalopelvic disproportion, it is important to recognize changes in fetal condition before permanent harm can occur. In many gravidas, the degree of disproportion becomes apparent when there is persistent delay in the rate of cervical dilation even when labor is augmented by oxytocin. This is easy to recognize. In others, the mechanical problem is revealed by the appearance of fetal heart rate changes and meconium in the amniotic fluid, or by failure of descent of the head, usually with increasing molding. These signs are not so easy to evaluate, but their early recognition is critical if fetal safety is to be ensured.

A simplified approach to molding assessment appears in Table 6.1. Although many clinicians believe that molding is normal, they rarely make a distinction in

Table 6.1 Types of Molding

Suture lines are
  0, normally separated
  1, touching (mild)
  2, overlapping but reducible (moderate)
  3, overlapping, not reducible (severe)

terminology. In general, physiologic molding is confined to the occiput, and pathologic molding is evidenced by changes in the parietal bones. The occurrence of both simultaneously is a sign of greater disproportion. This is often accompanied with statements by care providers that the position of the baby is difficult to determine.

Molding is graded as absent if the fetal skull bones are normally separated; mild if the suture lines are closed with no overlap; moderate where there is a bony overlap at the suture lines that can be reduced by digital pressure; and severe where there is an irreducible overlap at the suture lines. The amount of molding at the parietoparietal and parieto-occipital suture lines can then be interpreted together to provide some indication of the severity of disproportion.

To assist in clinical teaching and provide some greater understanding of the dynamic processes of labor, two systems or scoring techniques were devised. The scores are referred to as the *molding score* and *molding-labor score*.

The molding score is an excellent predictor of abnormal pelvic architecture. Because clinicians will rarely admit to the presence of severe molding and because molding always appears to be worse after the fact (i.e., after delivery), I have chosen a different grading system for molding that involves five criteria (Table 6.2). Physiologic molding only occurs over the occiput and is more ominous at a high station with a malposition.

Molding is graded as suspect, mild, or moderate. Grading each parameter as 0, 1, or 2, one then applies the rule of thirds for clinical interpretation, that is, normal, 8 to 10; intermediate, 4 to 7; abnormal, 3 or less. The molding score is outlined in Table 6.2.

The integration of the molding evaluation or score into clinical practice can be facilitated by the application of the molding-labor score (Table 6.3). The interpretation of this is identical to that used with the molding score and involves integration of other significant clinical findings. These concepts has proved to be helpful clinically and have been well received by practitioners.

Table 6.2 Molding Score

Score	0	1	2
Location	Parietal	Temporal	Occiput
Severity	Moderate	Mild	Suspect
Time in labor	Early (0–5 cm)	5–8 cm	Late
Station	−3	−2	−1
Position	Posterior	Transverse	Anterior

Table 6.3 Molding-Labor Score

Score	0	1	2
Labor	Arrest	Protraction	None
Meconium	Thick	Thin	None
Birthweight (g)	>4,000	>3,500	<3,500
Asynclitism/deflection	Present	Slight	None
Gestational age (wk)	>41	40–41	<40

Other clinical data are also important. Failure of the head to fill the posterior hollow of the sacrum is strong suggestion that the head remains high and has negotiated the midpelvis. Similarly, failure to easily pulsate the fetal ear also suggests a high station. Careful estimation of the amount of the fetal head that presents abdominally is also useful. In this technique, the extent of cranial descent into the pelvis is estimated in fifths using a palpation technique akin to the classic Leopold's maneuvers. Engagement of the fetal head has occurred when no more than one fifth of the fetal head remains palpable abdominally. Obviously anesthesia, patient size, and the skill and experience of the operator contribute to the success of the examinations [31].

Philpott [41–43] and O'Grady [31] describe an additional useful technique of gauging the extent of disproportion; in this method, the degree of cranial molding is estimated during pelvic examination by judging the overlap of the fetal cranial bones at the occipital-parietal and parietal junctions. The extent of this overlap and ease of reduction by simple digital pressure is noted. If the bones are overlapping and cannot be separated easily by simple digital pressure, molding is judged as advanced or extreme (+3), and true disproportion is likely present [31].

6.11 Clinical Pearls

> *The beginning of wisdom is to call things by their right names.*
> *—Chinese Proverb*

Many casual clinical comments, slang expressions, or unappreciated observations made in the delivery suite are often unrecognized signs of dystocia, or underrated in their clinical significance. We should be alert to such comments and listen to what we are saying to others. A list of such observations is detailed in Table 6.4. These clinical signs need to be appreciated and interpreted in view of the following interesting and clinically and legally significant comments from the literature (Table 6.5).

The evaluation of labor requires an understanding of factors other than the graph of cervical dilation and fetal descent, that is, pelvic architecture and fetal size and position. In our progressively mechanized society and labor rooms, we tend to give these other features only cursory attention. Clinical pelvimetry and Leopold maneuvers are not often applied. Although ultrasound examination is now commonly used in their stead, it provides a valuable role for understanding the fetal role in the progress of labor. Frequent uterine contractions on the fetal monitor are often inappropriately termed "good labor" despite the inability to predict progress in labor from uterine activity. Unfortunately, labor conduct is often a matter of watching a machine instead of a patient.

Schifrin and Cohen [1] state that we must not demean the progress that can be determined with a pencil and paper and believe that the graphic analysis of labor is the most reliable way of assessing progress and assisting in the communication thereof. We agree with Schifrin, who recommends universal adoption of the Friedman terminology and the graphic approach to the description

Table 6.4 Evidence of Cephalopelvic Disproportion

Cervical edema or swollen anterior lip
The head is coming through the cervix
Head not well applied to the cervix
Arrested labor
Molding (the best sign)
Severe caput
Deflexion
Asynclitism
Narrow arch
Early decelerations
"I can't feel the position"
"A fair size infant"/"a good size baby"
"A snug pelvis"
Wedging or fixation
Shrinking cervix after amniotomy
Head overriding symphysis
Premature pushing
Reverse Muller (receding head between contractions)
Poor thrust

Table 6.5 Quotes from the Literature

"0.5 cm decrease in BPD from molding is dangerous" (Oxorn and Foote [33])
"Molding is an educated guess" (Niswander [30])
"Molding is always worse at the time of CS" (O'Leary, personal observation)
"Any degree of CPD + arrest pattern = CS" (Friedman [26])
"Excessive molding equals fetal distress" (Stewart and Philpott [21])
"Any discernible evidence of CPD = no Pitocin" (Friedman [26])

BPD, biparietal diameter; CPD, cephalopelvic disproportion; CS, cesarean section.

of labor and further recommends abandoning the nondescript terms for labor progress that mire our communication and confound our understanding. Common parlance will help us to develop strategies to resolve pertinent clinical dilemmas facing contemporary obstetricians and perhaps avert attempts to understand uninterpretable data. It is important to understand more clearly the clinical diagnosis of dystocia and subscribe to an unequivocal communication of that information. Because many women with shoulder dystocia will show some evidence of labor abnormality, a clear understanding and use of accurate definitions is imperative.

6.12 Active Management of Labor

Active labor management represents a complete break with the traditional attitude of watchful expectancy. Acceleration of labor is effective and safe, restricts the duration of exposure to stress, and reduces the incidence of cesarean section. The actual acceleration procedure for a slow labor is both simple and safe. The main reason for failure to deal effectively with slow labor in the past has been the conflicting nature of the advice given and the vagueness of the restrictions, which were hinted at rather than defined. When a diagnosis of labor has been confirmed and progress is not satisfactory, augmentation is initiated in a routine manner 2 hours after admission. The aim is to achieve delivery within 8 hours of admission.

Active labor management has shown that the proposition that hypotonic and hypertonic uterine inertia represent distinct entities to be treated in opposite ways is not valid and that constriction ring, cervical dysfunction, and many other terms are objective expressions of the same phenomenon. The proliferation of these terms is a good illustration of the confusion in the past, and it would be a signal advance in obstetrics if "inefficient uterine activity" was substituted for all these terms.

Active management has effected a radical change in the interpretation of the mechanics of labor. Good uterine action has emerged as the dominant factor, and every case suspected of disproportion is now deemed worthy of a trial of labor.

Active management of labor, however, ensures that the propulsive force is adequate to the task and that the head readily descends and rotates; thus, the need for difficult extraction is eliminated. This has led to a sharp decline in the use of forceps to less than 2% of primigravidas, but, more significantly, it has almost eliminated the cases previously treated by rotation and strong traction. As a result, the forceps and the vacuum extractor can be discarded, and the small number of potentially difficult extractions remaining can be delivered by cesarean section.

One of the most important results of a policy of active labor management is the elimination of trauma, because delivery by propulsion is much safer than delivery by traction. The simple truth is that primigravidas do not inflict injury on themselves or on their babies; injury is inflicted by doctors, with instruments usually after slow labor. The practice by which residents in training are encouraged to cut their obstetric teeth on operative deliveries should be condemned. In the same context, a serious disadvantage of the extensive use of epidural anesthesia is the resulting high incidence of operative deliveries, usually in excess of 50% in primigravidas, and an increased incidence of shoulder dystocia.

6.13 Conclusion

The recognition of disproportion involves a careful review of all components pertaining to the passenger, passage, and the power.

Determination of the size and shape of the pelvis and the Muller-Hillis test are helpful in evaluating the passage. The presence of abnormal molding and caput are very significant findings as are asynclitism and deflection.

Arrest patterns in either descent or dilation should be considered disproportion until proven otherwise.

References

1. Schifrin B, Cohen W. Labor's dysfunctional lexicon. *Obstet Gynecol* 1989;74:121–124.
2. Hibbard LT. Shoulder dystocia. *Obstet Gynecol* 1969;34:424–429.
3. Mazzanti GA. Delivery of the anterior shoulder. *Obstet Gynecol* 1959;13:603–607.
4. Rubin A. Management of shoulder dystocia. *JAMA* 1964;189:835–839.
5. Heery RD. A method to relieve shoulder dystocia in vertex presentation. *Obstet Gynecol* 1963;22:360–361.
6. Chavis WM. A new instrument for the management of shoulder dystocia. *Int J Gynecol Obstet* 1979;16:331–332.
7. Woods CE. A principle of physics as applicable to shoulder delivery. *Am J Obstet Gynecol* 1943;45:796–804.
8. DeLee JB. *The Principles and Practices of Obstetrics* Philadelphia: W.B. Saunders; 1925:1043.
9. Barnum CG. Dystocia due to the shoulders. *Am J Obstet Gynecol* 1945;50:439–442.
10. Litt RL. Previous shoulder dystocia as an indication for primary cesarean section. *Coll Lett Int Corres Soc Obstet Gynecol* 1980;21:170.
11. Gonik B, Stringer CA, Held B. An alternate maneuver for management of shoulder dystocia. *Am J Obstet Gynecol* 1983;145:882–884.
12. Myerscough PR. Shoulder dystocia (chapter 13). *Monroe Kerr's Operative Obstetrics* London 3rd ed., England: Bailliere Tindall; 1982:347–354.
13. Hartfield VJ. Subcutaneous symphysiotomy–time for a reappraisal? *Aust N Z J Obstet Gynaecol* 1973;13:147–149.
14. Normal RJ. Six years experience of symphysiotomy in a teaching hospital. *Sfr Med J* 1978;52:1121–1124.
15. Acker DB, Sachs BP, Friedman EA. Risk factors for shoulder dystocia. *Obstet Gynecol* 1985;66:762–768.
16. Acker DB, Sachs BP, Friedman EA. Risk factors for shoulder dystocia in the average weight infant. *Obstet Gynecol* 1986;67:614–618.
17. Bassell GM, Humayun SG, Marx GF. Maternal bearing down efforts—another fetal risk? *Obstet Gynecol* 1980;56:39–41.
18. Beynon CL. The normal second stage of labor: A plea for reform in its conduct. *J Obstet Gynaecol Br Commonw* 1957;64:815–820.
19. Dierker LJ, Rosen M, Thompson K, Debanne S, Lynn P. The midforceps: Maternal and neonatal outcomes. *Am J Obstet Gynecol* 1985;152:176–183.
20. Greis JB, Bieniarz J, Scommengna A. Comparison of maternal and fetal effect of vacuum extraction birth forceps or cesarean deliveries. *Obstet Gynecol* 1981;52:571–577.
21. Stewart KS, Philpott RH. Fetal response to cephalopelvic disproportion. *Br J Obstet Gynaecol* 1980;87:641.
22. Quilligan EJ, Zuspan F. *Douglas-Stromme Operative Obstetrics* 4th ed. New York: Appleton-Century-Crofts; 1982.
23. Steer CM. *Moloy's Evaluation of the Pelvis in Obstetrics* 3rd ed. New York: Plenum Publishing; 1975.
24. Danforth DN. A method of forceps rotation in persistent occiput posterior. *Am J Obstet Gynecol* 1953;65:120.
25. Danforth WC. Forceps (chapter 12). In: Curtis AH, ed. *Obstetrics and Gynecology, II* Philadelphia: W.B. Saunders; 1933:232–239.
26. Friedman EA. Evaluation and management of pelvic dystocia. *Contemp Obstet Gynecol* 1976;7:155.
27. Friedman EA. *Labor: Clinical Evaluation and Management* New York: Appleton-Century-Crofts; 1967.
28. Friedman EA. Patterns of labor as indicators of risk. *Clin Obstet Gynecol* 1973;16:172.
29. Friedman EA. Trial of labor: Formulation, application and retrospective clinical evaluation. *Obstet Gynecol* 1957;10:1.

30. Niswander K. *Manual of Obstetrics: Diagnosis and Therapy*. 3rd ed. Boston: Little Brown; 1987.
31. O'Grady J, Gimovsky M, McIlhargie C. *Operative Obstetrics*. Baltimore: Williams & Wilkins; 1995.
32. Burke L, Rubin HW, Berenberg AL. The significance of the unengaged vertex in a nullipara at 38 weeks. *Am J Obstet Gynecol* 1958;76:132.
33. Oxorn H, Foote W. *Human Labor and Birth*. New York: Appleton-Century-Crofts; 1964.
34. Friedman EA, Sachtleben MR, Bresky PA. Dysfunctional labor, XII: long term effects on infant. *Am J Obstet Gynecol* 1977;127:779–785.
35. Hillis DS. Diagnosis of contracted pelvis. *Ill Med J* 1938;74:131–134.
36. Pritchard J, MacDonald P, Gant NF, eds. *Williams Obstetrics*. 17th ed. Norwalk, CT: Appleton-Century-Crofts; 1985:689.
37. Dunnihoo D. *Fundamentals of Gynecology and Obstetrics*. Second ed. Philadelphia: J.B. Lippincott; 357–359, 586.
38. DeCherney A, Pernoll M. *Current Obstetric and Gynecologic Diagnosis and Treatment*. 8th ed. 1994:353.
39. Nocon J. Shoulder dystocia (chapter 13). In: *Operative Obstetrics*. Baltimore: Williams & Wilkins; 1995;13, 233–256.
40. Bernard J, Dufour P, Vinatier D. et al. Fetal macrosomia: Risk factors and outcome. *European J Obstet Gynecol* 1998;77:51–59.
41. Stewart K, Philpott R. Fetal response to cephalopelvic disproportion. *Br J Obstet Gynecol* 1980;87:64–69.
42. Philpott R. Obstructed labour. *Clin Obstet Gynecol* 1982;9:663–683.
43. Philpott R. The recognition of cephalopelvic disproportion. *Clin obstet Gynecol* 1982;9:609–624.

Chapter 7
Delivery Techniques

James A. O'Leary

Summary The more severe the dystocia, the greater the need for additional maneuvers. Delivering of the posterior arm is the safest technique for the infant. Episiotomy is very important.

Keywords: McRoberts position · Rubin maneuver · suprapubic pressure · Woods maneuver

Contents

7.1	Overview	89
7.2	Current Practice	90
7.3	Treatment	91
7.4	Initial Techniques	92
7.5	Mild Dystocia (Grade I)	93
7.6	Moderate Dystocia (Grade II)	94
7.7	Severe Dystocia (Grade III)	97
7.8	Undeliverable Dystocia (Grade IV): Cephalic Replacement	98
7.9	Fundal Pressure	99
7.10	Comment	99
7.11	The Time Factor	101
7.12	Conclusion	103

7.1 Overview

Shoulder dystocia is undoubtedly one of the most frightening events in modern-day delivery rooms [1]. Having the father present, often with a video camera, only adds to the clinicians' anxiety. Because shoulder dystocia is an infrequent occurrence, clinicians have a limited chance to develop great expertise, compare various procedures, or become confident in their skills; thus, anxiety may lead to haste and even panic [2–8].

J.A. O'Leary

Professor Obstetrics & Gynecology (retired), University of South Florida, Tampa, Florida, USA

J.A. O'Leary (ed.), *Shoulder Dystocia and Birth Injury*,
DOI 10.1007/978-1-59745-473-5_7, © Humana Press, a part of Springer
Science+Business Media, LLC 2009

The best method for treating shoulder dystocia is no longer debatable. Many methods have been described, and the question of superiority is now generally accepted. The McRoberts maneuver, to be discussed later, continues to gain acceptance and is the most popular and effective current technique providing only gentle traction is used. The greatest current emphasis must be on prevention, identification of risk factors, anticipation, and proper evaluation. It is most noteworthy that the delivery of the posterior arm does not cause brachial plexus injuries.

Although it is important to deliver the infant quickly, excessive haste, overly aggressive manipulation, hyperflexion of the neck, and use of great force will result in injury. Much care is needed to effect the delivery of impacted shoulders without traumatizing the mother and baby. If a shoulder dystocia is anticipated and a vaginal delivery planned, an obstetrician who is experienced in dealing with the problem should be available, and the patient should be placed in the McRoberts position. If an individual is not experienced and a shoulder dystocia is anticipated, then a cesarean section is indicated.

The delivery of the head without the rest of the body does not cause immediate fetal compromise. Textbooks and other publications have emphasized for decades that delivery in the course of two separate uterine contractions is not a pathologic phenomenon. The fact that the face of the fetus turns blue during the intervening time may be unnerving for the uninitiated. The anxiety soon evaporates, however, when the next contraction expels the child in vigorous condition.

7.2 Current Practice

Contemporary practice standards permit the use of manipulative techniques to facilitate the delivery of the fetal body. However, they must be used with due attention to the physiology of the birthing process. Actions that are not in synchrony with the latter are counterproductive. It is critically important to avoid strong traction. The majority of brachial plexus injuries involve strong traction on the child's body within 3 minutes of the delivery of the head; that is, before the end of the next uterine contraction. Traction is not useful until the external rotation of the head has been completed. Thereafter, if used at all, it must be unerringly gentle.

Because the majority of shoulder dystocia follows spontaneous delivery of the fetal head and occurs without warning, a well-organized plan to deal with this obstetric emergency must be present and mentally rehearsed regularly by health care providers who deliver babies. The sequence of maneuvers chosen by the clinician should be based on the algorithm (see Chapter 14, Fig. 14.12 and Fig. 14.13) with which he or she is most familiar and which has proven successful in their hands.

Regardless of the sequence chosen, maternal pushing should be avoided and assistance should be requested. Some maneuvers require two assistants in addition to the obstetrician for optimal performance. Overzealous traction and fundal pressure should be avoided. Continued maternal pushing and desperate traction on the fetal head with or without fundal pressure will only increase the impaction of the anterior shoulder behind the pubic symphysis and impair resolution of the problem.

Although anticipation of shoulder dystocia and its prevention, when practical [9–18], is highly recommended and should be done by all, impaction of the anterior fetal shoulder can occur unexpectedly in the hands of even the most thoughtful obstetrician. When this happens, the fetus is immediately imperiled. Its oxygen supply may suddenly be restricted and delivery must be effected within the next several minutes if the baby's life is to be saved.

With a shoulder dystocia, there is little time for reflection or consultation. Assistance may occasionally, or even commonly, be available and should be called for, but neither its presence nor its quality can be relied on [9–19]. Consequently, anyone involved in obstetrics should prepare for this moment by developing and memorizing a sequence of maneuvers that he or she intends to use in this situation [20–23]. Those who have not done so will sweat and blunder, bringing a greater chance of traumatic injury to the pregnant woman and of hypoxic residua or death to the fetus [24].

7.3 Treatment

An understanding of the Kreitzer classification of shoulder dystocia is critical to proper management of this emergency (Table 7.1).

Treatment must be carefully preplanned and the mechanisms leading to the problem carefully understood by the obstetrician. The physician must be forewarned of the additional

"Three P's," these resulting from panic: pulling, pushing, and pivoting of the neck. Further pulling or traction will increase the impaction and cause injury to the child, and fundal pressure will do the same. Pivoting or twisting the neck does not help and only leads to neurologic damage. Adequate help must be obtained. Anesthesia assistance is important as is the presence of a pediatrician

Table 7.1 Kreitzer Classification of Shoulder Dystocia (see Chapter 14)

1.	Shoulder dystocia at cesarean section.
2.	Shoulder dystocia at vaginal delivery.
3.	Soft tissue dystocia after restitution.
4.	Bony dystocia after restitution.
5.	Bony dystocia due to failure of restitution.

and additional nursing care. The infant's airway must be cleared and nuchal cord ruled out. Rapid action is critical to grade the severity of the dystocia and to determine which procedure should be used. If possible, the distinction between a bilateral versus unilateral dystocia should be made (see Chapter 14, Fig. 14.8 and Fig. 14.11). We have not found vaginal lubricants useful, nor do we recommend their use. Although insertion of a Foley catheter is frequently mentioned, it is rarely necessary if a full bladder can be excluded.

7.4 Initial Techniques

Initially, most obstetricians apply gentle downward traction pressure to the head in an effort to dislodge the impacted anterior shoulder from under the pubic symphysis (see Chapter 14, Fig. 14.3A, B). This gentle downward pull is a standard maneuver for effecting delivery of the anterior shoulder in the otherwise normal vaginal delivery, so it is understandable why it is done so often for shoulder dystocia. We teach our residents that when shoulder dystocia is diagnosed, they must use only gentle traction on the baby's head. Pulling on the head risks brachial plexus injury. Continued traction is usually stronger traction.

Once the head has emerged, and it is evident that shoulder dystocia exists, several courses of action are available. First, it is essential that any possible interference from the soft tissues of the lower birth canal be eliminated by an adequate episiotomy. Whereas a deep mediolateral episiotomy is usually satisfactory, it risks extra blood loss, damage to the pubococcygeal muscles, and inadequate repair. Our experience shows that a deliberate perineotomy, which divides the anal sphincter and extends well up the rectovaginal septum, furnishes the needed space. It can be expected that a carefully repaired perineotomy will result in a better anatomic restoration of the vagina and perineum than will the repair of a wide mediolateral episiotomy.

In most cases, delivery can be accomplished without injury to the fetus if the physician is familiar with certain manipulative and operative techniques. Once the head has been delivered, the respiratory tract cleared of mucus and fluid, and the baby permitted a free airway, time becomes less important as long as the fetal heart is normal and shows no distress. Delivery of the impacted shoulders may then be performed unhurriedly and without panic. A scalp clip from the electronic fetal monitor will determine the urgency of delivery due to cord compression and manipulation.

When there is difficulty, the simplest and least traumatic measures should be attempted; for instance manipulative methods of extraction and strong pressure applied to the suprapubic area from above. We condemn the practice of effecting shoulder delivery by strong traction on the baby's head once it is delivered, for by such unwise pulling, injury to the brachial plexus or even to the cervical spine may result.

7.5 Mild Dystocia (Grade I)

This author prefers to grade shoulder dystocia based on the response to treatment, ranging from the easiest to a combination of more involved procedures (Table 7.2). The first and simplest step is direct suprapubic pressure in the midline. Using the palm (see Chapter 14, Fig. 14.15) of the hand, and not the fist, is preferable, with pressure directed slightly down and lateral away from the pubic bone as reported by Mazzanti [11]. This pressure should be to either side of the midline of the maternal abdomen to force the shoulders into an oblique diameter of the pelvis. The force should be directed so as to adduct the anterior shoulder. This is usually successful only with milder forms of shoulder dystocia.

With mild dystocia in which the above techniques fail, it has been our policy to perform a McRoberts maneuver. The procedure's only drawback is the requirement of two assistants, and it has been highly effective. Successful resolution of the dystocia has occurred in all but 4 of more than 40 cases at our institution. The McRoberts maneuver is easy and safe and can be rapidly performed [25] (Chapter 8 and Chapter 14).

Dr. McRoberts, in a letter to the editor, mentions his almost 40 years experience in using this procedure successfully [16]. We concur strongly with his recommendation that every obstetrician should know how to perform the maneuver. The McRoberts maneuver has been recommended by Benedetti [17] and Harris [19].

The McRoberts maneuver is currently recommended as the initial technique for the disimpaction of the anterior shoulder. In a retrospective review of 236 shoulder dystocia cases at Los Angeles County–University of Southern California Medical Center, this maneuver alone alleviated 42% of cases. Moreover, trends toward lower rates of maternal and neonatal morbidity were associated with the McRoberts maneuver. Objective testing has also shown that this

Table 7.2 Severity of Shoulder Dystocia and Suggested Treatment

Grade		Treatment
I.	Mild	McRoberts maneuver
		Suprapubic pressure with or without rotation
		Directed posterior (Mazzanti) [11]
		Directed to one side (Rubin) [4]
II.	Moderate	Rubin maneuver (reverse Woods) [1]
		Woods maneuver
		Posterior shoulder delivery [2]
III.	Severe	Fracture clavicle or humerus
		Repeat above with general anesthesia
IV.	Undeliverable	Cephalic replacement
		(Gunn-Zavanelli-O'Leary maneuver) [30]
		Abdominal rescue

maneuver may reduce fetal shoulder extraction forces and brachial plexus stretching [23,24].

The McRoberts maneuver involves exaggerated hyperflexion of the patient's legs, resulting in a straightening of the maternal sacrum relative to the lumbar spine with consequence cephalic rotation of the symphysis pubis [25]. The effects of this position enhance passage of the posterior fetal shoulder over the sacrum and through the pelvic inlet, positioning the plane of the pelvic inlet to its maximal dimension perpendicular to the maximum maternal expulsive force. Limitations to the technique include the need for two assistants and the extra time required to elevate and flex the patient's legs. Potential difficulty can also be encountered in moving the very obese patient or the patient with a dense epidural motor blockade.

The patient's legs are removed from the stirrups and sharply flexed against the abdomen. This straightens the sacrum relative to the lumbar spine, with rotation of the symphysis pubis cephalad and a decrease of the angle of inclination of the symphysis. Although this maneuver does not change the dimensions of the pelvis, the superior rotation of the symphysis trends to free the impacted anterior shoulder. As part of the McRoberts maneuver, if the shoulder is not released immediately, we combine the above techniques. The interested reader is referred to the next chapter for more in-depth discussion of the McRoberts technique.

7.6 Moderate Dystocia (Grade II)

The Woods screw maneuver (see Chapter 14, Figs. 14.16–14.18) or the Rubin [4] modification, which is a reverse rotation, should be applied next if the dystocia is moderate. These usually are unsuccessful in the more severe grades of dystocia, and one should not spend much time with them. Woods was one of the first to address this problem. He presented a wooden model to demonstrate that although an object might be too large to be delivered through the pelvis directly, it might be possible to effect the delivery by a screwing motion. He likened shoulder dystocia to the "crossed thread" of a bolt and nut. He therefore recommended that in shoulder dystocia, the screwing motion should be effected by exerting pressure on the anterior surface (clavicle) of the posterior shoulder of the infant [12]. It must be strongly emphasized that all rotational forces be done by pressure on the scapula and clavicle and never on the infant's head. Morris [13] also recommended pressure on the anterior surface of the posterior shoulder, specifically indicating that pressure should be exerted in the delto-pectoral triangle of the posterior arm and never on the head.

Rubin [4] emphasized the importance of having both of the infant's shoulders brought forward toward the chest. He referred to this as adduction of the shoulders and presented measurements to demonstrate that with the shoulders in this position, the circumference of the baby's body was less than when the shoulders were abducted. The latter would result from use of the Woods maneuver. Rubin recommended two maneuvers. First, the infant's shoulders are rocked from side to side by pushing on the mother's abdomen. If this does not disengage the anterior shoulder, one locates the baby's most readily available shoulder and uses the entire palm of the hand to push that shoulder 30 degrees toward the baby's chest. This results in adduction of both the baby's shoulders, and if they are at first located in the anteroposterior diameter of the pelvis, the maneuver displaces them into the longer oblique diameter of the pelvis. This maneuver is more successful if combined with suprapubic pressure in a direction that facilitates the vaginal rotation. The alliteration "shoving scapulas saves shoulders" may help the young student studying this problem. To be most effective, the clinician should use the right hand when attempting counterclockwise rotation (for Right Occiput Trauma (ROT) position) and the left hand when attempting clockwise rotation (for Left Occiput Trauma (LOT) position). This requires the attendant to supinate his or her forearm initially, directing the palm of the hand *outwardly* to place it behind the posterior aspect of the posterior shoulder (see Chapter 14, Fig. 14.9). Although initially awkward, this allows full use of the entire 180-degree rotational arc available, using one smooth continuous motion. Although more intuitive and comfortable initially, starting with the opposite hand would limit the degree of rotation achievable once the operator's forearm and elbow cross the midline. If more than 30 degrees of rotation is required, the operator would have to switch hands [26].

Beginning and completing the maneuver with the same-side hand as the fetal chest is facing (from the operator's perspective) during a posterior Rubin maneuver also allows for more natural palpation and support of the dorsal aspects of the fetus' posterior humerus and elbow. Pressing the humerus and elbow against the fetal chest should protect against frictional forces pinning the posterior arm behind the trunk during rotation, which would increase the risk for upper-extremity injury. This also positions the operator's hand in a better position to sweep the humerus and elbow across the fetal chest for delivery of the posterior arm (discussed below), particularly if the fetal elbow is extended [26].

When placing the hand into the posterior vagina, care should be taken to avoid decreasing the station already achieved by the posterior shoulder. One way to do this is to initially place the hand under the fetal shoulder and slide it behind the posterior aspect of the shoulder in much the way a blade from a pair of forceps would be applied to the side of the fetal head. As the posterior shoulder is being rotated, the operator should be applying traction simultaneously on the fetal trunk, guiding the posterior shoulder into the hollow of the sacrum in an effort to achieve the natural, forward-progressing winding motion. This can be done by grasping the acromion of the shoulder and being sure to couple this traction with rotation. It is especially important not to place a finger in the axilla, as direct axillary compression can produce radial nerve injury [26].

Either an anterior or posterior Rubin maneuver can be used prior to application of traction on the fetal head as an initial maneuver for shoulder dystocia. It also may be executed with or without simultaneous application of suprapubic pressure. If suprapubic pressure is used, it must be coordinated with the clinician's efforts to achieve the direction of rotation being attempted. Thus, for an anterior Rubin maneuver, suprapubic pressure is directed behind the shoulder away from the assistant, in the same direction as the clinician is attempting to rotate the shoulder. For a posterior Rubin maneuver, suprapubic pressure should be given from the anterior aspect of the anterior shoulder so that the direction of rotation being attempted is maintained. Unless the anterior shoulder moves easily in this circumstance, suprapubic pressure would only serve to abduct the shoulder, which could be counterproductive if the remainder of the thorax does not move easily, as it would increase rather than decrease the fetal shoulder width.

Hibbard [14] described a maneuver without any mention of outcome data in which pressure on the head results in directing it back into the vagina, and the infant's anterior shoulder is pushed toward the rectum to displace it from the symphysis. This requires an assistant capable of applying a sufficient amount of suprapubic and then fundal pressure. The steps are as follows: press firmly with a flattened hand against the infant's head, jaw, and upper neck, carrying the head and neck posteriorly toward the rectum and slightly upward to facilitate the release of the anterior shoulder; as the anterior shoulder moves away from the symphysis, the assistant is ready to apply suprapubic and then fundal pressure. When the anterior shoulder slips free of the superior surface of the symphysis, strong fundal pressure is applied at the same time, the continuing pressure against the jaw and neck is shifted slightly, aiming directly at the rectal area.

One must be careful not to acutely angulate the infant's neck, as this will lead to nerve injury (see Chapter 14, Fig. 14.4 A, B). However, it must be emphasized that *Williams Obstetrics* [27] feels this maneuver is contraindicated because of the high risk for nerve injury. The Hibbard maneuver [14] has not been accepted, and there is no published report describing a significant clinical experience. We have not used the maneuver at our institution.

A rather inventive method for shrinking the fetal shoulder width during shoulder dystocia was described long ago by Jacquemier and later in the United States by Barnum [26]. By delivering the posterior arm before the shoulders, the bisacromial diameter is reduced to the axilloacromial diameter. The technique begins much the same way as the authors have described the posterior Rubin maneuver and the modified Woods screw maneuvers above. The operator places an upturned hand beneath the acromion of the posterior shoulder. Again, for maximal operator flexibility, it is preferable to use the same-side hand as the fetal chest is facing (from the operator's perspective) [26].

A number of authors have written about delivery of the posterior arm to overcome shoulder dystocia. Schwartz and Dixon [15] reported on the management of 48 patients with shoulder dystocia. Traction was employed to deliver 31 babies, and in this group 9 babies died and 7 were damaged. Extraction of the posterior arm was used for 17 babies; no infants died, 4 were damaged. These authors understandably favor delivery of the posterior arm. I also favor delivery of the posterior arm as one of the most efficacious and expeditious means of over-coming moderate shoulder dystocia (see Chapter 14, Fig. 14.19 and Fig. 14.20).

The method I use is the following. The definitive move is to introduce one hand into the vagina posteriorly to determine the reason for difficulty. If the infant's back is on the mother's right, the right hand is employed, and vice versa. If shoulder dystocia is due to a very large baby, the true pelvis is tightly filled with the baby's torso, and it will be impossible or extremely difficult to insert the examining hand very far into the vagina. Sliding the hand along the dorsal aspect of the humerus and pressing it against the fetal chest to avoid fracture, the clinician then palpates the elbow. If the elbow is already flexed, the hand is guided around the elbow to grasp the fetus' forearm and wrist. If the elbow is extended, the operator should grasp the elbow and gently press his or her thumb in the brachial fossa while flexing the elbow using his or her fingers along the dorsal aspect of the forearm. Once the elbow is flexed, the operator continues to guide the hand around the elbow to grasp the forearm and wrist [26]. After grasping the forearm and wrist, the operator pulls the forearm over the chest and across the infant's face, extending the arm at the elbow and shoulder to deliver through the introitus. All motions should be directed medially toward and across the fetal chest, supporting and pressing the humerus against the chest to avoid pulling the arm against lateral resistance [26].

If the baby's large torso fills the pelvis, the baby's posterior hand is located and pulled across the chest. It has been recommended that pressure be applied in the antecubital space to flex the arm and make the hand more accessible (see Chapter 14, Fig. 14.19 A, B). I have found that this is difficult when the arm and hand are tightly wedged in the pelvis. It may be possible to get an index finger around the wrist and/or possibly on the elbow and then force the arm anterior across the chest. As the posterior hand is brought down across the baby's chest, the posterior arm and shoulder deliver outside the vagina and the remainder of the delivery can usually be completed without undue difficulty.

The Barnum maneuver can be used alone or as a natural extension of either a posterior Rubin maneuver or a modified Woods screw maneuver. Delivery of the posterior arm also can be used as the initial maneuver for shoulder dystocia; in Canada, this is not an uncommon approach, with lower injury rates reported than those encountered when maternal maneuvers are used beforehand [26]. Although humerus fracture is almost exclusively associated with delivery of the posterior arm compared with other fetal maneuvers, the relative morbidity must be considered. Skeletal fractures will always heal, whereas 10% of brachial plexus nerve injuries result in permanent dysfunction of the affected arm.

7.7 Severe Dystocia (Grade III)

Deliberate fracture of the clavicle sometimes has been considered necessary to accomplish delivery of the impacted shoulder, although it is difficult to do in a large fetus with well-calcified bones. Some have advocated cutting the clavicle, but this is particularly risky for both mother and fetus. It is a good medicolegal practice to announce a deliberate fracture beforehand. Deliberate fracture of the clavicle is often mentioned but has never been substantiated with a statistical analysis of efficacy. Purposeful fracturing of the clavicle on the side of the impaction has been described as a practical technique for overcoming shoulder dystocia. Although sound theoretically, the technique is difficult and particularly so in a macrosomic fetus whose bones are strong. Thus, it remains an approach that only a few practitioners dare to use.

We have had no experience with the shoehorn-like instrument, symphysiotomy, or the Heery [18] technique of forming a groove for the anterior shoulder using the index and middle fingers palm-up behind the pubic bone, or its variant, palm-down. When all of the above fail, the dystocia must be considered undeliverable, or a grade IV. As soon as this determination can be made, cephalic replacement must be performed.

7.8 Undeliverable Dystocia (Grade IV): Cephalic Replacement

After the diagnosis of irreducible or undeliverable bilateral severe shoulder impaction dystocia is made, the following steps should be taken: prepare for abdominal delivery, initiate tocolysis if necessary (subcutaneous terbutaline 0.2 mg), monitor the fetal heart rate, and rapidly perform a cephalic replacement. The episiotomy repair can be deferred and hemostats placed on any major bleeding vessels. The head is easily replaced by constant but firm pressure with the palm of the hand after rotating it back to the occiput anterior (OA) position. The head must be "reflexed" and kept in the position of flexion, then the vertex is pushed as far cephalad as possible (usually zero station) and held in that position by an assistant if necessary (see Chapter 9 for more details).

The push procedure, or cephalic replacement, was easy to carry out in each of our four cases. All infants initially experienced a prolonged deceleration of 60 to 70 beats per minute for 2 to 4 minutes but rapidly returned to a normal baseline rate with good short and long variability. The cesarean sections in every instance were routine for patients who normally would undergo abdominal delivery at full dilation. The infants were delivered in good condition and with no difficulty. The bilateral shoulders impaction may prevent the head from becoming wedged deep into the pelvis as is so frequently encountered with cesarean sections for cephalic disproportion.

As a last resort, rapid cephalic replacement, tocolysis, and abdominal delivery seems to offer the infant, the mother, and the obstetrician the best outcome. This technique should be used only when continued persistence at vaginal manipulation would lead to a predictably poor outcome for all concerned. There must be a reasonable chance of a safe delivery for the mother and a good outcome for the baby. At present, it is not recommended for routine use until the more classic procedures have failed.

7.9 Fundal Pressure

The timing of fundal pressure is critically important in the definition, management, and legal defense of shoulder dystocia. Gross et al. [28] define true shoulder dystocia as any delivery requiring maneuvers to deliver the shoulders in addition to downward traction and episiotomy. Fundal pressure in the absence of other maneuvers resulted in a 77% complication rate and was strongly associated with orthopedic and neurologic damage. The use of fundal pressure delayed the implementation of more effective techniques and further impacted the anterior shoulder into the pubic bone, leading to more traction and greater risk to the brachial plexus.

Historically, application of fundal pressure was advocated for assistance with fetal manipulation. In his original paper, Woods [12] describes using fundal pressure as an ancillary technique to increase the forward progression of the fetal trunk as it is being wound through the "threads" of the maternal pelvis. As long as the impaction is cleared, applying fundal pressure does in fact advance the fetus in the birth canal. However, if an impaction still exists, fundal pressure only serves to increase it.

Although this phenomenon was recognized as early as 1970 [29,30], it was not until the early 1980s that the notion of fundal pressure being counterproductive during shoulder dystocia entered mainstream obstetrics [31]. In 1987, Gross et al. [28] determined that shoulder dystocia deliveries in which fundal pressure and traction were used were associated with a 70% incidence of fetal injury. Thereafter, fundal pressure became contraindicated in the management of shoulder dystocia.

Although not practiced today, requesting fundal pressure during a rotational maneuver was standard practice through the 1960s [31]. Today, use of more than one shoulder dystocia maneuver (other than fundal pressure), especially when exercised simultaneously by more than one operator, must be carefully coordinated to achieve the intended objective. The primary clinician must be aware of the effectiveness or ineffectiveness of assistants' efforts and redirect their actions or adjust his or her own accordingly. Communication and continuous feedback regarding progress is essential. Otherwise, the cross-purposeful actions of two or more team members can, albeit unintentionally, increase the risk for injury.

7.10 Comment

The first step is anticipation of shoulder dystocia, including recognition of the previously described antepartum and intrapartum risk factors. Every effort should be made to prepare a rapid, ingrained, and well-coordinated stepwise plan. When fetal macrosomia is suspected, the patient should be thoroughly counseled as to the risks and benefits of a trial of vaginal delivery. Prophylactic cesarean section may be strongly considered when the estimated fetal weight is greater than 4,500 g or 4,000 g in the diabetic patient, or in a patient with a prior history of shoulder dystocia. Operative vaginal delivery should be avoided in the setting of macrosomia and/or an abnormal labor pattern. Delivery should be performed in the delivery room rather than in the labor room.

Shoulder dystocia is usually heralded by the classic "turtle sign" (see Chapter 14, Fig. 14.9). After the fetal head delivers, it retracts back onto the maternal perineum. As maternal efforts to expel the fetal body continue, the fetal shoulders become further impacted behind the symphysis pubis. Having diagnosed a shoulder dystocia, it is extremely important to avoid feelings of panic. If the physician is alone, immediate obstetric assistance should be called for. Anesthesia, additional nursing support, and nursery staff should also be contacted. Do not attempt to relieve a tight nuchal cord. The mother should be instructed to stop pushing. All attendants should refrain from applying fundal pressure, as this has been shown to worsen the impaction and increase the chance of brachial plexus injury.

Our experience indicates an improving prognosis as a result of earlier detection of macrosomia by ultrasound, a higher index of suspicion as a result of routing glucose screening, and a more liberal policy of cesarean section in this group of women when they show signs of dysfunctional labor.

The prevention of shoulder dystocia begins with the first prenatal visit, where all the preconceptual and prenatal risk factors except for total pregnancy weight gain can be determined. Early identification and proper counseling, and perhaps induction of labor at term, will help to reduce the severity of this problem. However, it must be emphasized that even under optimal circumstances and in the best of hands, an unexpected shoulder dystocia can occur in a nonmacrosomic infant. Thus, it behooves us to have well-defined treatment plans committed to memory.

A detailed medical record of the findings and the sequence of maneuvers leading to resolution of a shoulder dystocia is very important. It is regrettable that until recently, many institutions commonly failed to write detailed descriptions of the maneuvers that were used in cases of shoulder dystocia. This failure to document makes legal defense difficult and tends to aid the plaintiff's case.

To reiterate, no single maneuver has been found to be consistently successful for the relief of shoulder dystocia; this may result from the fact that fetal attitude and positions differ from case to case. However, posterior arm delivery is the safest! It is agreed by all who practice obstetrics that the presence in their repertoire of only one or two maneuvers is inadequate for the potential problems that exist with different types of shoulder dystocia. Most clinicians react to this by mentally accumulating the entire array of maneuvers or at least a significant portion thereof.

Is there a definable benefit to clinical experience? Acker et al. [32] noted that experience must be of some benefit. Nevertheless, we see relatively inexperienced junior residents deal effectively and competently with shoulder dystocia at the delivery table, whereas some older, ostensibly more experienced clinicians may not do as well. Some young practitioners acquire admirable competence after only a few cases, whereas others never become truly skillful regardless of their exposure. When we examined the record of our staff obstetricians, we found a few seasoned and experienced clinicians had conducted deliveries in which the baby developed an Erb palsy as a result of a shoulder dystocia. Thus, the element of experience may not be as important as we think it should be. [32]

As cesarean section rates have increased at our institution, the number of shoulder dystocia cases appears to have decreased. As a result, one important criterion for a safe vaginal delivery is becoming increasingly difficult to fulfill: residency training programs that provide sufficient opportunity to acquire adequate experience. In-depth teaching, memorizing a plan of action, and periodically reviewing these procedures (a so-called fire drill) are imperative. The author has used an antepartum and intrapartum scoring system as a teaching tool and a clinical aid in identifying and quantitating risk factors. The antepartum shoulder dystocia score has been valuable in our hands. It alerts the staff to the proper and organized review of the significant risks of macrosomia, maternal weight gain, obesity, glucose intolerance, and gestational age. When the risk factors are evaluated by a scoring system (Chapter 4), it is possible to separate the high-risk from the low-risk patient.

At our institution, the women with a good or high score (8 to 10) did not frequently experience shoulder dystocia, and if they did it was usually mild. However, with a low score (0 to 3), the results were less reliable. It appears that this scoring system is valuable for screening patients who are not likely to develop a shoulder dystocia. Women with low (0 to 3) or intermediate (4 to 7) scores are analyzed with the intrapartum shoulder dystocia score (Chapter 4). Our preliminary results with this tool show good specificity (a high true-negative rate) but a somewhat reduced sensitivity (a lower true-positive rate). The doubling of our primary cesarean section rate in the past 4 years has led to a fourfold reduction in shoulder dystocia.

7.11 The Time Factor

Shoulder dystocia management is paradoxically time sensitive. The two competing issues are the amount of time needed to resolve a shoulder dystocia without asphyxial insult and how quickly to progress from one maneuver to the next in order to minimize the risk of peripheral nerve injury.

A frequent question is, how much time do I have before brain damage will occur? More than 30 years ago, Wood et al. [10] described serial pH determinations between delivery of the head and trunk. The pH declined at the ratio of 0.04 U per minute. Thus, there is adequate time to proceed in a well-organized manner, knowing that cephalic replacement is ultimately available. Delays greater than 7 to 10 minutes may be associated with low Apgar scores and prenatal asphyxia.

A rapidly reduced shoulder impaction usually implies excessive haste [26]. When an injury occurs in a nonmacrosomic infant who is delivered rapidly after an impaction, the injury is probably a result of excessive angulation, but may also be secondary to rapid traction. It is most likely that these mothers have a platypelloid pelvis. Some authors [26] recommend waiting for the next contraction before initiating treatment. It is an appropriate way to allow resolution of the dystocia, after clearing the airway and checking for a nuchal cord.

The prevailing thinking is that the time window in which to resolve a shoulder dystocia before asphyxial insult (not injury) is likely is about 4 minutes. This is based on a 1973 study by Wood et al. [10] in which the decline in cord pH was mathematically calculated for different time intervals from just before the head delivers to when the head emerges and then finally after the trunk delivers [26]. In this study, the cord pH is calculated to drop by 0.04 units per minute during the head-to-body interval. It is this precipitous drop that has caused the authors of the consensus statement on cerebral palsy and neonatal encephalopathy to liken the risk of asphyxia during shoulder dystocia to that of cord prolapse, in which there is near complete or complete occlusion of the cord [26].

However, this time frame was extrapolated retrospectively from only 22 deliveries, none of which were complicated by shoulder dystocia. Rather, the study of Woods et al. compared two groups: spontaneous deliveries from natural uterine contractions without traction applied and deliveries where traction was applied immediately upon emergence of the head. Indeed, the study found that the average cord pH at delivery was still normal at about 7.25, which did not differ significantly between the two delivery groups [26].

Five studies present data from more than 200 shoulder dystocia deliveries with a recorded head-to-body interval, a 5-minute Apgar score, and/or a measured cord pH. These included permanently injured and uninjured children who were all products of shoulder dystocia deliveries, with a range of head-to-body intervals up to 15 minutes on the perineum [26]. Not only were there no permanent CNS sequelae before 8 minutes, but also the rate of decline in pH was not significantly different from the overall average pH of 7.24 over that 8-minute interval in either the injured or uninjured groups [26]. An 8-minute window of time should help reduce clinician anxiety during actual shoulder dystocia events. Clinicians should not be as concerned if they find that additional time is needed to perform alternative maneuvers [26].

There appeared to be more time in which to resolve shoulder dystocia than what is conventionally perceived, however, it was also determined that time must be used wisely [26]. By dividing the number of shoulder dystocia maneuvers performed by the head-to-body interval, the maneuver rate (measured in maneuvers per minute) was found to be inversely related to the severity of resultant brachial plexus palsy. For shoulder dystocia deliveries resulting in permanent brachial plexus injury, fewer than two maneuvers were used per minute during head-to-body interval, whereas deliveries with no or only temporary injury were resolved using two or more maneuvers per minute [26].

When performed at a fixed rate, the relative risk of brachial plexus injury when fetal maneuvers are not used is significantly lower, but only if fetal maneuvers are resorted to within the first 2 minutes, after that the risk of injury is no different than when only maternal maneuvers are used, suggesting that by that time, the injury has probably already occurred. Thus, if one maneuver fails to resolve shoulder dystocia within 30 seconds, another maneuver—preferably a fetal maneuver—should be attempted [26].

7.12 Conclusion

A high level of suspicion for shoulder dystocia is a reasonable indication for cesarean section if founded on a solid database of known risk factors. The mnemonic "A DOPE" (age of mother, diabetes, obesity, postdatism, and excessive fetal weight or maternal weight gain) identifies women at greatest risk. Placing a patient in the McRoberts position improves the results with all techniques. If suprapubic pressure and the McRoberts position are unsuccessful, and simple rotational maneuvers and delivery of the posterior arm do not work, cephalic replacement must be attempted.

The Barnum maneuver (posterior arm delivery) is the safest and most effective maneuver.

It should be emphasized that "delivery of the posterior arm" does not equate with delivery of the posterior shoulder using upward traction on the fetal head. This latter maneuver is often performed either consciously or unconsciously after downward traction fails to deliver the anterior shoulder early on in the shoulder dystocia encounter [26]. However, such action, if it fails to resolve the dystocia quickly and easily and the upward-directed force is too great and/or too lateralized, places the posterior brachial plexus at the same risk for stretch injury as downward traction does for the anterior brachial plexus [26].

Fetal manipulation appears to be the best method for atraumatic resolution insofar as it takes better advantage of pelvic geometry and requires less traction to complete the delivery than do maternal maneuvers. It can eliminate the need to repeat traction on the fetal head, by instead applying the traction to the fetal trunk. Fetal manipulation also does not depend on the skill or presence of an assistant and can reasonably be practiced at all shoulder dystocia deliveries and even at routine deliveries, as was done a generation ago [26].

Fetal maneuvers can reduce the incidence of brachial plexus palsy (as was demonstrated 50 years ago). Fetal maneuvers are both safe and effective: They were described earlier than maternal maneuvers, and when they were the prevailing standard for shoulder dystocia management, they resulted in a fourfold reduction in neonatal injury. When used as the sole management strategy, fetal manipulation is actually associated with a very low rate of injury compared with maternal maneuvers or traction alone. Because of these advantages, training in fetal maneuvers should be emphasized and should be prioritized in shoulder dystocia management algorithms.

References

1. Mazzanti G. Delivery of the anterior shoulder: A neglected art. *Obstet Gynecol* 1959;13:603–607.
2. Dignam W. Difficulties in delivery, including shoulder dystocia and malpresentations of the fetus. *Clin Obstet Gynecol* 1976;19:3–12.
3. Pritchard J, McDonald P, Gant N. ,*Williams Obstetrics* 17th ed. Norwalk, CT: Appleton-Century-Crofts; 1985:668.
4. Rubin A. Management of shoulder dystocia. *JAMA* 1964;189:835–844.
5. Hopwood H. Shoulder dystocia: Fifteen years' experience in a community hospital. *Am J Obstet Gynecol* 1982;144:162–168.
6. Benedetti T. Managing shoulder dystocia. *Contemp Obstet Gynecol* 1979;14:33–39.
7. Klebanoff M, Mills J, Berendes H. Mothers birth weight as a predictor of macrosomia. *Am J Obstet Gynecol* 1985;153:253–258.
8. O'Shaughnessy R, Russ J, Zuspan F. Glyucosylated hemoglobins and diabetes mellitus in pregnancy. *Am J Obstet Gynecol* 1979;135:783–789.
9. Seigworth G. Shoulder dystocia. *Obstet Gynecol* 1966;28:767–771.
10. Wood C, Ng K, Hounslow D, Benning H. Time: An important variable in normal delivery. *J Obstet Gynaecol Br Commons* 1973;80:295–299.
11. Mazzanti G. Delivery of the anterior shoulder. *Obstet Gynecol* 1959;13:603–609.
12. Woods C. A principle of physics as applicable to shoulder delivery. *Am J Obstet Gynecol* 1943;45:796–812.
13. Morris W. Shoulder dystocia. *J Obstet Gynaecol Br Commonw* 1955;62:302–308.
14. Hibbard L. Coping with shoulder dystocia. *Contemp Obstet Gynecol* 1982;20:229–233.
15. Schwartz B, Dixon D. Shoulder dystocia. *Obstet Gynecol* 1969;28:764–769.
16. McRoberts W. Maneuvers for shoulder dystocia. *Contemp Obstet Gynecol* 1984;24:17–21.
17. Benedetti T, Gabbe S. Shoulder dystocia: A complication of fetal macrosomia and prolonged second stage of labor with midpelvic delivery. *Obstet Gynecol* 1978;52:526–529.
18. Heery R. A method to relieve shoulder dystocia in vertex presentation. *Obstet Gynecol* 1963;22:360–366.
19. Harris B. Shoulder dystocia. *Clin Obstet Gynecol* 1984;27:106–111.
20. O'Leary J, Gunn D. Cephalic replacement for shoulder dystocia. *Contemp Obstet Gynecol* 1986;27:157–159.
21. O'Leary J. Shoulder dystocia. *Contemp Obstet Gynecol* 1986;27:78–82.
22. O'Leary J, Pollack N. The McRobert's maneuver for shoulder dystocia. *Surg Forum* 189;40:467–468.
23. O'Leary J. Clinical opinion—shoulder dystocia: Prevention and treatment. *Am Obstet Gynecol* 1990;162:5–9.
24. Sandberg E. The Zavanelli maneuver: A potentially revolutionary method for the resolution of shoulder dystocia. *Am J Obstet Gynecol* 1985;152:479–483.
25. McRoberts W. Maneuvers for shoulder dystocia. *Contemp Obstet Gynecol* 1984;24:17.
26. Gurewitsch E, Allen R. Fetal manipulation for management of shoulder dystocia. *Mat-Fetal Med Rev* 2006;17:239–280.
27. Cunningham G, MacDonald P, Gant N, eds. *Williams Obstetrics*. 18th ed. New York: Appleton and Lang;1989.

28. Gross S, Shime J, Farine D. Shoulder dystocia: Predictors and outcome. A five-year review. *Am J Obstet Gynecol* 1987;156:334–336.
29. Lynn J. Shoulder dystocia. *J Am Osteo Assoc* 1970;69:70–76.
30. Chez R, Bennedetti T. How to manage shoulder dystocia during delivery. *Cont Obstet Gynecol* 1982;19:208–209.
31. Ramieri J, Iffy L. Shoulder dystocia. In: *Operative Obstetrics*. 3rd ed. London and New York: Taylor & Francis; 2006.
32. Acker DB, Sachs BP, Friedman EA. Risk factors for shoulder dystocia. *Obstet Gynecol* 1985;66:762–768.

Chapter 8
The McRoberts Maneuver

James A. O'Leary

Summary The McRoberts position, or maneuver, is a good first-line technique. If combined with more than gentle traction, a brachial plexus will occur. It usually requires additional strong suprapubic pressure.

Keywords: McRoberts position/maneuver · suprapubic pressure · thigh hyperflexion

Contents

8.1	Introduction	107
8.2	Literature Review	108
8.3	Technique	109
8.4	Suprapubic Pressure: The Mazzanti Maneuver	111
8.5	Delivery	112
8.6	Effects of the McRoberts Maneuver	113
8.7	Research	113
8.8	Improper McRoberts Maneuver	114
8.9	Clinical Experience	114
8.10	Conclusion	116

8.1 Introduction

The McRoberts maneuver [1–7] deserves a prominent place in all obstetric textbooks. The delivery of the head without the rest of the body does not cause immediate fetal compromise. Textbooks and other publications have emphasized for decades that delivery in the course of two separate uterine contractions is not a pathologic phenomenon [8]. The fact that the face of the fetus turns blue during the intervening time may be unnerving for the uninitiated. The anxiety soon evaporates, however, when the next contraction expels the child in vigorous condition [9].

J.A. O'Leary
Professor Obstetrics & Gynecology (retired), University of South Florida, Tampa, Florida, USA

J.A. O'Leary (ed.), *Shoulder Dystocia and Birth Injury*,
DOI 10.1007/978-1-59745-473-5_8, © Humana Press, a part of Springer
Science+Business Media, LLC 2009

Although originally described in the 19th century in France, and presented in American texts as early as 1914, it was not until the early 1980s that the McRoberts maneuver was reintroduced to mainstream obstetrics [10]. Since that time, maternal manipulation has become the first-line treatment for shoulder dystocia. There are several reasons for this: First, and most simply, it is often effective. Used alone, the McRoberts position successfully resolves up to 40% of shoulder dystocia deliveries without injury, although success rates in some reports are higher. In an often incompletely understood laboratory model, McRoberts positioning proved to result in fewer clavicle fractures and less brachial plexus stretch for some shoulder dystocia deliveries compared with lithotomy. However, as the shoulder dystocia became more severe, McRoberts positioning had no benefit over lithotomy in terms of neonatal morbidity [1].

There is also the perception, based on retrospective studies, that fetal maneuvers actually increase the risk of fetal injury. This bias has led to the false recommendation that fetal manipulation be reserved for only those shoulder dystocia deliveries where maternal manipulation has already failed [8].

Contemporary practice standards permit the use of fetal manipulative techniques to facilitate the delivery of the fetal body. However, they must be used with due attention to the physiology of the birthing process. Actions that are not in synchrony with the latter are counterproductive. It is critically important to avoid strong traction. The majority of brachial plexus injuries involve extraction of the child's body within 3 minutes of the delivery of the head; that is, before the end of the next uterine contraction. Traction is not useful until the external rotation of the head has been completed. Thereafter, if used at all, it must be unerringly gentle [9]. This method maintains the axis of the cervical spine as close as possible to that of the thoracic spine, thus avoiding stretching of the brachial plexus.

Smeltzer [2], in an excellent review of shoulder dystocia, notes that the McRoberts position has essentially eliminated the need for other maneuvers in more than 5,000 deliveries. He believes that its use is more effective before the anterior shoulder has been wedged into the inlet.

We believe it is best to think of the McRoberts maneuver as the McRoberts position (see Chapter 14, Fig. 14.14). It is also best to think of the McRoberts position as possibly the preferred initial position to deal with a shoulder dystocia. We believe that all obese women and those with other risk factors for shoulder dystocia should be delivered in this position.

The term *prophylactic McRoberts maneuver* is now common parlance in many hospitals and many teaching institutions. Many authorities advocate its use as a first, not final, resort [10].

8.2 Literature Review

Many contemporary reviews promote the McRoberts maneuver as the primary technique to resolve shoulder dystocia. However, it was first described by Greenhill in 1955. The McRoberts maneuver, as originally named by Gonik and co-workers [1], involves exaggerated flexion of the patient's legs, similar to a knee-chest position. This results in straightening of the sacrum relative to the lumbar spine and consequent rotation of the symphysis pubis cephalad, with a decrease in the angle of inclination. This maneuver is not reported to change the dimensions of the true pelvis but rather rotates the symphysis superiorly thus freeing the impacted anterior shoulder without manipulation of the fetus. In a laboratory model [8], the McRoberts maneuver decreased shoulder extraction forces, brachial plexus stretching, and the incidence of clavicular fracture.

The McRoberts maneuver is currently recommended as the initial technique for the disimpaction of the anterior shoulder. Moreover, trends toward lower rates of maternal and neonatal morbidity were associated with the McRoberts maneuver.

In a series of 250 cases of shoulder dystocia, the McRoberts maneuver alone successfully alleviated 42 percent of the cases [10]. The combination of the McRoberts maneuver, suprapubic pressure, and/or proctoepisiotomy relieved 54 percent of shoulder dystocias [11]. The need for additional maneuvers is associated with greater birthweight, longer active phase, and longer second stages. The group requiring additional procedures to relieve shoulder dystocia also had a trend toward an increased incidence of postpartum hemorrhage and brachial plexus injury [11].

Dr. McRoberts of Houston, Texas, refers to his technique as one that can be done rapidly and as one that results in a safe delivery [4]. He recommends it as the first technique and one that every obstetrician should know how to perform. He notes that it has been used successfully for almost 40 years at Hermann Hospital and the University of Texas Medical School in Houston. He emphasizes the need for "sharply" flexing the thighs against the maternal abdomen. McRoberts refers the interested reader to the paper by Gonik et al. [8] Unfortunately, McRoberts does not provide us with a statistical analysis of his clinical experience or the total number of cases [4].

Rosenzweig [3] describes a 25-year experience with the McRoberts maneuver without a single fracture of the clavicle or humerus. As does McRoberts, he emphasizes the need to flex both thighs as much as possible against the abdomen. However, he does not mention the total number of women treated and fails to comment on nerve injuries.

8.3 Technique

Ideally, the preparations for possible shoulder dystocia should begin before the delivery of the head [9]. If the patient is not already in the lithotomy position, or if the delivery begins with the mother on a labor bed, the patient must be placed immediately at the edge of the table. It is very important that the buttocks be off the end of the table.

The first step is anticipation of shoulder dystocia, including recognition of the previously described antepartum and intrapartum risk factors. Every effort should be made to prepare a rapid, ingrained, and well-coordinated stepwise plan. When fetal macrosomia is suspected, the patient should be thoroughly counseled as to the risks and benefits of a trial of vaginal delivery. Prophylactic cesarean section may be strongly considered when the estimated fetal weight is greater than 4,500 g or 4,000 g in the diabetic patient, or in a patient with a prior history of shoulder dystocia. Operative vaginal delivery should be avoided in the setting of macrosomia and/or an abnormal labor pattern.

Shoulder dystocia is usually heralded by the classic "turtle sign." After the fetal head delivers, it retracts back onto the maternal perineum. As maternal efforts to expel the fetal body continue, the fetal shoulders become further impacted behind the symphysis pubis. Having diagnosed a shoulder dystocia, it is extremely important to avoid feelings of panic. If the physician is alone, immediate obstetric assistance should be called for. Anesthesia and pediatric and additional nursing support should be obtained. Do not attempt to immediately suction the nares or relieve a tight nuchal cord. The mother should be instructed to stop pushing. All attendants should refrain from applying fundal pressure, as this has been shown to worsen the impaction and increase the chance of brachial plexus injury.

Sharp hyperflexion of the patient's legs against her abdomen had been found useful for facilitating the delivery long before Gonik and McRoberts re-emphasized its importance [12]. Traditionally, it was used only during contractions. Thus, a cooperative parturient, laboring without conduction anesthesia, could implement it without any assistance. Under the circumstances of threatening or existing shoulder dystocia, this position needs to be maintained for a prolonged period of time. Therefore, it requires two assistants. The position aligns the sacrum with the lumbar spine and rotates the symphysis pubic to a blunt angle, thus facilitating the passage of the shoulder underneath. According to one report, the McRoberts maneuver alone resolved all cases of shoulder dystocia without the use of any other technique [2]. This finding confirms that the nonintervention until the next uterine contraction drastically reduces the occurrence of serious shoulder dystocia.

Smeltzer [2] stated that the simplicity of application of this technique (as shown in Fig. 14.14 of Chapter 14) hides an elegant complexity of the physical and mechanical forces that it invokes. It simultaneously reverses almost all the factors tending to cause shoulder dystocia created by the dorsal lithotomy position. First, the McRoberts maneuver elevates the anterior shoulder of the fetus with respect to the mother. This both carries the fetus anteriorly and flexes the fetal spine toward the anterior shoulder. The lifting and flexion push the fetal posterior shoulder over the sacrum and through the inlet. Second, the maneuver straightens the maternal lumbar and lumbosacral lordosis. This essentially removes the sacral promontory as an obstruction to the inlet. Third, the maneuver removes all weight-bearing forces from the sacrum, the main pressure point of the pelvis in the lithotomy position. This permits the inlet to open to its maximum dimension. Fourth, the inlet is brought into the plane perpendicular to the maximum maternal expulsive force [13].

This elegant maneuver optimally improves the passageway and motive forces for delivery of the posterior shoulder in the dorsal position and manipulates the fetus for delivery of that shoulder as well [2]. If this is the first maneuver to attempt, it should be maintained through further maneuvers because it facilitates them. It can be relaxed during induction of general anesthesia, if this should be necessary, and repeated if unsuccessful on the first attempt.

The success of the maneuver is signaled by relaxation of the inward traction on the fetal head as the posterior shoulder traverses the inlet, permitting normal delivery of the anterior shoulder. If adequate regional anesthesia is present, placement of the operator's hand at the infant's back to palpate the posterior shoulder, scapula, and spine during the maneuver will help one appreciate the genius of this maneuver, verify that the delivery of the posterior shoulder has occurred, and, if it fails, make it possible to proceed immediately or simultaneously with the Rubin maneuver [2].

Often, the uterine contraction continues after the delivery of the head [12]. If so, it rotates the shoulders into the anteroposterior diameter of the pelvis. At this point, gentle traction at an angle of about 30 degrees to 45 degrees under the horizontal, combined with suprapubic pressure, may facilitate the delivery of the body.

8.4 Suprapubic Pressure: The Mazzanti Maneuver

Suprapubic pressure is the simplest maneuver to use and often the one most often improperly performed (see Chapter 14, Fig. 14.15). At the request of the operator, suprapubic pressure, described in 1955, is applied by another member of the health care team [12]. The birth attendant must know the relative position of the shoulders so that she or he may instruct the provider of suprapubic pressure as to the location of the posterior aspect of the shoulder. This can only be ensured by the delivering clinician's direct palpation of the fetal shoulder behind the head. Reliance upon the direction in which the head is facing to identify the posterior aspect of the shoulder can be misleading, as restitution may be incomplete or "incorrectly" directed owing to the mechanical obstruction to delivery.

Suprapubic pressure is generally applied by an assistant. With one fist or preferably the palms of the hands one hand on top of the other hand, immediately over the symphysis pubis, the anterior shoulder is depressed with a lateral bias toward the infant's face to facilitate rotation of the shoulders into the oblique diameter in order to allow its passage under the pubic arch. For the most effective use of this approach, the bladder must be empty. Ideally, bearing-down effort by the mother, suprapubic pressure by the assistant, and light traction by the physician should be applied simultaneously. This well-orchestrated effort must be pursued with awareness of the fact that delivery of the head and the body during the same uterine contraction is not necessary [9,14].

The use of suprapubic pressure is often the first maneuver and then combined with the McRoberts maneuver. The pressure must be very strong and directed down and lateral. Direct downward pressure toward the floor is not as effective as pushing the shoulder laterally into the much larger oblique diameter of the inlet. Once shoulder orientation is confirmed by the birth attendant, the assistant stands on the same side of the mother as the posterior aspect of the shoulder, places his or her closed fist on the mother's abdomen just behind the pubic symphysis, and directs steady pressure in a 45-degree downward angle away from himself or herself. The goal is to transmit this pressure to the posterior aspect of the anterior fetal shoulder that is lying below the assistant's fist. Pressure must be sufficient to produce adduction of the anterior shoulder toward the fetal chest and assist in rotating the shoulder to the physiologic oblique orientation in the pelvis. To achieve sufficient leverage, the assistant should begin with a flexed elbow and be able to sharply extend the forearm as firm pressure is applied.

Using the palm of the hand is much more preferable than fingertips or fist. Moderate suprapubic pressure may work, but macrosomic infants usually require strong force.

8.5 Delivery

After the delivery of the head, the next uterine contraction may be slightly delayed. This time offers an opportunity for optimizing the effect of the next one. The mother can be placed into a favorable position for delivery, and the assistants can move to the sides of the parturient. Meanwhile, the physician can suction the mouth and nose of the child and check for nuchal cord. When present, it should be eased around the head of the fetus if it can be done without difficulty. Causing avulsion of the cord at its umbilical insertion may lead to catastrophe. Besides, its handling can reduce the still existing circulation through the umbilical vessels. Facilitated by the McRoberts maneuver, with suprapubic pressure and gentle downward traction, but most of the time even without, the next contraction expels the shoulders and then the body of the fetus [9].

The effects of this position enhance passage of the posterior fetal shoulder over the sacrum and through the pelvic inlet, positioning the plane of the pelvic inlet to its maximal dimension perpendicular to the maximum maternal expulsive force. Limitations to the technique include the need for two assistants and the extra time required to elevate and flex the patient's legs. Potential difficulty can also be encountered in moving the very obese patient or the patient with a dense epidural motor blockade.

The patient's legs are removed from the stirrups and sharply flexed against the abdomen. This will decrease the angle of inclination of the symphysis. Although this maneuver does not change the dimensions of the pelvis, the superior rotation of the symphysis trends to free the impacted anterior shoulder. As part of the McRoberts maneuver, if the shoulder is not released immediately, we combine it with stout suprapubic pressure.

8.6 Effects of the McRoberts Maneuver

1. The anterior shoulder is elevated.
2. The fetal spine is flexed.
3. The posterior shoulder is pushed over the sacrum.
4. Maternal lordosis is straightened.
5. The sacral promontory is removed as a point of obstruction.
6. The weight-bearing force is removed from the sacrum.
7. The inlet is opened to its maximum.
8. The inlet is brought perpendicular to the maximum expulsive force.

8.7 Research

An x-ray analysis of the McRoberts position has been published by Gonik et al. [1] in which the symphysis was noted to rotate superiorly by a distance of 8 cm. Likewise, they observed that the angle of inclination was reduced from 26 degrees to 10 degrees. The researchers concluded that this rotation of the symphysis superiorly frees the impacted anterior shoulder without any fetal manipulation.

In Gonik's experience [8], this freeing of the impaction seems to allow a spontaneous delivery of the infant. Our experience indicates that additional maneuvers are almost always required, such as suprapubic pressure, gentle rotation and/or traction, and subsequent terminal fundal pressure after the impaction is released. Occasionally, rotational maneuvers or other techniques are required. Spontaneous fetal expulsion is the exception and not the rule.

The basic research experiments conducted by Gonik and colleagues [1] suggest that, in addition to the axially oriented fetal neck forces, a component of flexion (lateral force) is present. As the difficulty of shoulder delivery increases, the impact of these inadvertent flexion forces becomes most pronounced at the brachial plexus level [8]. This is the first study to reproducibly measure shoulder extraction forces in a laboratory model for shoulder dystocia and to describe the pathophysiology of specific neonatal injuries from a force perspective. The force data generated with this modeling system are consistent with previously measured *in situ* extraction forces for both routine and difficult deliveries. These data demonstrate that as more force is needed to extract the fetal shoulders, a significant increase is noted in lateral flexion, which selectively augments stretching within the anterior brachial plexus. Clavicle fracture is directly associated with increasing traction forces; thresholds for fracture are in the range of 100 N (about 20 lb). Using this modeling system, Gonik et al. [8] objectively documented that McRoberts positioning reduces shoulder extraction forces, brachial plexus stretching, and clavicle fracture.

8.8 Improper McRoberts Maneuver

Mistakes are frequently made in an attempt to properly perform the McRoberts position. The patients buttocks must be pulled down on the delivery table so that they hang off of the end of the table. The thighs must be hyperflexed straight back toward the head of the patient, as far as they can go. It is a major mistake to simply pull the knees and thighs out to the side (laterally). This accomplishes nothing. This author has reviewed 27 videotaped births of shoulder dystocia. More than half (16 patients) received an improper McRoberts maneuver.

8.9 Clinical Experience

A 3-year retrospective study of 28,122 consecutive deliveries described a total of 174 shoulder dystocias [6]. Two study groups were analyzed: one in which the McRoberts maneuver was the initial technique, and a second group in which it was not.

Not unexpectedly, there was an increase in macrosomia and overall birthweight in the shoulder dystocia group compared with the normal population. The average birthweight and percentage of macrosomic children were similar in both groups. Other relevant data relating to parity, gestational age, and postdate pregnancies were similar in both groups, as was the method of delivery of the fetal head. It could not be determined how the various maneuvers were chosen, and no significant trends were identified. In the non–McRoberts group of 119 patients, the Woods screw maneuver was used on 85 women, 21 were treated with delivery of the posterior arm, and in 13 the method of delivery was not clearly delineated. The maneuvers were distributed evenly throughout the four teaching hospitals and between private and nonprivate patients.

Fetal morbidity was evaluated in this study on the basis of Apgar scores and the frequency of clavicular fracture and Erb palsy [6]. These assessments were made in the delivery room and in the newborn nursery by the pediatrician in attendance. This analysis revealed a minimal variation in Apgar scores at 1, 5, and 10 minutes between the two groups. The McRoberts maneuver group showed slightly higher Apgar scores overall. Comparing low Apgar scores from McRoberts deliveries versus non–McRoberts deliveries showed no statistical difference at a 95% confidence interval. Relative risks were calculated for 1-minute and 5-minute Apgar scores showing 1.2 and 1.1 for the non–McRoberts' group, respectively. The McRoberts group had a relative risk of 1.0.

A distinct difference was noted in the frequency of fetal injury in the two groups [6]. In the non–McRoberts' group, 13% of the babies suffered a fractured clavicle compared with none when the McRoberts maneuver was used. Partial Erb palsy occurred slightly more frequently in the non–McRoberts deliveries; however, this was not statistically different. The overall trauma in the McRoberts group was 3.6%, whereas in the non–McRoberts group it was 16%. The population total of 174 had 23 injuries, a mean injury rate of 13.2% (combining both McRoberts group and non–McRoberts' group). An injury rate of 3.63% (2 of 55 in the McRoberts group) verifies that the McRoberts frequency of injury would not come from the combined or control population with a probability of greater than 0.99 (P = .01) with a standard deviation of 4.8.

These statistics indicate that the McRoberts maneuver may reduce the subsequently identified trauma to a significant extent when compared with groups not using the McRoberts maneuver. However, these data suggest that the McRoberts maneuver merits more study for its potential effect on trauma. Relative risk analysis revealed trauma to be 4.4 times more likely in the non–McRoberts group of infants.

The success rate using the McRoberts maneuver as the initial mode of treatment for shoulder dystocia was 90%, or 50 of 55 patients. The remaining 5 births were then effected by delivery of the posterior arm.

Few obstetricians have suggested alternative first-line approaches to shoulder dystocia that involve less fetal manipulation. The McRoberts maneuver is extremely effective and is probably most effective before the anterior shoulder has been wedged into the inlet. In a well-respected review, Harris [13] recommends it as the first maneuver.

The results of using the McRoberts maneuver as the initial treatment have not been well described in the literature; however, several authors have made favorable comments [13,14]. Our study [6,7] supports the idea that the McRoberts technique for the delivery of impacted shoulders is a reasonable approach to the initial management of a shoulder dystocia. The success rate is higher and the injury rate is lower than that of other methods that involve fetal manipulation rather than maternal manipulation.

The success of the maneuver is apparent by relaxation of the traction on the fetal head as the posterior shoulder traverses the inlet, permitting normal delivery of the anterior shoulder. Placement of the hand on the infant's back to palpate the posterior shoulder, scapula, and spine during the maneuver will help verify that the delivery of the posterior shoulder has occurred, or that there is a need to proceed immediately or simultaneously with other maneuvers. In our current medicolegal environment, concern for the brachial plexus requires that alternative maneuvers designed to lessen fetal trauma (posterior arm delivery) and allow more room for delivery (episiotomy) should be resorted to somewhat more quickly than before; and the McRoberts position should be used for the initial maneuver [9].

8.10 Conclusion

The optimal method or position for treating shoulder dystocia no longer remains debatable. While many methods have been described and the question of superiority is clouded by the undeniable fact that no clinic has had enough patients to statistically validate a given approach, the McRoberts maneuver continues to gain acceptability. The need for strong suprapubic pressure must be emphasized. Despite this advance, current emphasis must still be on fetal manipulation in the treatment of shoulder dystocia.

Fetal manipulation appears to be the best method for atraumatic resolution insofar as it takes better advantage of pelvic geometry and requires less traction to complete the delivery than do maternal maneuvers. It can eliminate the need to repeat traction on the fetal head, by instead applying the traction to the fetal trunk. Fetal manipulation also does not depend on the skill or presence of an assistant and can reasonably be practiced at all shoulder dystocia deliveries and even at routine deliveries, as was done a generation ago [15].

Fetal maneuvers can reduce the incidence of brachial plexus palsy (as was demonstrated 50 years ago). Fetal maneuvers are both safe and effective. They were described earlier than maternal maneuvers, and when they were the prevailing standard for shoulder dystocia management, they resulted in a fourfold reduction in neonatal injury. When used as the sole management strategy, fetal manipulation is actually associated with a very low rate of injury compared with maternal maneuvers or traction alone. Because of these advantages, training in fetal maneuvers should be emphasized and should be prioritized in shoulder dystocia management algorithms.

References

1. Gonik B, Stringer C, Held B. An alternate maneuver for the management of shoulder dystocia. *Am J Obstet Gynecol* 1983;145:882–888.
2. Smeltzer J. Prevention and management of shoulder dystocia. *Clin Obstet Gynecol* 1986;29:299–308.
3. Rosenzweig W. Comment: *Contemp Obstet Gynecol* 1984;24:17.
4. McRoberts W. Maneuvers for shoulder dystocia. *Contemp Obstet Gynecol* 1984;24:17.
5. O'Leary J, Gunn D. Cephalic replacement for shoulder dystocia. *Contemp Obstet Gynecol* 1986;27:157.
6. O'Leary J. Shoulder dystocia–an ounce of prevention. *Contemp Obstet Gynecol* 1986;27:78.
7. O'Leary J, Leonetti H. Shoulder dystocia. Prevention and treatment. *Am J Obstet Gynecol* 1990;162:5–10.
8. Gonik B, Allen R, Sorab J. Objective evaluation of the shoulder dystocia phenomenon: Effect of maternal pelvic orientation on force reduction. *Obstet Gynecol* 1989;74:44–48.
9. Ramieri J, Iffy L. Shoulder dystocia (chapter 21). In: *Operative Obstetrics*. Third ed. London and New York: Taylor & Francis; 2006:253–263.
10. Gherman R. Shoulder dystocia (chapter 40). In: *Management of Common Problems in Obstetrics & Gynecology*. Fourth ed. London: Blackwell Publishing 2002;153–156.

11. Gilstrap L, Cunningham F, Vandorsten J. *Operative Obstetrics*. Third ed. New York: McGraw-Hill; 2002:207.
12. Greenhill J. *Obstetrics*. 11th ed. Philadelphia: W.B. Saunders; 1955:278.
13. Harris B. Shoulder dystocia. *Clin Obstet Gynecol* 1984;27:106–111.
14. Resnik R. Management of shoulder girdle dystocia. *Clin Obstet Gynecol* 1980;23:559–566.
15. Bager B. Perinatally acquired brachial plexus palsy: A persisting challenge. *Acta Pediatr* 1997; 86:1214–1219.

Chapter 9
Cephalic Replacement:
The Gunn-Zavanelli-O'Leary Maneuver

James A. O'Leary

Summary Cephalic Replacement is a reasonable alternative when standard maneuvers for shoulder dystocia are unsuccessful.

Keywords: cephalic replacement · severe shoulder dystocia · Zavanelli maneuver

Contents

9.1 Introduction   119
9.2 Initial Clinical Experience   120
9.3 Technique and Results   121
9.4 Survey.   122
9.5 Discussion.   124
9.6 Abdominal Rescue   126
9.7 Conclusion   126

9.1 Introduction

Williams Obstetrics states that cephalic replacement is "reasonable to attempt" after usual techniques fail; however, adequate clinical experience has yet to be reported [1].

The concept of cephalic replacement, also known as the Zavanelli maneuver, was not conceived and used in desperation, as described by Sandberg [2], but on the contrary was developed in anticipation of the undeliverable bilateral shoulder dystocia. This technique was first performed by David Gunn in 1976 and subsequently reported by O'Leary and Gunn, who recommended the use of terbutaline and an internal scalp electrode [3]. Unaware of Gunn's experience, Sandberg attributed the first performance of the technique to Dr. William

J.A. O'Leary
Professor Obstetrics & Gynecology (retired), University of South Florida, Tampa, Florida, USA

J.A. O'Leary (ed.), *Shoulder Dystocia and Birth Injury*,
DOI 10.1007/978-1-59745-473-5_9, © Humana Press, a part of Springer
Science+Business Media, LLC 2009

Zavanelli in 1978 [4]. The fetal head was returned to its previous intravaginal location, and the fetus was extracted by cesarean section.

Sandberg has published the results of 12 years of experience with the Zavanelli maneuver with 103 total cases (92 cephalic, 11 breech) [2]. Cephalic replacement was successful in 84 (91%) cases, and breech replacement was successful in all 11 cases. Six of the successful cephalic replacement cases were accomplished after uterine relaxation. Eight attempts were unsuccessful with vaginal delivery, six were accomplished after symphysiotomy, and two were accomplished by manipulation through a hysterotomy incision. There were eight neonatal deaths (seven in cephalic replacement, one in breech replacement) and six intrauterine deaths (all in cephalic replacement). Ten neonates suffered significant neurologic sequelae, all in the cephalic replacement group. Three uterine ruptures and four lacerations of the lower uterine segment/upper vagina were the most serious maternal complications encountered.

Cephalic replacement has great appeal because of its simplicity and ease of performance [5,6]. Its uniqueness, along with physician inexperience and temerity, has delayed its general acceptance. Experience is easy to obtain at the time of delivery of term stillbirths if there is adequate analgesia and/or anesthesia and informed consent.

The early successes with this maneuver has helped to overcome its divergence from traditional obstetric teaching. The dramatic nature of this innovative technique will be overcome in time, a common phenomenon in the history of obstetric procedures. O'Leary and Gunn concluded that it was a reasonable alternative; thus we recommended that this procedure be called the Gunn-Zavanelli-O'Leary maneuver. We are confident that others will continue to test its feasibility, especially when there is an early recognition of a bilateral impaction of the shoulders. Sandberg is to be congratulated on his wisdom and foresight in immediately recognizing the significant potential and broad application of cephalic replacement [7].

As mentioned in the discussion of Sandberg's paper [8], the fetal replacement procedure has also been reported by Iffy and by Varga. The total number of cephalic replacements continues to increase, along with positive comments on its expediency, simplicity, and effectiveness. Although it was initially denied thoughtful inquiry because its performance is so contrary to age-old obstetric dicta, it has proved to be a useful alternative when routine maneuvers fail.

9.2 Initial Clinical Experience

In 1986, we reported four successful cephalic replacements in women who had bilateral shoulder impaction [6]. The clinical and demographic data of our report are outlined in Table 9.1. There were no unusual prenatal complications

Table 9.1 Successful Cephalic Replacement

Age (y)	Parity	No. of Weeks	Prenatal Problems	Labor	Anesthesia	Delivery	Fetal Weight (g)
18	0	41	P.I.H*	Protracted dilation	Epidural	Elective low forceps	4,501
17	1	40	None	Normal	Pudendal	Indicated manual rotation and midforceps fetal distress	3,684
27	1	37	Diabetes	Normal	Pudendal	Indicated midforceps fetal distress	4,260
36	5	41	No care	Normal	Pudendal	Spontaneous	3,781

*Pregnancy induced hypertension

in these four women, except that one was a noncompliant insulin-dependent gestational diabetic. All patients were at term, and none were postdate. The labors were all normal except for one with a mildly protracted active phase. The second stages were not prolonged. Two indicated midforceps deliveries were performed for significant terminal fetal distress.

9.3 Technique and Results

Prior to employing cephalic replacement, each of the four patients was subjected to at least three distinctly different techniques for reduction of the bilateral shoulder dystocia. Once it became apparent that the situations were hopeless, a fetal scalp electrode was used in each instance, and subcutaneous terbutaline 0.25 mg was administered to three of the four patients.

We recommended that after the diagnosis of bilateral severe shoulder impaction dystocia is made and classic methods have failed, the following steps should be taken: the McRoberts maneuver, preparation for abdominal delivery, initiation of tocolysis, and electronic or auditory monitoring of the fetal heart rate.

The head is easily replaced by constant but firm pressure on the occiput with the palm of the right hand so as to flex the head while depressing the posterior vaginal wall with the left hand. The vertex is pushed as far cephalad as possible, close to zero station where it will usually remain without the need of an assistant. Insertion of a Foley catheter is recommended after completion of the maneuver (see Chapter 14, Fig. 14.14 and Fig. 23A, B).

The entire head is replaced in the vagina (see Chapter 14, Fig. 14.14 and Fig. 24A, B). Great pressure is not required. If the head has undergone rotation to the side, it must be rotated to the occiput anterior position. The episiotomy repair may be delayed until the cesarean section is completed providing

Table 9.2 Clinical Outcome

Interval to Cesarean Section (min)	Electronic Fetal Monitor	Apgar Score	Complications	Transfusions	Discharge Day
60–70	Normal	6 and 8	Postoperative anemia	2	6
60	Early decelerations	4 and 8	Bandl ring around shoulders	1	8
65	Severe variable decelerations	8 and 8	Nuchal arm	4	6
45	Severe variable decelerations	8 and 9	Very thick lower uterine segment	0	6

homeostasis has been attained. In our cases, the cephalic reduction was easy to carry out. All four infants initially experienced a prolonged deceleration of 60 to 70 beats per minute for 2 to 4 minutes. The decelerations were rapidly followed by a return to a normal baseline rate with good short-term and long-term variability.

The cesarean sections in every instance paralleled those for patients undergoing abdominal delivery at full dilation. The infants were delivered without difficulty and in good condition, with normal Apgar scores and no injuries. The clinical outcome is shown in Table 9.2. The bilateral shoulder impaction prevents the infant's head from becoming wedged deep into the pelvis, as is so frequently encountered with cesarean sections for cephalopelvic disproportion, carried out at full dilation.

The blood loss at the time of cesarean section was not unusual. There was no trauma to the lower uterine segment, bladder, vagina, cervix, or uterine vessels. Three women received transfusions for postoperative anemia because of the blood loss from an episiotomy and cesarean section, plus the presence of preoperative hemoglobin levels less than 11.0%. None of the women had intraoperative problems.

Premature placental separation was not encountered in any case. There was no maternal morbidity, and all patients and their infants left the hospital in 4 to 5 days. Antibiotics were administered for prophylaxis. All infants were normal at 2 years of age.

9.4 Survey

Since the initial report, a registry for cephalic replacement cases was established [4]. A direct mailing went to all chairmen of obstetrics and gynecology departments and to program directors of all teaching hospitals with residencies in obstetrics and gynecology in the United States. Members of the Society of Perinatal

Obstetricians were also notified in writing about the Cephalic Replacement Registry. Two announcements were placed in the monthly newsletter of the American College of Obstetricians and Gynecologists (ACOG). Finally, cases were reported directly to the author by word of mouth, letter, or submission of original medical records. A total of 59 cases were collected.

The key clinical features collected were Apgar scores, neonatal complications, time elapsed before replacement of the head, ease of replacement, interval to cesarean delivery, type of anesthesia, gestational age, delivery techniques, and maternal and fetal complications.

Nineteen women had postdate pregnancies, and six delivered before 40 weeks. Midpelvic delivery was used in 16 women, whereas 14 had low forceps or low vacuum delivery, and 29 delivered spontaneously. Some confusion existed with respect to the type of operative delivery because a few physicians used the traditional textbook definition of midpelvic delivery, whereas others chose the newer and more liberal ACOG definition, and some were unsure. It could not be determined whether the mode of delivery contributed to the dystocia.

The time interval for replacement of the infant's head was a "best estimate" given by the delivering physician as it appeared in the operative notes. A majority (38, or 64.4%) of the replacements were recorded as performed in 5 to 10 minutes, 9 before 5 minutes, and 12 after 10 minutes. The recorded times from replacement of the infant's head to cesarean delivery are shown in Table 9.1. In 42 of the 59 women, delivery was successful within 20 minutes. Only seven patients were delivered after 30 minutes. The three longest intervals, 41, 60, and 70 minutes, resulted from the unavailability of an anesthesiologist; these infants were born in good condition.

The ease of replacement is difficult to quantitate and can only be a subjective evaluation by the delivering physician. The physician's assessment of the degree of cephalic pressure required for the replacement was categorized as mild, moderate, or strong. Forty-two of 59 (71.2%) of the cephalic replacements required only mild pressure and were reported as being simple, easy, or uncomplicated. The degree of force applied to the fetal head was described as moderate in 12 instances, and the replacement was considered difficult and required strong cephalic pressure in 5 cases.

There were six failed cephalic replacements. The reasons for the failures could not be determined. Two occurred in the moderate-force group. After the induction of general anesthesia, the cephalic replacement was considered easy in both cases. The four remaining failures were described as difficult and required strong cephalic pressure for replacement; three required symphysiotomy and were delivered vaginally, and one needed a low transverse hysterotomy. After hysterotomy, the anterior shoulder was rotated into the oblique diameter, and the infant was delivered vaginally.

Thirty women were delivered with either epidural or spinal anesthesia. The remaining 29 received a local block, and six of these were given general anesthesia for the cephalic replacement. Infant Apgar scores were recorded at 1 and

5 minutes (Table 9.2). As expected, the 1-minute scores were much lower than the 5-minute scores. A total of 42 (71.2%) infants were placed in the 0 to 3 range at 1 minute, and only 8 (13.5%) were considered normal. After resuscitation, only 16 infants demonstrated a clinical state that placed them in the Apgar range of 0 to 3. Umbilical cord gases were not obtained.

The neonatal complications were few. Four infants with complications subsequently were noted to have seizures during their nursery course; two infants may have had a permanent neurologic injury. Two macrosomic infants died, one from gastric hemorrhage and the other from severe hypoxic-ischemic encephalopathy. It could not be determined whether the injuries resulted from the delivery techniques, the interval between delivery and reinsertion, or both. Erb palsy was noted in 12 infants, and permanent palsy remained in only five infants.

Fourteen women received terbutaline to prevent further uterine contractions. An internal scalp electrode was used in seven instances, and variable decelerations were noted in five patients.

Several important maternal complications were reported. Two patients suffered a ruptured uterus from a Bandl ring and required hysterectomy, three patients had a lower uterine segment laceration; however, most physicians described the cesarean as easy to perform and without major technical difficulties. Six (10.2%) women required transfusion. All patients received prophylactic antibiotics, and only 13.5% had morbid postoperative courses. In two women, the episiotomy required repair in the recovery room.

Three patients redelivered the infant's head because of continued uterine contractions and maternal pushing. Repeat cephalic replacement was successful in two cases. One of these infants was stillborn at the time of cesarean, presumably because of an occult cord prolapse. The third infant delivered vaginally without a dystocia!

9.5 Discussion

The concept of cephalic replacement was developed by Dr. David Gunn [5] in anticipation of the undeliverable shoulder dystocia. The use of terbutaline to stop further uterine activity and the application of an internal scalp electrode to assess fetal welfare was reported as helpful. Sandberg [2,4] recognized and reported the important potential and possible broad application of cephalic replacement and chose the term *Zavanelli maneuver*. He was unaware of Gunn's experience.

In view of the experience described in this chapter, it is hoped that others will test the feasibility of cephalic replacement, especially when there is early recognition of bilateral impaction of the shoulders or signs of a difficult extraction. Failed cephalic replacements can occur from inadequate anesthesia; after the induction of general anesthesia, repeat attempts may be successful. A similar observation has been reported by Dimitry [9].

The cesarean deliveries included in this review were described as easy and less difficult than those performed in patients undergoing abdominal delivery at full dilation with a deeply engaged head. Bilateral shoulder dystocia, as manifested by a positive "turtle sign," failure of external rotation, and absence of the posterior arm in the hollow of the sacrum, prevents the infant from becoming wedged deep in the pelvis, as is so common with cesarean sections for suspected fetopelvic disproportion carried out at full dilation. Therefore, it is not difficult to extract the infant's head.

There were no unusual complications directly related to the cesarean operation, though exceptions have been reported. The infants were extracted with minimal effort and were usually in fair to good condition; a few had serious permanent injuries. The maternal clinical outcomes were excellent. Few of the women had significant intraoperative or postoperative problems or morbidity related to the cephalic replacement. The blood loss at surgery was not unusual. There was no trauma to the bladder, vagina, cervix, or uterine vessels. However, cephalic replacement ruptured a constriction ring and resulted in the need for hysterectomy in two cases. Six women received transfusions because of blood loss from an episiotomy and cesarean delivery, as well as preoperative anemia. Premature placental separation, cord prolapse, or cervical lacerations after reinsertion of the head were not encountered.

The technique of cephalic replacement should be considered and performed early when continued persistence at vaginal manipulation will lead to a predictably poor outcome for all concerned and before the infant becomes severely asphyxiated. An interval of 2 to 3 minutes is more than sufficient to realize that further attempts at delivery would be futile. Because time is of the essence, rapid cephalic replacement, tocolysis, delayed repair of the episiotomy, and abdominal delivery offers the infant, mother, and obstetrician the best outcome.

In the rare situation when an experienced care provider is unavailable, early cephalic replacement may be worthy of consideration, although at present there is no clinical experience to support this speculation. When delivery occurs in bed, in the emergency room, or in an ambulance, cephalic replacement could be considered as an immediate solution. In addition, whenever a positive "turtle sign" occurs, bilateral dystocia is very likely, and therefore cephalic replacement needs immediate consideration.

Comments received as part of the survey indicate that cephalic replacement is clearly a reasonable solution to difficult cases and should receive greater consideration. The critical question facing clinicians is whether they can safely deliver an infant vaginally with persistent manipulation or whether they should choose the second option of cephalic replacement [10–13]. In the past, rigid thinking dictated an all-or-none philosophy of vaginal delivery at all costs. Because the true incidence of complications are not excessive, the results of this study support a new alternative that should be incorporated into our teaching and practice.

Because the applicability of this technique is becoming better known, we recommend that all persons performing deliveries consider adding cephalic replacement to the array of procedures for severe or unremitting dystocia. Most writers described the procedure as simple, easy, and gratifying.

The cephalic replacement maneuver has particular appeal because of its simplicity and its ease of performance. It offers not only the potential of an additional therapeutic maneuver for a difficult problem but also a window into a new realm of obstetric thought.

Whereas it is apparent to all that initial successes prove little, the 20-year results of the cephalic replacement maneuver as a revolutionary, or at the least an ancillary, approach to the treatment of shoulder dystocia remains unassailable. The maneuver has been used successfully without traumatic injury to the fetus or the pregnant woman in circumstances in which other maneuvers failed. Thus, every individual who assists at a childbirth should seriously consider adding the maneuver to his or her list of available methods for the management of shoulder dystocia, especially that which is severe and unremitting.

9.6 Abdominal Rescue

O'Leary and Cuva described *abdominal rescue* [14] after failed cephalic replacement as a final effort in delivery of the fetus, whereby low transverse hysterotomy is performed and the fetal shoulder is assisted below the symphysis pubis, followed by vaginal delivery of the infant. The abdominal rescue had previously been described in the context of breech delivery with entrapment of the aftercoming fetal head [13].

Recently, Vollebergh and van Dongen reported a case of a failed Zavanelli maneuver followed by a hysterotomy and failed abdominal rescue [8]. They then performed a breech extraction through the hysterotomy with a repeat Zavanelli maneuver, which was successful. Although the neonatal outcome was poor, this offers another approach for catastrophic shoulder dystocia when all other options fail.

O'Shaughnessy [15] described a hysterotomy facilitation of vaginal delivery of the posterior arm after all other maneuvers, including manipulation of the fetal shoulder, failed. After vaginal delivery of the posterior arm, transabdominal shoulder rotation and vaginal extraction were accomplished.

9.7 Conclusion

Cephalic replacement and abdominal rescue have made an impact on obstetric thinking. Despite the dramatic nature of the procedures and the emotions evoked by a shoulder dystocia, acceptance has been gratifying. There is already widespread evidence to support a willingness to try this new approach. In those situations when classic maneuvers [7] fail to rapidly resolve the problem of bilateral dystocia, the clinician has no other alternative than an attempt at cephalic reduction. Because time is of the essence, rapid cephalic replacement, tocolysis, delayed repair of the episiotomy, and abdominal delivery seem to offer the infant, mother, and obstetrician the best outcome. The technique should be performed when continued persistence at vaginal manipulation will lead to a predictably poor outcome but before the infant has been severely asphyxiated.

References

1. Cunningham F, MacDonald P, Gant N, eds. Dystocia due to abnormalities in presentation. In: *Williams Obstetrics*. appleton Lange: Connecticut 18th ed. 1989:371.
2. Sandberg E. The Zavanelli maneuver: A potentially revolutionary method for the resolution of shoulder dystocia. *Am J Obstet Gynecol* 1985;152:479–483.
3. O'Leary J, Gunn D. Cephalic replacement for shoulder dystocia. *Am J Obstet Gynecol* 1985;153:592–595.
4. Sandberg E. The Zavanelli maneuver: 12 years of recorded experience. *Obstet Gynecol* 1999;93:312.
5. O'Leary J, Gunn D. Cephalic replacement for shoulder dystocia. *Contemp Obstet Gynecol* 1985;27:157–159.
6. O'Leary J. Shoulder dystocia. *Contemp Obstet Gynecol* 1986;27:78–82.
7. Iffy L. Comment in Gross TL, Sokol RJ, Williams T, Thompson K. Shoulder dystocia: A fetal physician risk. *Am J Obstet Gynecol* 1987;156:1416–1423.
8. Vollebergh J, van Dongen P. The Zavanelli maneuver in shoulder dystocia. *Eur J Obstet Gynecol Reprod Biol* 2000;89:81.
9. Dimitry E. Cephalic replacement: A desperate solution for shoulder dystocia. *J Obstet Gynecol* 1989;10:49–50.
10. O'Leary J, Pollack N, Leonetti H, Hratko J. The McRoberts maneuver for the initial treatment of shoulder dystocia. *Am J Gynecol Health* 1991;5:21–24.
11. Graham J, Blanco J, Wan T, Magee K. The Zavanelli maneuver: A different perspective. *Obstet Gynecol* 1992;79:883–884.
12. Swartzer J, Bleker O, Schutte M. The Zavanelli maneuver applied in locked twins. *Am J Obstet Gynecol* 1992;166:532.
13. Iffy L, Apuzzio J, Cohen-Addad N. Abdominal rescue after entrapment of the aftercoming head. *Am J Obstet Gynecol* 1986;154:623.
14. O'Leary J, Cuva A. Abdominal rescue after failed cephalic replacement. *Obstet Gynecol* 80;514–516.
15. O'Shaughnessy M. Hysterotomy facilitation of the vaginal delivery of the posterior arm in a case of severe shoulder dystocia. *Obstet Gynecol* 1998;921:693.

Chapter 10
Infant Injury

James A. O'Leary

Summary Nontraction, nonstretch injuries to the brachial plexus are uncommon. The causes of these injuries are very easy to identify. Birth-related brachial plexus palsies are low-velocity and low-impact injuries compared with adult brachial plexus injuries (e.g., vehicular accidents), which are high velocity and high impact.

Keywords: avulsion · axonotmesis · Erb palsy · Klumpke palsy · neurapraxia · neuroma · neurotmesis

Contents

10.1	Introduction	129
10.2	Classification of Injuries	130
10.3	Incidence and Prognosis	132
10.4	Pathophysiology	133
10.5	Anatomy of a Peripheral Nerve	134
10.6	Vulnerable Fetuses	135
10.7	Clinical Presentation	135
10.8	Mortality and Morbidity	136
10.9	Causation	138
10.10	Cesarean Injuries	141
10.11	Mechanism of Labor and Injury	141
10.12	Conclusion	141

10.1 Introduction

The incidence of brachial plexus injury is rising, a phenomenon that may require reevaluation of present-day treatment [1].

Obstetric brachial plexus palsy results from iatrogenic (physician induced) strong traction or stretch injury to the cervical roots C5-8 and T1, thus the risk

J.A. O'Leary
Professor Obstetrics & Gynecology (retired), University of South Florida, Tampa, Florida, USA

J.A. O'Leary (ed.), *Shoulder Dystocia and Birth Injury*,
DOI 10.1007/978-1-59745-473-5_10, © Humana Press, a part of Springer
Science+Business Media, LLC 2009

of permanent injury is high. The reported incidence of palsy is 0.5% to 2.7% of all births. In cases of shoulder dystocia, the risk of palsy has been estimated to be as high as 58% [1]. The primary or main cause is stretching of the nerves during a difficult delivery of the shoulders (i.e., traction). Developments in obstetrics over the past 20 years have been directed largely at avoiding birth asphyxia and trauma [2–11]. Comparison of birth asphyxia and trauma in the same obstetric service during periods 20 years apart shows some reassuring and some disquieting findings [12–21]. Liberalized use of cesarean section, electronic monitoring of the fetal heart in labor, and replacement of opiate sedation by epidural anesthesia have had their beneficial effect.

Currently, a major hazard for shoulder dystocia in the term infant is the use of forceps and vacuum extraction along with the increased use of pain relief by continuous epidural anesthesia. The increased incidence of shoulder dystocia with regional anesthesia is now well accepted [22–32].

However, the two studies that come closest to the "ideal" study show a tendency toward some 20% to 30% residual deficits in contrast with the optimistic view of more than 80% complete or almost complete recovery, which is often encountered [33].

The universally respected textbook *Child Neurology* by Menkes et al. in its most recent edition [34] has once again addressed the issue of brachial plexus palsy causation: traction at the time of delivery of the shoulders by the care provider.

Brachial plexus injuries result from stretching of the plexus owing to turning the head away from the shoulder in a difficult cephalic presentation of a large infant. The condition has been reported in a few instances after delivery by cesarean section. However, whatever scant evidence exists for a classic brachial plexus injury resulting from intrauterine maladaptation is principally based on faulty interpretation of Electromyography (EMG). When intrauterine palsies do occur, they are characterized by limb atrophy and abnormal dermatoglyphics at birth.

In most instances, the brachial plexus stretching leads to compression by hemorrhage and edema within the nerve sheath. Less often there is an actual tear of the nerves, or avulsion of the roots from the spinal cord occurs, with segmental damage to the gray matter of the spinal cord. With traction, the fifth cervical root gives way first, then the sixth, and so on down the plexus. Thus, the mildest plexus injuries involve only C5 and C6 and the more severe involve the entire plexus.

10.2 Classification of Injuries

The U.S. National Institute of Neurological Disorders and Stroke describes four types of brachial plexus injuries: avulsion, the most severe type, where the nerve is torn from the spinal cord; rupture, where the nerve is torn but not at the spinal attachment; neuroma, where healing has occurred with fibrosis, putting pressure on the injured nerve and preventing nerve conduction; and neurapraxia, the most common type, where the nerve has been damaged but not torn.

The site and type of brachial plexus injury determine the prognosis. For avulsion, there is no hope for recovery. For rupture injuries, there is no potential for recovery unless surgical reconnection is made in a timely manner. For neuromas and neurapraxias, the potential for recovery varies. Most patients with neurapraxias recover spontaneously with a 90% to 100% return of function [16].

The degree and extent of dysfunction depends on the specific location of injury. The palsies can be grossly categorized as upper, intermediate, lower, or total plexus injuries. With upper plexus injury (Erb palsy), which usually involves C5 and C6 (and sometimes C7), the neonate presents with "waiter's tip" posture (abduction, internal rotation of the shoulder, extension and pronation of the elbow, wrist flexion with over-pull of the wrist and finger flexors). Also, an associated atrophy of the deltoid, trapezius, or latissimus dorsi muscles can be seen with later presentations. The intermediate type involves injury to C7 and sometimes C8–T1. Klumpke palsy, involving C8 and T1, is purely a lower brachial plexus palsy that presents as paralysis of the hand with function at the shoulder and elbow. Pure lower plexus palsy is very infrequently encountered among brachial plexus injury patients. Newborns who have complete brachial plexus palsy present with a limp, dangling appendage, without any trace of movement. In time, this is accompanied by atrophy of the hand. Erb palsy and total plexus palsy are by far the two most common types of injury.

Brachial plexus injury occurs from traction on the head and neck in the vertex delivery, not from arm traction. The classic descriptions of brachial plexus palsy have identified lesions affecting the upper plexus (Erb palsy, C5, C6) and lesions affecting the lower plexus (Klumpke palsy, C8, T1). However, recent statistics on incidence do not reflect such a clear separation. Erb palsy comprises 58% to 72% of the cases, with the entire plexus being involved in up to 25% of cases, and isolated Klumpke palsy being involved only rarely. Bilateral brachial palsy is uncommon, occurring in 8% to 22% of cases.

Because of an associated involvement of higher cervical roots (C4 to C5) from which the phrenic nerve arises, diaphragmatic paralysis on the same side as the brachial plexus may occur in 5% to 9% of the cases. In middle (C7) and lower (C8, T1) plexus injury, the weakness primarily affects the forearm and hand, particularly the flexors of wrists and fingers, and the intrinsic muscles of the hand. Horner syndrome may coexist with these lower brachial plexus injuries.

Brachial plexus injuries based on predicted functional recovery can be grouped into four neurologic categories for the purpose of evaluation. A pure upper trunk involves muscles supplied by the C5 and C6 nerve roots, an Erb lesion involves the same territory as a pure upper lesion and also includes muscles supplied by the C7 nerve root; a posterior cord/middle trunk lesion involves only muscles supplied by the C7 nerve root and middle trunk; and a combined lesion includes all nerve roots mentioned above together with muscles supplied by the C8 nerve root, the lower trunk, or both.

10.3 Incidence and Prognosis

Figures based on a study carried out in Denmark reported respective annual incidences of one brachial plexus injury per 1,000 births and 0.7 per 1,000 births [35]. The incidence of birth-related brachial plexus injuries in The Netherlands is reported to be 2 per 1,000 births, of which only 37 or 38 cases need active treatment per year [35]. Correlation of the Dutch study with the Danish birth figures indicates a range of 80 to 160 new cases per year in Denmark; 90% of these, according to the Dutch experience, will recover spontaneously, leaving a maximum of 8 to 16 cases requiring active treatment annually [35].

Wagner et al. [36] describe Haase's experience with approximately 18,600 deliveries from 1990 through the end of 1994; 18 cases of birth-related brachial plexus injuries were seen for an incidence of 1 in 1,000. Only two (11%) of the cases needed prolonged follow-up. Similar figures were seen in the Fyn Island study over a 14-year period, with 39 cases or 85% attaining good results spontaneously and 15% requiring follow-up [36].

McCall [15] studied 105 cases of shoulder dystocia. After delivery, 8 babies died, 2 as a direct result of difficulty in delivery. Twenty-one of the remaining 97 babies had neonatal asphyxia and/or injury to the brachial plexus. Of the infants who survived, 46 were traced. Two were mentally retarded, 5 more were below their expected school grade, and 7 had speech defects.

Gordon et al. [4] studied 59 children with neonatal brachial paralysis. At 4 months of age, 6 of 52 (12%) children examined were still paralyzed; at 12 months, 4 of 52 (8%) children were paralyzed; and at 48 months, 3 of 41 (7%) children were paralyzed. Erb-Duchenne (upper brachial plexus) paralysis was observed more frequently than the Klumpke (lower brachial plexus) type. Psychological tests were performed at 8 months and at 4 years of age and compared with a control group. The distribution of test scores was similar for both groups at 8 months and at 4 years.

Eng [21] followed 20 newborn infants with brachial plexus palsy. Six babies had recovered with a minimum deficit at 6 months of age. Of the remainder, 11 infants demonstrated moderate dysfunction and required 1 year to resume normal function. Fourteen infants had severe deficits, including total brachial plexus paralysis, and one had a Horner syndrome.

Hardy [5] reviewed 36 infants who had sustained birth injuries to the brachial plexus. Shoulder dystocia had occurred in 10 instances. No child with signs at age 13 months recovered completely, and no improvement was seen after age 2 years. Among 5 children with residual damage who were delivered vaginally from cephalic presentation, the mean birthweight was 4,576 g.

In three studies in which a control group of term-size neonates born during the study period were compared with neonates weighing 4,500 g or more at birth, the perinatal mortality was at least five times higher for the macrosomic group. The incidence of maternal, fetal, and neonatal complications was also high, suggesting that many of those large neonates experienced difficult deliveries. This conclusion has prompted some authors to propose that delivery by cesarean section may prevent many of the problems associated with the excessively large fetus. Parks and Ziel [20] suggested that macrosomia alone may be an indication for primary cesarean section. However, all fetuses weighing less than 4,500 g at delivery were included in their study as the control group. Because this group includes premature fetuses, who are known to have higher mortality, the validity of comparisons on the basis of mortality is questionable.

In a retrospective study by Modanlou et al. [8] comparing 287 macrosomic neonates with 284 appropriate weight term-size neonates, macrosomia occurred in 1.3% of annual deliveries, with a male-to-female ratio of 2.3 to 1. This excess neonatal morbidity in the macrosomic neonates was predominately caused by the traction during the delivery process.

The prognosis for recovery of function varies with the severity of the injury. In studies of infants with brachial plexus injury where all cases were followed, 70% to 92% showed complete recovery, and most of the remaining infants demonstrated some degree of improvement [8]. Collective experience from the literature indicates that, in the infant who does recover completely, some improvement will be seen by 2 weeks, and most infants will achieve full recovery by 1 month and no later than 5 months [3–5]. With infants who show partial recovery, improvement may begin after 2 weeks, but it may be delayed as much as 4 to 6 weeks, with decreasing intensity of improvement over the following 12 to 24 months. Improvement after 2 years is not known to occur.

10.4 Pathophysiology

Because the nervous system is not fully developed immediately after birth, the functional anatomy of the brachial plexus differs between children and between adults. Birth-related brachial plexus lesions, which are of low velocity and low impact origin, are thus considered an entity quite different from brachial plexus injuries, which occur later in life and are the result of high-velocity and high-impact trauma after vehicular accidents and falls.

Excessive lateral traction on the neck can cause a variety of stretch injuries to the brachial plexus, with injury increasing in severity from upper to lower plexus roots. Ruptures (*neurotmesis*), complete or incomplete, are a form of laceration that occur to the postganglionic nerve. Both the neuronal and sheath elements are disrupted and should be repaired in certain situations for optimal return of function. *Neuromas*, which are a disorganized collection of fibrous tissue and nerve endings, form when rupture occurs and the nerve attempts to grow and meet the distal end. *Axonotmesis* occurs when the neuronal element is damaged, but the sheath remains intact. This type of injury allows the nerve to use the sheath as a guide for growth and recovers without surgical intervention within 4 to 6 weeks. *Neurapraxia* is a temporary conduction defect, which is not associated with any permanent structural damage, and recovery occurs quickly.

These different types of lesions occur as the nerve rootlets coalesce to form the mixed nerve root that traverses and exits the root canal. Trunks, divisions, cords, and peripheral nerves may suffer the same trauma as the nerve roots, including rupture or neurotmesis, axonotmesis, neurapraxia, and neuroma in continuity.

These conditions are treatable, but not all injuries are amenable to direct surgical repair. Avulsions, for example, occur when the nerve rootlets, before they form the ganglion, are torn from the spinal cord. At present, these cannot be successfully reconnected to the spinal cord, and fortunately, this type of injury does not occur very often. New techniques of surgical nerve transfer, however, do help to restore function through appropriate functional reorganization of intact donor nerve.

The classification system for traumatic nerve injuries is universally accepted and ranges from neurapraxia through avulsion [23]. Various combinations of these lesions may be present after traumatic nerve injuries. Avulsion occurs when nerve rootlets are traumatically detached from the spinal cord; the spinal cord itself may sometimes be damaged during the avulsive process. Avulsed nerve rootlets will not recover function, and their surgical reconnection is not possible. Differential avulsions involving either the posterior or anterior rootlets, or both, are seen in brachial plexus injury.

Neurotmesis, or rupture, is similar to nerve laceration, involving interruption of both the neuron sheath and the axons. Partial or complete rupture may evolve into a neuroma in continuity as the sprouting neurons of the growth bulb of the proximal damaged end form a mass of fibrous tissue and disorganized neurons (neuroma) in their attempt to reach the distal stump. Nerve conduction through the neuroma depends on the number of neurons making the correct connection distally. Recovery is usually incomplete in this instance. Axonotmesis is the disruption of the internal neural elements (axons) while the sheath elements remain intact. The proximal nerve growth bulb usually reconnects to the distal disconnected neural elements within the neural sheath. Recovery of function with axonotmetic lesions usually takes place 4 to 6 months after injury. Neurapraxic lesions are temporary nerve conduction blocks without permanent structural damage or transection; recovery takes place quickly, usually within a month, and is complete.

10.5 Anatomy of a Peripheral Nerve

A peripheral nerve is composed of myelinated axons embedded in endoneurium and bound in fascicles by the perineurium. These groups of fascicles are in turn loosely bundled together by connective tissue called the interstitial epineurium; all the fascicles are wrapped in the circumferential epineurium and together constitute a peripheral nerve. More than 50% of a nerve is connective tissue, which serves as the nerve's skeletal framework. The number of fascicles changes throughout the length of the nerve. The more distal the nerve, the greater the differentiation of axons with grouping of motor or sensory axons for the same muscle or region. For example, whereas all axons of the brachial plexus are mingled, in the more distal ulnar nerve, one fascicle will be almost entirely dedicated to motor function and another to sensory function.

The elastic epineurium allows some mobility of the nerve, which is secured only where branching occurs. Inside the epineurium, the perineurium surrounds groups of nerve fibers, forming fascicles. The blood supply of a peripheral nerve is longitudinal, beginning at root level with collaterals entering through a vasa vasorum. Intraneural vessels are numerous, and dissection that follows the vasa vasorum can usually be carried for long distances (up to 10 cm) without impairing nerve function. The central nucleus for motor neurons is situated in the anterior horn of the spinal cord; for the sensory nerves, it is located in the spinal ganglion close to the spinal foramen but outside the spinal canal.

10.6 Vulnerable Fetuses

Some fetuses may be more vulnerable to damage from stretching than others, for example, preterm and/or growth-restricted infants. Those who are hypoxic, it has been speculated, might have relatively poor muscle tone and thus not provide sufficient resistance to a strain imposed on the plexus during a normal delivery. This speculation remains unproven. These possibilities can be identified, and health care providers at delivery have to take this into consideration when applying traction to the fetal head. In all cases, this should be gentle and of short duration and should cease as soon as it is realized that the uterine contractions and maternal effort are failing to achieve descent of the shoulders [27].

10.7 Clinical Presentation

Symptomatology of birth-related brachial plexus lesions is usually first observed by the obstetrician, midwife, or in the infant's family shortly after birth. The injuries are more common after difficult deliveries with forcible head traction during head and breech presentations [35]. Clearing the shoulders in a difficult delivery of a vertex presentation or in a breech presentation carries the risk of a plexus trauma.

The majority of children who present with birth-related brachial plexus injuries demonstrate classic Erb-type upper-plexus lesions of roots C5 and C6. The arm is clinically limp, the shoulder abducted with its upper part internally rotated, the elbow extended, and the forearm pronated with flexed wrist and fingers. Other levels of involvement can include C7, which causes triceps paresis and some insufficiency of wrist and finger extension. A C4 root lesion causes phrenic nerve palsy with accompanying respiratory problems. In contrast with radiculopathies, brachial plexus neuritis, and tumors among adults, the birth-related brachial plexus syndrome does not usually include pain [34]. Classic

Klumpke patients, a variety rarely seen today, present with flexion in the elbow and extended wrist without finger movement; this syndrome is based on C8 and T1 root involvement, often with avulsion. The presence of Horner syndrome is diagnostic of C8- and T1-level lesions. Dysfunction of the dorsal scapular (rhomboid muscle) nerve or the long thoracic (anterior serratus muscle) nerve indicates a root-level injury. A lesion of the suprascapular (supraspinatus and infraspinatus muscles) nerve indicates an upper-trunk lesion. Combined total plexus lesions from C5 to T1 constitute the remaining cases [35].

10.8 Mortality and Morbidity

Death at delivery from shoulder dystocia has recently been studied. A total of 56 cases were analyzed where the injuries and cause of death resulted from delivery techniques. There were no adverse affects from labor forces, intrauterine causes, or other so-called spontaneous events rarely associated with brachial plexus injuries. Less than 50% of the cases had a fundal height measurement. Obesity and macrosomia were significantly increased. Traction was recorded in 24 of 56 cases, and 3 charts did not describe any technique. Surprisingly, only 64% (36 cases) of the women had an episiotomy. Fundal pressure was used in six cases. Autopsy revealed hypoxia in 95% and birth trauma in 24%.

The head to body delivery time was less than 5 minutes in 21 (47%), and only 9 (20%) had an interval greater than 10 minutes. The mechanism of injury with a short interval may be from cord prolapse or compression of the neck resulting in cerebral venous obstruction or from excessive vaginal stimulation.

Neonatal death from shoulder dystocia is reported from 21 to 290 per 1,000 cases, and neonatal morbidity has been reported to be immediately obvious in 20% of infants. Brachial plexus injury, clavicular fracture, facial nerve paralysis, asphyxia, central nervous system (CNS) injury, neuropsychiatric dysfunction, and death after shoulder dystocia are all described [36].

Reports of neonatal asphyxia and CNS injury resulting from shoulder dystocia are confounded by a variety of factors, including vaginal delivery methods, fetal heart rate and labor abnormalities, the presence or absence of meconium, and differences in infant birth weight. Perinatal death resulting from shoulder dystocia seems to be related to the diagnosis-to-delivery interval and the difficulty involved in reducing the dystocia [36]. Good neonatal outcomes have been reported with diagnosis-to-delivery intervals of up to 70 minutes.

Empirically, the extent of fetal injury is related to both the degree of shoulder impaction and the procedures necessary to resolve it [36,37]. For example, the sole use of fundal pressure in treating shoulder dystocia was found by Gross to result in a 75% complication rate, primarily resulting in orthopedic and neurologic injury.

All investigators have documented increased perinatal morbidity and mortality with the diagnosis of shoulder dystocia. Mortality has varied from

21 to 290 per 1,000 when shoulder dystocia impaction occurred, and neonatal morbidity has been reported to be obvious immediately in 20% of infants overall. Boyd et al. [16] reviewed 131 macrosomic infants and found that one half of all cases of brachial palsy in macrosomic infants were accompanied by the diagnosis of shoulder dystocia. Severe asphyxia was observed in 143 of 1,000 births with shoulder dystocia compared with 14 of 1,000 overall. Fetal morbidity is not always apparent immediately. McCall [15] found that 28% of infants born with shoulder dystocia demonstrated some neuropsychiatric dysfunction at 5- to 10-year follow-up. Fewer than one half of these children had immediate morbidity.

Does vaginal delivery of a macrosomic infant change the outcome for delivery of a subsequent fetus weighing more than 4,500 g at birth? An unusual article gives us the answer. This retrospective study by Lazer et al. [38] included 525 infants who weighed more than 4,500 g. Prior experience decreases the risk of maternal injury in such cases, but the fetal risks remain excessive. The incidences of perinatal mortality, brachial plexus injury, and low Apgar scores were significant. This is clearly noted in pregnancies where women who had delivered infants weighing more than 4,500 g birthweight in the past were compared with normal controls.

Results of the study showed that the rates of grand multiparity, diabetes mellitus, pregnancy-induced hypertension, deliveries in women above 35 years of age, placenta previa, and weight gain of more than 15 kg were higher than in a control group weighing 2,500 to 4,000 g. The rates of delivery with instruments and cesarean section were also significantly higher. The main indication for cesarean section in the study group was cephalopelvic disproportion, whereas in the control group it was repeat cesarean section. Rates of postpartum hemorrhage, shoulder dystocia, oxytocin augmentation of labor, and tears in the birth canal far exceeded those in the control group. Maternal and fetal morbidity and perinatal mortality were significantly higher than in the control group. The complications were due to a difficult second stage of labor. Clearly, the fetal risks where birthweight equals or exceeds 4,500 g are large enough to make abdominal birth preferred, regardless of prior obstetric experience.

The risk of traumatic injury and low Apgar score was studied by Wikstrom et al. [39] in 473 infants with a birthweight of 4,500 g or more at term, and in 473 infants with normal weight (birthweight ± 1 standard deviation of the mean for the respective gestational age). The large for gestational age (LGA) group comprised 3.2% of all infants delivered during a 5-year period. Traumatic injuries were observed in 8.0% of the large infants versus 0.6% of the normal-size group. In the LGA group, there were 28 fractured clavicles, 4 fractured humeri, and 12 brachial plexus injuries. Six of the large infants had multiple injuries. The injuries in the normal infants were three fractured clavicles. All infants with traumatic injuries were delivered vaginally. Contributory obstetric factors for traumatic injury were forceps, postterm pregnancy, and vacuum extraction. High birthweight and postterm pregnancy correlated with a low Apgar score at 1 minute.

In three studies in which a control group of term-size neonates born during the study period were compared with neonates weighing 4,500 g or more at birth, the perinatal mortality was at least five times higher for the macrosomic group. The incidence of maternal, fetal, and neonatal complications was also high, suggesting that many of those large neonates experienced difficult deliveries. This conclusion has prompted some authors to propose that delivery by cesarean section may prevent many of the problems associated with the excessively large fetus. Parks and Ziel [20] suggested that macrosomia alone may be an indication for primary cesarean section. However, all fetuses weighing less than 4,500 g at delivery were included in their study as the control group. Because this group includes premature fetuses, who are known to have higher mortality, the validity of comparisons on the basis of mortality is questionable.

10.9 Causation

Regarding causation in 2007, Allen et al., using a sophisticated birthing simulator and fetal model, demonstrated that "SD [shoulder dystocia] itself does not pose additional brachial plexus stretch" to the anterior shoulder over naturally occurring deliveries unaffected by shoulder dystocia. They also found that the degree of stretch in the posterior brachial plexus was greater during routine deliveries than in shoulder dystocia deliveries and concluded that the degree of brachial plexus stretch demonstrated by their study "would be unlikely to cause injury in neonates independent of additional, externally applied force [40]."

The occurrence and extent of nerve injury depends on the magnitude, direction, and rate at which that delivery force is applied [41]. Clinical studies reveal that neurapraxic injury and fracture may occur at about 20 lb of traction, if applied quickly. To sustain axonal disruption requires more than 30 lb of traction; higher magnitudes of force are needed to produce the more severe mechanical disruptions, such as rupture or avulsion [41].

Experimentally and clinically measured clinician-applied delivery forces typically reach up to 10 lb of traction force during routine deliveries. As expected, clinician-applied traction increases with difficulty of the delivery.

However, in addition to magnitude, the direction of force is also a critical determinant of injury. Forceps studies conducted in live births in the 1960s, as well as other cadaveric studies, have shown that the fetal neck and spinal cord can withstand traction forces up to 90 lb before injury occurs, provided the force is applied axially, with the cervical and thoracic vertebrae aligned [41]. With axially applied traction, the brachial plexus, which is oriented nearly perpendicular to the spine near the base of the neck, is least stretched [41].

Torsion increases the vulnerability of the brachial plexus during the application of traction [41]. If the head is twisted away from the contralateral shoulder and then traction is applied, the resultant tension produced in the brachial plexus is higher than when the head remains in neutral position. This emphasizes the importance of confirming the relative position of the head and shoulders after restitution, before applying traction. And finally, the rate at which force is applied also affects likelihood of injury. Jerky or rapidly applied force is less tolerated by the brachial plexus than is force of comparable magnitude and direction applied in a smooth, slow manner [41]. In a clinical study that included two shoulder dystocia deliveries with similar-weight children delivered with similar magnitude of force, one resulted in an injury and one did not. The temporary brachial plexus injury occurred after the delivery in which the force was applied three times more quickly than in the other delivery [41]. The strain reached approximately 15% in shoulder dystocia and routine deliveries, well below the 50% elastic limit of fetal nerve [41]. Although there have been mathematically calculated uterine forces that approach 200 lb, this level of force is neither scientifically sound nor clinically evident [41].

To date, the maximum uterine force that has been clinically measured is around 35 lb. Interestingly, this magnitude of uterine force occurred only during Valsalva combined with McRoberts positioning, the latter of which increased intraabdominal pressure further than maternal effort alone [41].

Although this magnitude of uterine force alone appears to be sufficient to cause injury, because uterine forces are axially transmitted, they typically do not produce the lateral deviation of the head from the shoulders needed to stretch the brachial plexus beyond its elastic limit. Such deviation is more likely to result from uterine maladaptation (e.g., transverse lie or asynclitism) than from uterine forces themselves. Because of this, it is imperative to apply the least amount of traction to the head in any delivery—most especially, during shoulder dystocia [41].

A 1983 review of the deliveries at Johns Hopkins [27] included 17 documented cases of Erb palsy for an incidence of 0.725 per 1,000. The incidence of Erb palsy remained the same despite an increasing cesarean section rate. Of the 17 cases of Erb palsy, there were three cases with birthweights greater than 4,000 g. Eight of the 17 cases had shoulder dystocia. Four of the 17 cases were midforceps deliveries. There were three cases of prolonged second stage of labor, two of which were delivered by midforceps. Shoulder dystocia accompanied two of these three cases. There were three cases of persistent neurologic deficits. Two of these three cases were simple uncomplicated Erb paralysis diagnosed at delivery. The other case was complicated by diaphragmatic paralysis and a partial Horner syndrome. All of these were the result of a traumatic delivery.

A 2006 Johns Hopkins article has added further insight to the cause of brachial plexus injuries from shoulder dystocia [40]. In this study of brachial plexus palsy (BPP) after cephalic vaginal delivery, shoulder dystocia (SD) emerged as the injury's predominant antecedent; they found that BPP was 75 times more likely to occur after SD delivery (21.6%) than after a non-SD delivery (3 per 1,000). These rates were comparable with those most often reported among general populations and within SD cohorts [40]. Among permanent injuries, the rate of SD in both data sets exceeded 90%, confirming the near universal association found in most articles addressing the topic [40]!

They further established that in the rare deliveries not recorded as shoulder dystocia but where BPP is permanent, the residual deficit was nearly always mild, whereas nerve root avulsions and/or complete brachial plexus impairment (C5-C8, T1) occurred almost exclusively with antecedent shoulder dystocia [40].

They also found that temporary injury associated with SD was highly correlated with clinicians in training completing SD deliveries that were classified as mild by objective criteria. This may reflect a supervising clinician's difficulty in assessing the amount of traction exerted by a trainee and/or the trainee's inexperience at recognizing milder SD at its onset [40]. Such factors may have increased the risk for injury; fortunately, the effect was transient. They found that neonatal outcomes were dissimilar between SD and non-SD deliveries involving temporary palsy; it is unlikely that the non-SD deliveries in this stratum universally represent undiagnosed or unreported SD events, as previously suggested [50].

Among non-SD deliveries [40], the rate of palsy among instrumented deliveries was greater than six times that among noninstrumented deliveries—almost triple the difference in the rate of SD between these types of deliveries. Because operative delivery is a risk factor for permanent injury, axial traction with the instrument is unlikely to cause a palsy. It is likely that factors associated with instrumented delivery rather than operative delivery itself contribute to temporary non-SD injuries. Asynclitism and a narrow pelvis that slows progress in the second stage are often managed with operative delivery. These abnormalities can also predispose to lateral deviation of the head relative to the neck during descent [40].

Despite limited available data, they have found that involvement of the posterior shoulder with BPP is unusual. Thus, their marginal finding that non-SD BPP affects the posterior shoulder more commonly than does SD BPP further supports that the two injuries are probably mechanistically distinct. Except in the most severe cases in which both shoulders are impacted, forward progress during a birth that culminates with SD usually involves unimpeded motion of the posterior shoulder until customary downward traction is met with failure to deliver the anterior shoulder [40].

The Hopkins investigation [40] supports that intrauterine and intrapartum phenomena can rarely contribute to the mechanism of birth-related palsy. Fortunately for the affected children, temporary palsies that arise from non-SD deliveries are clinically benign. They conclude that non-SD palsy is real, though very uncommon, and is likely mechanistically distinct from SD palsy. Contributors to the mechanism of this temporary injury include asynclitism, posterior shoulder involvement, and decreased muscle tone from fetal acidoms [40]. The Johns Hopkins researchers concluded that it appears reasonable to conclude, that if it occurs at all, brachial plexus injury unrelated to the process of delivery is a rare phenomenon with little bearing upon the overall problem of SD at birth.

Using a statistical model involving three urban teaching hospitals, Dyachento [41] was able to identify an adverse combination of risk factors for neonatal injury after a clinical recognition of SD. The model included maternal height and weight as well as gestational age and parity. The score identified 50.7% of the SD and brachial plexus injuries (BPI) injuries, along with a low false-positive rate of 2.7%. These authors concluded that contrary to some current opinions, a portion of SD with injury can be predicted without undue increase in false-positive detections.

10.10 Cesarean Injuries

See Chapter 17 for discussion of brachial plexus injuries at cesarean section.

10.11 Mechanism of Labor and Injury

The mechanism is determined by the shape of the maternal pelvis and of the fetal head and shoulders. The head normally enters the pelvis in the widest diameter of the pelvic inlet, rotates in the pelvic cavity, and emerges through the widest diameter of the pelvic outlet.

While the head is being born in the anteroposterior diameter, the fetal shoulders normally enter the pelvic brim in the transverse or oblique diameter. They then rotate in the cavity and emerge through the anteroposterior diameter of the outlet [42].

When the head has emerged from the pelvic outlet and has undergone external rotation, the anterior aspect of the fetal neck is flexed under the symphysis pubis.

The depth of the symphysis pubis is about 4 cm, and there is virtually no fat above, behind, or below the joint. The posterior wall of the pelvis, the sacrum, is curved and measures about 7 cm. The neck of a fetus of average weight is normally about 5 cm long.

Therefore, even when the anterior shoulder is fixed above the symphysis after the birth of the head, the brachial plexus that is lying anteriorly should not be under significant tension [37]. Traction at this time causes stretching of the brachial plexus; if there is a 20% stretch, the nerve fibers will begin to tear.

10.12 Conclusion

Early recognition and evaluation of risk factors for macrosomia are the keys to success in avoiding trauma to the brachial plexus.

Physician-induced traction or stretch injuries will occur in 8% to 20% of infants with shoulder dystocia. The majority of injured children will have significant improvement in 6 to 24 months; beyond this time, the injury will be permanent. Traction or stretch injuries can and do occur at cesarean delivery from excessive pulling by the surgeon when the incision(s) are too small.

References

1. Bager B. Perinatally acquired brachial plexus injury: A persisting challenge. *Acta Paediatr* 1997;86:1214–1219.
2. Sack RA. The large infant. *Am J Obstet Gynecol* 1969;104:195–204.
3. Levine MG, Holroyde J, Woods JR, et al. Birth trauma: Incidence and predisposing factors. *Obstet Gynecol* 1984;63:792–797.
4. Gordon M, Rich H, Deutchberger J, Green M. The immediate and long term outcome of obstetric birth trauma. Brachial plexus paralysis. *Am J Obstet Gynecol* 1973;117:51–57.
5. Hardy AE. Birth injuries of the brachial plexus. *J Bone Joint Surg Br* 1981;63:98–102.
6. Curran JS. Birth associated injury. *Clin Perinatol* 1981;1:111–114.
7. Golditch IM, Kirkman K. The large fetus: Management and outcome. *Obstet Gynecol* 1978;52:26–30.
8. Modanlou HD, Dorchester WL, Thorosian A, Freeman RK. Macrosomia—maternal, fetal, and neonatal implications. *Obstet Gynecol* 1980;55:420–424.
9. Boome RS, Kaye JC. Obstetric traction injuries of the brachial plexus: Natural history, indications for surgical repair and results. *J Bone Joint Surg Br* 1988;70:571–574.
10. Johnstone NR. Shoulder dystocia: A study of 47 cases. Royal Women's Hospital, Melbourne. *Aust N Z J Obstet Gynaecol* 1979;19:28–31.
11. Byers RK. Spinal cord injuries during birth. *Dev Med Child Neurol* 1975;17:103–110.
12. McFarland LV, Raskin M, Daling JR, Benedetti TJ. Erb-Duchenne's palsy: A consequence of fetal macrosomia and method of delivery. Obstet Gynecol 1986;68:784–788.
13. Wood C, Ng KH, Hounslow D, Benning H. Time—an important variable in normal delivery. *J Obstet Gynaecol Br Commonw* 1973;80:295–300.
14. Harris BA. Shoulder dystocia. *Clin Obstet Gynecol* 1984;27:106–111.
15. McCall JO Jr. Shoulder dystocia. A study of after effects. *Am J Obstet Gynecol* 1962;83:1486–1491.
16. Boyd ME, Usher RH, McLean FH. Fetal macrosomia: Prediction, risks proposed management. *Obstet Gynecol* 1983 61:715–720.
17. Niebyl J, Repke J, King T. Brachial plexus injury. *Proc Soc Perinat Obstet* 1984;8:146.
18. Simcha L, Yigal B, Mosme M, Herman L, Vaclav I. Prior experience decreases the risk of maternal injury. *J Reprod Med* 1986;31:501–505.
19. Borten M, Friedman E. *Legal Principles and Practice in Obstetrics and Gynecology.* Vol. 1. Chicago: Yearbook Medical Publishers; 1989.
20. Parks DG, Ziel HK. Macrosomia, a proposed indication for primary cesarean section. *Obstet Gynecol* 1978;52:407–412.
21. Eng GD. Brachial plexus palsy in newborn infants. *Pediatrics* 1971;48:18–22.
22. Acker DB, Gregory KD, Sachs BP, Friedman EA. Risk factors for Erb-Duchenne palsy. *Obstet Gynecol* 1988;71:389–392.
23. Griffin PP. Orthopedics in the newborn. In: Avery GB, ed. *Neonatology Pathophysiology and Management of the Newborn.* 2 nd ed. Philadelphia: JB Lippincott; 1981:906.
24. Soni AL, Mir NA, Kishan J, et al. Brachial plexus injuries in babies born in hospital: An appraisal of risk factors in a developing country. *Ann Trop Paediatr* 1985;5:69–73.
25. Baerthlein WC, Moodley S, Stinson SK. Comparison of maternal and neonatal morbidity in midforceps delivery and midpelvic vacuum extraction. *Obstet Gynecol* 1986,67:594–597.
26. Cohen AW, Otto SR. Obstetric clavicular fractures. A three year analysis. *J Reprod Med* 1980;25:119–122.
27. Cohen W. Influence of the duration of second stage labor on perinatal outcome and puerperal morbidity. *Obstet Gynecol* 1977;49:266–269.
28. Friedman EA, Niswander KR, Sachtleben MR. Dysfunctional labor, XI: Neurologic and development effect on surviving infants. *Obstet Gynecol* 1969;33:785–791.
29. Friedman EA, Niswander KR, Sachtleben MR, Naftaly N. Dysfunctional labor, X: Immediate results to infant. *Obstet Gynecol* 1969;33:776–784.

30. Friedman EA, Sachtleben MR, Bresky PA. Dysfunctional labor, XII: Long term effects on infant. *Am J Obstet Gynecol* 1977;127:779–783.
31. Greis JB, Bieniarz J, Scommengna A. Comparison of maternal and fetal effect of vacuum extraction birth forceps or cesarean deliveries. *Obstet Gynecol* 1981;52:571–577.
32. Katz M, Lunenfeld E, Meizner I, Bashan N, Gross J. The effect of the duration of second stage of labor on the acid-base state of the fetus. *Br J Obstet Gynaecol* 1987;94:425–430.
33. Pondaag W, Thomas R. Natural history of obstetric brachial plexus palsy. *Devel Med Child Neurol* 2004;46:138–144.
34. Menkes J, Sarnat H, Maria B. Child Neurology. 7th ed. New York: Lippincott, Williams & Wilkins; 2006.
35. Laurent J. Brachial plexus trauma and other peripheral nerve injuries of childhood. In: *Principles and Practice of Pediatric Neurosurgery*. New York: Thieme Medical Publishers;1999:897–913.
36. Wagner R, Nielsen P, Gonik B. Shoulder dystocia. *Obstet Gynecol Clin North Am* 1999;26:371–383.
37. Stirrat G, Taylor R. Mechanisms of obstetric brachial plexus palsy. *Clin Risk* 2002;8:218–222.
38. Lazer S, Biale Y, Mazor M, Lewenthal H, Insler V. Complications associated with the macrosomia fetus. *J Reprod Med* 1986;31:501–505.
39. Wikstrom I, Axelsson O, Bergstrom R, Meirik O. Traumatic injury in large-for-date infants. *Acta Obstet Gynecol Scand* 1988;67:259–264.
40. Gurewitsch E, Johnson E, Hamzehzadeh S, Allen R. Risk factors for brachial plexus injury with and without shoulder dystocia. *Am J Obstet Gynecol* 2006;194:486–492.
41. Dyachenko A, Ciampi A, Fahey J, Mighty H, Oppenheimer L, Hamilton E. Prediction of risk for shoulder dystocia with neonatal injury. *Am J Obstet Gynecol* 2006;195:1544–1549.
42. Allen RH, Cha SL, Kranker LM, Johnson TL, Gurewitsch ED. Comparing mechanical fetal response during descent, crowning, and restitution among deliveries with and without shoulder dystocia .AM J Obstet Gynecol 2007;196:539–541.

Part III
Clinical Considerations

Chapter 11
In Utero Causation of Brachial Plexus Injury: Myth or Mystery?

James A. O'Leary

Summary *In utero* causation is a manufactured theory based on speculation that contradicts known anatomic and physiologic principles. Brachial plexus injury (BPI) is a very-low-velocity and very-low-impact injury. Adult BPI is a high-velocity and high-impact injury. Labor forces are compressive and expulsive, not traction or stretching. "Using a statistical model it is possible to identify adverse combinations of factors that are associated with shoulder dystocia and neonatal injury [1]."

Keywords: labor forces · traction

Contents

11.1	Overview	147
11.2	Controversies Concerning Etiology	148
11.3	*In Utero* Research	150
11.4	The Johns Hopkins Rebuttal	154
11.5	Engineering Research	156
11.6	Fundal Dominance: The Uterine Injury?	157
11.7	Intraabdominal Forces	159
11.8	Discussion	159
11.9	Conclusion	161

11.1 Overview

Since Sever first proved that permanent brachial plexus palsy (BPP) cannot occur as a result of labor forces, many others have been intrigued by how commonly brachial plexus palsy occurs, how severely, and by what mechanism [2]. Because stout traction applied during shoulder dystocia (SD) is a well-established mechanism of injury, traditionally, brachial plexus palsy

J.A. O'Leary
Professor Obstetrics & Gynecology (retired), University of South Florida, Tampa, Florida, USA

J.A. O'Leary (ed.), *Shoulder Dystocia and Birth Injury*,
DOI 10.1007/978-1-59745-473-5_11, © Humana Press, a part of Springer
Science+Business Media, LLC 2009

noted at birth has been attributed to antecedent shoulder dystocia, and those brachial plexus palsies occurring without recorded shoulder dystocia have been touted as failure to recognize the complication [2]. Neonatal brachial plexus palsy has many reported causes, though mechanisms unrelated to the birth process are extremely rare [2].

11.2 Controversies Concerning Etiology

Apart from being devastating for many of its victims, cases of shoulder dystocia have affected the professional lives of obstetricians. Consequently, this entity has often been discussed in the medicolegal context [3]; in this process, a series of pseudoscientific papers appeared recently suggesting that, in many cases, brachial plexus injury is a prenatal event, unrelated to the arrest of the shoulders at birth [3]. Based on the information that evidence of denervation in adult subjects is not detectable by electromyography until 10 to 14 days after the insult, evidence of denervation within a few days after birth in affected newborns was interpreted as proof that the injuries had been sustained *in utero* before the onset of labor. This concept had to be discarded when a pertinent study showed that neuromuscular deficits develop much faster in fetal than in adult pigs [3]. An alternative hypothesis, namely, that brachial plexus injury is frequently caused during the labor process by uterine forces, still prevails. However, because the maternal forces mobilized during labor and delivery are expulsive in nature, it is impossible to perceive a natural mechanism that could imitate the effect of traction injuries. The latter have been proved to be associated with forceful extraction of the shoulders.

Rare cases of brachial plexus damage attributed to spontaneous *in utero* injury have been reported [2]. However, if an *in utero*-acquired Erb palsy is relatively frequent, it should occur often among neonates delivered abdominally, as the rate of cesarean sections has been at the range of 25% during the past two decades. It is a matter of interest, therefore, that in a published series of more than 200 brachial plexus injuries, only one of the affected children was delivered by (a repeat) cesarean section [2]. The delivery of this macrosomic baby had been preceded by two failed extraction attempts and involved the Zavanelli maneuver (cephalic replacement). Thus, there is serious doubt whether even this single case can be attributed to forces other than those used during the delivery attempts. Even a casual review of the literature (Table 11.1) proves that brachial plexus palsy follows shoulder dystocia. It appears reasonable to conclude, therefore, that, if it occurs at all, brachial plexus injury unrelated to the process of delivery is a very rare phenomenon with little bearing upon the overall problem of shoulder dystocia at birth [1].

Intrauterine malposition has also been posited as a cause of brachial plexus injury. However, such an etiology would necessarily result in atrophic change in the muscles innervated by the plexus at the time of birth [2].

Table 11.1 Relationship of BPI and SD: Summary of Selected Studies [30]. of Cephalic Vaginal Births Resulting in Brachial Plexus Injury

Study	Year	No. of Deliveries	Injury Type (No.)	Recorded SD (%) [30]
Acker	1988	32,068	U 22	100
Allen	2002	103	P 103	94
Morrison	1992	37,000*	T 75	100
			P 7	100
Ouzounian	1997	63	P 63	90
Crecin	1995	102	P 102	100
Wolf	2000	9,912	T 56	88
McFarland	1986	210,000	P 106	100
Backen	1995	40,518	P 33	100

T, temporary; P, permanent; U, unknown.
*Approximate number of deliveries.

Reports of brachial plexus injury (BPI) in the absence of recorded shoulder dystocia began to appear in the American literature in 1992 [3]. Jennett, from Phoenix, Arizona, reported a series of 39 infants diagnosed as having incurred brachial plexus impairment. Seventeen were associated with recorded diagnosis of shoulder dystocia, whereas 22 had no such recorded association. The authors commented [3] :

> It has been postulated that intrauterine pressures associated with uterine anomalies could be a factor. Although the presence of such anomalies *could not* be determined from the available data, uterine maladaptation associated with young maternal age and multiparity *might* well be associated with a higher incidence of intrauterine pressures resulting in nerve impairment. Spontaneous vaginal delivery was more than twice as common in the non-shoulder dystocia group, suggesting less probability of difficulty in delivery. Certainly, the brachial plexus impairment in a 2572 gm infant delivered by cesarean section from a transverse lie would have a high probability of intrauterine maladaptation as a cause [4].

The theory in Phoenix, therefore, was that some form of uterine "maladaptation" was responsible for those cases of brachial plexus injury that could not be explained by shoulder dystocia. Hankins and Clark suggested an alternative theory when they reported a single case in which brachial plexus injury had occurred in the posterior shoulder without the recording of shoulder dystocia [5]. They speculated on the mechanism that the posterior shoulder may become temporarily lodged behind the sacral promontory, yet delivery of the head results from maternal expulsive efforts or use of instruments. These two authors were not involved with the delivery of the 11-lb baby but base their publication and conclusion on physician testimony.

Other authors have reported brachial plexus injury without shoulder dystocia but without suggesting a mechanism. Sandmire and DeMott [6] reported a retrospective study from 1985 to 1994 and reported 19 brachial plexus injuries associated with shoulder dystocia and a further 17 in cephalic deliveries in the absence of recorded dystocia; newborns with shoulder dystocia–associated brachial plexus injury were larger than those having the same injury without shoulder dystocia. They did not consider failure to diagnose as an option.

Other authors [5, 6] also reported brachial plexus injury without recorded shoulder dystocia but again did not suggest a mechanism. A group from Los Angeles [7] published a paper whose purpose was to determine whether Erb palsies occurring in the absence of shoulder dystocia differ from those occurring after shoulder dystocia. They found that the characteristics of the children concerned did differ in certain respects: smaller birthweight and an increased incidence of both precipitate labor and clavicular fracture. The authors speculated that "pressure of the fetal shoulder against the symphysis pubis during the antepartum period may also lead to clavicular fracture." This is a highly unlikely event, physiologically impossible, and one that has not been previously reported. In a term-size fetus, the only opportunity for the anterior shoulder to impact upon the symphysis pubis is when the fetal head is already delivered and not before.

Most of these *in utero* reports have as their logical basis the failure of reported shoulder dystocia in the births of babies found later to be suffering from Erb palsy. The danger of drawing conclusions from matters not recorded is self-evident. A further difficulty was pointed out by a correspondent in the *American Journal of Obstetrics and Gynecology* following the papers by Gherman et al. [8]:

> In their article Gherman et al. [Refs. 4 and 7] found that 17 of 40 (42.5%) cases of Erbs palsy occurred "without shoulder dystocia" and that these infants had more fractured clavicles and were more likely to be permanently injured. The authors concluded that this group of injuries occurred from "an in utero insult" and not neck traction.
>
> The authors define the "shoulder dystocia" group on the basis of "the need for ancillary obstetric maneuvers other than gentle downward traction after delivery of the fetal head."
>
> Another explanation for their results is very possible. What if the operator experienced shoulder dystocia and managed it by pulling hard on the infant's neck to achieve delivery? In a retrospective review of hospital charts that type of case would not be classified as "shoulder dystocia," because no other maneuvers were performed. The excessive neck traction could result in more fractures and permanent Erb's palsy than occur in infants who were managed by applying classic shoulder dystocia maneuvers.
>
> Although the authors have attempted to further understand the etiology of Erb's palsy, these retrospective data do not do that [8].

These authors in reply conceded, "We agree that there is inherent ascertainment bias in our retrospective study [8]."

11.3 *In Utero* Research

11.3.1 Jennett Theory

Jennett's first article [3] in 1992 included two references that did not support his theory [9,10]. He assumed that if shoulder dystocia and strong traction were not recorded, they did not happen. His most recent article has accepted traction as a cause [11]. A letter to the editor [8] regarding Jennett's research points out that others' experience differs, as noted in the world literature. He compares brachial plexus injury at birth with motorcycle and sports accidents and draws false conclusions. The former is a low-impact and low-velocity injury and the latter are high-impact and high-velocity injuries. He postulates but does not prove that "the irregular contour of the pelvis could cause an injury [8]."

The first study by Jennett [3] used a large, computer-generated, retrospective obstetric database to point out that the incidence of shoulder dystocia and the incidence of brachial plexus palsy were not related. In their series, 56% of babies born with Erb-Klumpke palsy did not have the diagnosis of shoulder dystocia written in the chart at the time of delivery. This finding is consistent with the 71% of unreported brachial plexus injuries reported by Gonik et al. [9,12] in 1991, which were not associated with the diagnosis of shoulder dystocia. The papers by Jennett [11] ignore the known underreporting of shoulder dystocia. The early data presented by Gonik [12] indicate that the concept of an intrauterine cause of many cases of brachial plexus palsy is unlikely. Dr. Gonik and associates have clearly shown that electromyographic evidence of nerve injury occurs much earlier in the neonate than in the adult, most likely related to the length of nerves involved, and is evident by 24 to 48 hours after injury [12].

11.3.2 Gherman Theory

This research is speculation based on the absence of a recorded shoulder dystocia [14–17]. He uses an inaccurate definition of shoulder dystocia: the need for "additional maneuvers" to establish the diagnosis. He does not permit any possible causes of brachial plexus injury in the first 1 minute of the shoulder dystocia. It is well-known that many infants are injured in the first 60 seconds of traction [18]. Gherman admits to "inherent ascertainment bias in his retrospective studies [13]." He ignored his own references, relied on falsely interpreted cesarean section data, made no mention of the causative pressures or forces [14–17], and did not consider failure to diagnose, poor record-keeping, and/or attempts to conceal. He expects physicians to always record strong traction in their delivery notes [7, 14–17], which is well-known not to occur.

Gherman reviewed 126 cases of shoulder dystocia among 9,071 vaginal deliveries [15]. He identified 40 cases of Erb palsy. Of those 40 cases, he indicated 17 did not have an identifiable shoulder dystocia while 23 were associated with shoulder dystocia. Gherman goes on to state:

> Moreover, as many as 50% of brachial plexus injuries *may* be attributable to unavoidable intrapartum or antepartum events and not to shoulder dystocia. Many of the factors that predispose to shoulder dystocia *may* place increased tension on the brachial plexus before delivery of the fetal head [emphasis added].

It is interesting that Gherman:

Acknowledge that among the cases of Erb's palsy occurring without shoulder dystocia, there may have been instances of non-recognition or incomplete documentation of a difficult delivery. Concern over medico/legal implications, however, would probably have led to an even better documentation of maneuvers. . . .

He further goes on to state that:

Many permanent brachial plexus injuries *may* be due to in utero forces that precede the actual delivery. Before the recognition of the shoulder dystocia, a significant degree of stretch or pressure *may* have already been applied to the brachial plexus. Moreover, even when a brachial plexus injury is associated with shoulder dystocia it *may* have occurred independent of traction applied by the obstetrician.

It is interesting to note how many times the word *may* appears in the preceding discussion. William Spellacy, MD, in his letter to the editor regarding the Gherman article, posits that [19]:

Another explanation for their results is very possible. What if the operator experienced a shoulder dystocia and managed it by pulling hard on the infant's neck to achieve delivery? In a retrospective review of hospital charts that type of case would not be classified as "shoulder dystocia" in this study because no other maneuvers were performed.

Spellacy concludes by stating that: "Although the authors have attempted to further the understanding of the etiology of Erb's palsy, these retrospective data do not do that."

It is interesting to note that in his reply, Gherman states that he has already acknowledged that "some of the 'no shoulder' brachial plexus injuries may have represented non-recognition or incomplete documentation of antecedent shoulder dystocia [13]." He further agrees that there is an "inherent ascertainment bias" in their retrospective study. The authors explain that:

Because there is no current accepted method to objectively quantify "excessive lateral traction," the mere occurrence of brachial plexus injuries should not therefore be taken as prima facia evidence of medical negligence.

Gherman has also studied [15,16]:

- 58,565 total deliveries: 8,451 by cesarean sections.
- 303 shoulder dystocia (0.61%) and 48 brachial plexus injuries (0.096%).
- 17 brachial plexus injuries after cesarean section, 9 with breech delivery and 2 with operative report of difficulty in delivery of the fetal head. Six others remained, with cesarean section and brachial plexus injuries without clear breech or head impaction. Six out of 48 brachial plexus injuries.

Something is wrong here: they had more than one third of the total brachial plexus injuries occurring in cesarean sections. That simply does not make sense. Only 14% of all deliveries were cesarean sections. This means that a brachial plexus injury was twice as likely to occur in a cesarean section than via vaginal delivery.

A critical look at these articles shows that the vast majority of brachial plexus palsies in patients with shoulder dystocia are caused by the way it is handled to a probability of 95% to 98%. This data actually shows that Erb palsy in the absence of shoulder dystocia is a very rare event and that shoulder dystocia itself is a risk factor for Erb palsy at a 50- to 200-times level.

In sum:

1. The number of patients with shoulder dystocia in Gherman's review was 126; the number of patients without shoulder dystocia was 8,945.
2. Therefore, the incidence of Erb palsy in patients with shoulder dystocia was $23/126 = 18.25\%$.
3. The incidence of Erb palsy in patients without shoulder dystocia was $17/8,945 = 0.19\%$.
4. The relative risk for Erb palsy associated with shoulder dystocia is 96.05.
5. Otherwise put, by these advocate's own data, you are 95 times more likely to get an Erb palsy if you have shoulder dystocia than if you do not.
6. Further analyzed, this data means that if you have a shoulder dystocia, and end up with an Erb palsy, the likelihood that it would have occurred in the absence of the shoulder dystocia is $0.19/18.25 = 1.04\%$ and the likelihood that it is related to the shoulder dystocia is 98.96%.

The data from authors who seem to minimize the relationship of shoulder dystocia and the way it is handled with Erb palsy prove the opposite of what the authors try to convey. That the authors never did this simple analysis of their own numbers is telling in and of itself.

11.3.3 Gonik Theory

Gonik's research since 1999 has used dummy models, mathematical formulas, but never human or animal subjects [19–21]. The computer simulation did not allow for intercase variability and did not account for dissipation of force in pelvic soft tissues and various lubrication properties (amniotic fluid and vaginal mucous). No statistical significance could be determined. The protective effect of the amniotic fluid (bag of water), fetal muscle, and the uterine muscle were ignored. All of these factors do play a critical role. He wisely concluded that "there is no direct application of these results to the clinical arena [20,21]."

The research model assumed maternal pushing causes stretching. He [20,21] assumes that force on the shoulder is equal to the force on the brachial plexus: an unproven statement. He assumes that the head pulls the body, as opposed to the body pushing the head. This is false.

Gonik's research (Table 11.2) violated the basic principles of Newton's law of equilibrium and this led to a very significant miscalculation of the endogenous forces [21]. He falsely concluded that 180 lb of force on the neck was required, as opposed to the accurate determination of 18 lb, in order to cause an injury [25, 26]!

Table 11.2. Outline of Gonik's Research

Gonik no. 1	Mathematical model only. No patients.
A.J.O.G. 2000;172:689–691	Measured piston (engine) area.
	"Mathematical exercise."
	Doesn't account for soft tissue effect.
	No data to quantify traction threshold.
	Only compressive forces!
	Under normal conditions, not SD.
Gonik no. 2	No patients.
A.J.O.G. 2003;188:1068–1072	Crash dummy model (high-velocity, high-impact).
	Downward traction >30% increases brachial plexus stretch.
	No validation in humans.
	Numerous limitations.
	"*Cannot* be applied to clinical arena."
Gonik no. 3	"Model refinements are necessary."
A.J.O.G. 2003;189:1168–1172	Measured compression not stretching forces.
	Does not include a brachial plexus component.
	Unable to measure stretch.
	Measures compression of shoulder not nerve.
	Couldn't calculate statistical significance.
	No data for compression injuries.
	Cannot be applied to the clinical arena.

11.3.4 Sandmire Theory

The Sandmire theory [6,23,24] is based on his review and reinterpretation of the literature. He has performed no research, and admits his opinions are based solely on "indirect evidence [24]." These writings rely on speculation in arriving at his disproportionate propulsion theory (DPT), or disproportionate descent theory. His conclusions are based on the absence of recorded shoulder dystocia in medical records. He speculates that once the baby's body stops moving (stuck shoulder), some "unknown force" leads to further movement of the head. Looked at another way: the head pulls the body. His DPT, according to Sandmire himself, is based on "indirect evidence." The very excellent 2006 clinical research from Johns Hopkins does not include his writings in their review [1].

11.4 The Johns Hopkins Rebuttal

A 2006 Johns Hopkins article has added great insight into the cause of brachial plexus injuries from shoulder dystocia [2]. In this study of BPP after cephalic vaginal delivery, SD emerged as the injury's predominant antecedent; they found that BPP was 75 times more likely to occur after SD delivery (21.6%) than after a non-SD delivery (3 per 1,000). These rates were comparable with those most often reported among general populations and within SD cohorts. Among permanent injuries, the rate of SD in both data sets exceeded 90%, confirming the near universal association found in most articles addressing the topic [2]!

They further established that in the rare deliveries not recorded as shoulder dystocia, but where BPP is permanent, the residual deficit was nearly always mild, whereas nerve root avulsions and/or complete brachial plexus impairment (C5-C8, T1), occurred almost exclusively with antecedent shoulder dystocia.

They also found that temporary injury associated with SD was highly correlated with clinicians in training completing SD deliveries that were classified as mild by objective criteria. This may reflect a supervising clinician's difficulty in assessing the amount of traction exerted by a trainee and/or the trainee's inexperience at recognizing milder SD at its onset [2]. Such factors may have increased the risk for injury; fortunately, the effect was transient. They found that neonatal outcomes were dissimilar between SD and non-SD deliveries involving temporary palsy; it is unlikely that the non-SD deliveries in this stratum universally represent undiagnosed or unreported SD events, as previously suggested [1].

Among non-SD deliveries [2], the rate of palsy among instrumented deliveries was greater than six times that among noninstrumented deliveries—almost triple the difference in the rate of SD between these types of deliveries. Because operative delivery is a risk factor for permanent injury, and axial traction versus the instrument is unlikely to cause a palsy, it is again likely that factors associated with instrumented delivery rather than operative delivery itself contribute to temporary non-SD injuries. Asynclitism and a narrow pelvis that slows progress in the second stage are often managed with operative delivery. These abnormalities can also predispose to lateral deviation of the head relative to the neck during descent.

They have found that involvement of the posterior shoulder with BPP is unusual. Thus, their marginal finding that non-SD BPP affects the posterior shoulder more commonly than does SD BPP further supports that the two injuries are probably mechanistically distinct. Except in the most severe cases in which both shoulders are impacted, forward progress during a birth that culminates with SD usually involves unimpeded motion of the posterior shoulder, until customary downward traction is met with failure to deliver the anterior shoulder [2].

The Johns Hopkins investigation supports that intrauterine and intrapartum phenomena can rarely contribute to the mechanism of birth-related palsy [2,25]. Fortunately for the affected children, temporary palsies that arise from non-SD deliveries are clinically benign. They conclude that non-SD palsy is real, though very uncommon, and is likely mechanistically distinct from SD palsy. Contributors to the mechanism of this temporary injury include asynclitism, posterior shoulder involvement, and decreased muscle tone from fetal acidosis [2]. These researchers concluded that it appears reasonable to conclude therefore, that if it occurs at all, brachial plexus injury unrelated to the process of delivery is a rare phenomenon with little bearing upon the overall problem of shoulder dystocia at birth.

11.5 Engineering Research

Intrauterine causation is a manufactured theory. This theory is not accepted by obstetricians outside the United States and is not accepted by non-obstetricians inside the United States as a reliable or established theory.

Studies conducted by Allen [8,17,26] included attaching force monitoring equipment during actual deliveries, including deliveries in which shoulder dystocia occurred. The forces exerted by 39 obstetricians during simulated delivery of babies for three perceived categories of delivery (normal, difficult, and shoulder dystocia) were measured, both in magnitude and direction. The forces applied by the physicians in the simulated shoulder dystocia situations were close to double those applied by the same physicians for normal deliveries, both as to total axial force and to the force of neck bending. There were substantial differences among the physicians in force exerted to accomplish the same task, and the physicians themselves did not appreciate the substantial differences in forces exerted. Peak forces varied almost threefold between normal and shoulder dystocia deliveries. Many physicians applied substantial upward traction on the neck, as well as downward traction on the neck, a phenomenon that may well explain the occurrence occasionally of posterior shoulder injury after shoulder dystocia. Neck bending was often significant and inadvertent [2,8,25,26].

Fractures of the clavicle have been proven to occur with peak forces of 100 N or more; this is considered a fracture threshold. It is reasonable to assume that a traction sufficient to cause clavicular fractures is more than enough to cause brachial plexus injury. The peak forces in this model were very close to the peak forces measured in actual clinical conditions; the model is valid [25,26].

The retraction forces on the fetal head ("turtle sign") have been described as strong by Sandmire, who provides no information or research to support the word *strong*. So-called positive evidence does not exist. In reality, this is a passive movement approaching 1 cm in length. Engineering studies have demonstrated that the brachial plexus must be stretched 20% to be injured [24].

There is no proof that the slowly applied force of uterine contractions and maternal pushing is of sufficient strength, torque, or duration to cause an Erb palsy. The underreporting of shoulder dystocia is well-known and well documented. Such a finding does not strongly suggest a biologic phenomenon rather than underreporting. The statement that infants with Erb palsy who do not have shoulder dystocia have a higher permanency rate (41.2% vs. 8.7%) is just a reflection of failure to diagnose and properly treat the dystocia. This failure to diagnose leads to use of improper techniques and therefore more damage. It does not suggest some magical other cause.

11.6 Fundal Dominance: The Uterine Injury?

Is the uterus the culprit injuring the brachial plexus? Compressive forces come from the upper two-thirds of the uterus, the only portion that contracts. Excessive compression would affect the umbilical cord and lead to heart rate decelerations and ultimately bradycardia, long before muscle or nerve compression.

Severe compression would cause the entire fetal body to be black and blue; the skin and muscle would be injured prior to nerve injury. Bones would break before well-protected and deeply placed nerves.

Severe compression (uterine tetany) would cause fetal pain and thus increase in heart rate and cause accelerations with contractions. Cord compression would precede any nerve compression and thus lead to fetal bradycardia and fetal distress. The bag of water absorbs the forces and protects the baby. The uterine muscle would injure itself before a deeply placed nerve in the neck and would cause the placenta to be separated and bleed.

11.6.1 Differentiation of Uterine Activity

During this uterine phase of parturition, the uterus differentiates into two distinct parts. The actively contracting upper segment becomes thicker as labor advances; the lower portion comprising the lower segment of the uterus and the cervix is relatively passive compared with the upper segment, and it develops into a much more thinly walled passage for the fetus. The lower uterine segment is analogous to a greatly expanded and thinned-out isthmus of the uterus of nonpregnant women, the formation of which is not solely a phenomenon of labor. The lower segment develops gradually as pregnancy progresses and then thins remarkably during labor. By abdominal palpation, even before rupture of the membranes, the two segments can be differentiated during a contraction. The upper uterine segment is quite firm or hard, whereas the consistency of the lower uterine segment is much less firm. The former represents the actively contracting part of the uterus; the latter is the distended, normally much more passive and protective portion [27,28].

If the entire sac of uterine musculature, including the lower uterine segment and cervix, were to contract simultaneously and with equal intensity, the net expulsive force would be decreased markedly. Herein lies the importance of the division of the uterus into an actively contracting upper segment and a more passive lower segment that differ not only anatomically but also physiologically. The upper segment contracts, retracts, and expels the fetus; in response to the force of the contractions of the upper segment, the ripened lower uterine segment and cervix dilate and thereby form a greatly expanded, thinned-out muscular and fibromuscular tube through which the fetus can be extruded, and without compressing the brachial plexus [28].

The tension, however, remains the same as before the contraction. The effect of the ability of the upper portion of the uterus, or active segment, to contract down on its diminishing contents with myometrial tension remaining constant is to take up slack, that is, to maintain the advantage gained with respect to expulsion of the fetus, and to maintain the uterine musculature in firm contact with the intrauterine contents. As the consequence of retraction, each successive contraction commences where its predecessor left off, so that the upper part of the uterine cavity becomes slightly smaller with each successive contraction. Because of the successive shortening of its muscular fibers with each contraction, the upper uterine segment becomes progressively thickened throughout the first and second stages of labor and tremendously thickened immediately after delivery of the fetus. The phenomenon of retraction of the upper uterine segment is contingent upon a decrease in the volume of its contents. For its contents to be diminished, particularly early in labor when the entire uterus is virtually a closed sac with only a minute opening at the cervix, there is a requirement that the musculature of the lower segment stretch, permitting increasingly more of the intrauterine contents to occupy the lower segment [27,28].

The relaxation of the lower uterine segment is by no means complete relaxation, but rather the opposite of retraction. The fibers of the lower segment become stretched with each contraction of the upper segment, after which these are not returned to the previous length but rather remain relatively fixed at the longer length; the tension, however, remains essentially the same as before. The musculature still manifests tone, still resists stretch, still contracts somewhat on stimulation, and remains protective.

The successive lengthening of the muscular fibers in the lower uterine segment, as labor progresses, is accompanied by thinning, normally to only a few millimeters in the thinnest part. As a result of the thinning of the lower uterine segment and the concomitant thickening of the upper, the boundary between the two is marked by a ridge on the inner uterine surface, the physiologic retraction ring. From quantitative measurements of the difference in behavior of the upper and lower parts of the uterus during normal labor, it was found that there is normally a gradient of diminishing physiologic activity from the fundus to the cervix. Thus, there are no abnormal endogenous forces on the brachial plexus.

It is evident from muscle tracings that the intensity of each contraction is greater in the fundal zone than in the midzone and greater in the midzone than lower down. Equally noteworthy is the differential in the duration of the contractions; those in the midzone are much briefer than those above, whereas the contractions in the lower zone are extremely brief and sometimes absent. This lessening of contractions in the midzone, at a time when the upper zone is still contracting, is indicative that the upper part of the uterus throughout a substantial portion of each contraction comes to exert pressure caudally on the more relaxed parts of the uterus [27,28].

11.7 Intraabdominal Forces

After the cervix is dilated fully, the force that is principally important in the expulsion of the fetus is that produced by increased intraabdominal pressure created by contraction of the abdominal muscles simultaneously with forced respiratory efforts with the glottis closed. In obstetrical jargon, this is usually referred to as pushing. The nature of the force produced is similar to that involved in defecation, but usually the intensity is much greater. The important role that is served by intraabdominal pressure in fetal expulsion is most clearly attested to by the labors of women who are paraplegic. Such women suffer no pain, although the uterus may contract vigorously. Cervical dilatation measures the result of uterine contractions acting on a ripened cervix. Expulsion of the infant is rarely possible except when the woman is instructed to bear down and can do so at the time of uterine contractions. Although increased intraabdominal pressure is required for the spontaneous completion of labor, it is futile until the cervix is fully dilated. In other words, it is a necessary auxiliary to uterine contractions in the second stage of labor, but pushing accomplishes little in the first stage, except to fatigue the mother. At no time does the uterus stretch the brachial plexus [27,28].

11.8 Discussion

Regarding causation in 2007, Allen et al. [26], using a sophisticated birthing simulator and fetal model, demonstrated that "SD itself does not pose additional brachial plexus stretch" to the anterior shoulder over naturally occurring deliveries unaffected by SD. They also found that the degree of stretch in the posterior brachial plexus was greater during routine deliveries than in SD deliveries and concluded that the degree of brachial plexus stretch demonstrated by their study "would be unlikely to cause injury in neonates independent of additional, externally applied force."

There are three studies in the literature that appear to support the concept of intrauterine brachial plexus injury. The first of these, by Koenigsberger [10] in 1980, was an abstract that presented two cases. One of these infants had evidence of denervation injury on day 4 of life. The other infant reportedly had electromyographic evidence of denervation injury, but unfortunately the abstract does not say how long after birth the studies were performed, although presumably by day 4. Therefore, at least one and perhaps both of these could have been the result of injuries at delivery, according to the author's data. Gonik has refuted this study [9]. The second study is a case report by Dunn and Engle [29] in 1985 that is really not pertinent to the discussion of injuries that might be caused by shoulder dystocia because it involved a case of a uterine malformation leading to a long-term chronic compression injury of the fetal neck. That baby was born with a left brachial plexus palsy, phrenic nerve palsy, and Horner syndrome as well as subcutaneous fat necrosis in the left side of the neck, distortion of the first four ribs, and an undergrown left arm. Clearly, this was a chronic intrauterine injury, however, because of the uterine malformation, it really is not pertinent to a discussion of injuries potentially related to shoulder dystocia.

The third study is an article by Jennett [3], who in 1992 used a large, computer-generated, retrospective obstetric database to point out that the incidence of shoulder dystocia and the incidence of brachial plexus palsy were not related. In his series, 66% of babies born with Erb-Klumpke palsy did not have the diagnosis of shoulder dystocia written in the chart at the time of delivery. This finding is comparable and consistent with the 71% of unreported brachial plexus injuries reported by Gonik et al. in 1991 [9], which were not associated with the diagnosis of shoulder dystocia. The papers by Jennett [11] ignore the known underreporting of shoulder dystocia. Nevertheless, these three reports, plus data from electromyographic studies of brachial plexus nerve injuries in adults, have led to some favorable medicolegal verdicts for physicians.

The arguments against *in utero* causation are summarized in Table 11.3.

Table 11.3 Arguments Against *In Utero* Causation

1.	Only U.S. obstetricians believe this is an *in utero* causation.
2.	No neurology literature or texts supports *in utero* causation.
3.	Uterine forces are in upper two-thirds of uterus and not low down near neck.
4.	*In utero* reports are frequently written by defense experts.
5.	*In utero* causation is based on:
	a. Failure to record dystocia.
	b. Unproven theory (disproportionate propulsion, e.g., head pulls body).
	c. It happens at C.S. (which is really a traction force).
	d. A pressure injury (but there is no pressure injury on overlying skin, fat, or muscle of the infant).
	e. An injury to the posterior arm (no evidence for impact or compression injury, it is a traction injury).
	f. Engineering studies used for *in utero* are invalid and have not withstood peer review.
6.	Neurosurgical intraoperative findings confirm stretch injury.
7.	Incidence figures support traction.
8.	Improved delivery techniques have reduced injury rate fourfold.
9.	Statistical analysis of *in utero* causation disproves the theory.
10.	The failure to diagnose SD group of mothers has the worst injury rate.
11.	Evidence of fetal pain with so-called *in utero* injuries has not been reported.
12.	The injury rate is directly related to fetal size; the larger the baby, the greater the injury.
13.	The injury rate is directly related to the number of maneuvers used to treat the dystocia.
14.	The bag of water protects the baby.
15.	Labor forces are uniform throughout the world: the injury incidence is not.
16.	Other causes of injury are easily diagnosed.
17.	Incidence of SD is 0.15% to 1.7%. Not random.
18.	Incidence of injury increases 2 to 10 times with forceps/vacuum births. Therefore not random.
19.	Seventy-five percent to 90% of injuries occur in large babies.
20.	Amount of force to injury is not generated *in utero*.

11.9 Conclusion

In utero causation of brachial plexus injury is neither a myth nor a mystery! *It is the traction!* Using a statistical model, it is possible to identify adverse combinations of factors that are associated with shoulder dystocia and neonatal injury [30].

References

1. Dyachenko A, Ciampi A, Fahey J, Mighty H, Oppenheimer L, Hamilton E. Prediction of risk for shoulder dystocia with neonatal injury. *Am J Obstet Gynecol* 2006;195:1544–1549.
2. Gurewitsch E, Johnson E, Hamzehzadeh S, Allen R. Risk factors for brachial plexus injury with and without shoulder dystocia. *Am J Obstet Gynecol* 2006;194:486–492.
3. Jennett R. Brachial plexus palsy: An old problem revisited. *Am J Obstet Gynecol* 1992;166:1673–1677.
4. Gherman R, Goodwin T. Shoulder dystocia. Current opinion. *Obstet Gynecol* 1998;10:459–463.
5. Hankins G, Clark S. Brachial plexus palsy involving the posterior shoulder at spontaneous vaginal delivery. *Am J Perinatol* 1995;12:44–45.
6. Sandmire H, DeMott R. The physician factor as a determinant of cesarean birth rates for the large fetus. *Am J Obstet Gynecol* 1996;174:1557–1564.
7. Gherman R, Ouzounian J, Miller D, Kwak L, Goodwin T. Spontaneous vaginal delivery: A risk factor for Erbs palsy? *Am J Obstet Gynecol* 1998;178:423–427.
8. Allen R. Severe brachial plexus injury in the posterior arm: An alternative explanation [letter]. *Am J Obstet Gynecol* 2002;186:1377–1378.
9. Gonik B, Hollyer V, Allen R. Shoulder dystocia Recognition. *Am J Perinatol* 1991;8:31–34.
10. Koenigsberger M. Brachial plexus palsy at birth: Intrauterine or due to birth trauma [abstract]? *Ann Neurol* 1980;8:228.
11. Jennett R, Tarby T. Diffuse asteoporosis as evidence of brachial plexus palsy due to intrauterine fetal maladaption. *Am J Obstet Gynecol* 2001;185–237.
12. Gonik B, McCormick E, Verwey B, et al. The timing of congenital brachial plexus injury: A study of electromyography findings in the newborn piglets. *Am J Obstet Gynecol* 1998;178:688–695.
13. Gherman R. Spontaneous vaginal delivery: A risk factor for Erb's palsy. *Am J Obstet Gynecol* 1998;178:423–427.
14. Gherman R. Brachial plexus palsy associated with cesarean section: An in-utero injury? *Am J Obstet Gynecol* 1997;177:1162–1164.
15. Gherman R. Shoulder dystocia. *The Female Patient* 1998;23:79–90.
16. Gherman R. A comparison of shoulder dystocia-associated transient and permanent brachial plexus palsies. *Am J Obstet Gynecol* 2003;102:544–548.
17. Allen R, Gurewitsch E, Shoukas A. Computer modeling of shoulder dystocia. *Am J Obstet Gynecol* 2003;188:1804–1805.
18. Spellacy W. Erb's palsy without shoulder dystocia [letter]. *Am J Obstet Gynecol* 1998;179:561.
19. Gonik B. Walker A, Grimm M. Mathematic modeling of forces associated with a shoulder dystocia. *Am J Obstet Gynecol* 2000;182:689–691.
20. Gonik B, Zhang N, Grimm M. Defining forces that are associated with shoulder dystocia: The use of a mathematic dynamic computer model. *Am J Obstet Gynecol* 2003;188:1068–1072.

21. Gonik B, Zhang N, Grimm M. Prediction of brachial plexus stretching during shoulder dystocia using a computer simulation model. *Am J Obstet Gynecol* 2003;189:1168–1172.
22. Allen R, Edelberg S. A problematic model to predict intrauterine forces during shoulder dystocia. *Am J Obstet Gynecol* 2001;182:689–691.
23. Sandmire H, DeMott R. Erb's palsy causation: A historical perspective. *Birth* 2002;29:52–54.
24. Sandmire H, DeMott R. Erb's palsy: Concepts of causation. *Obstet Gynecol* 2000;95:941–942.
25. Allen R, Edelberg S. Brachial plexus palsy causation [letter]. *Birth* 2003;30:141–143.
26. Allen RH, Cha SL, Kranker LM, Johnson TL, Gurewitsch ED. Comparing mechanical fetal response during descent, crowning, and restitution among deliveries with and without shoulder dystocia. *Am J Obstet Gynecol* 2007;196:539–541.
27. Creasy R, Resnik R. *Maternal Fetal Medicine.* 5th ed. Philadelphia: Saunders; 2004;79–87.
28. Cunningham FG, MacDonald PC, Gant NF, Leveno KJ, Gilstrap III LC, eds. *Williams Obstetrics.* appleton & Lange 19th ed. Norwalk, CT: 1993:297–363.
29. Dunn D, Engle W. Brachial plexus palsy: Intrauterine onset. *Pediatr Neurol* 1985;1:367–369.
30. Allen R, Edelberg S. Erb's palsy: Concepts of causation. *Obstet Gynecol* 2000;96:801–802.

Chapter 12
Recurrent Shoulder Dystocia

James A. O'Leary

Summary Prior shoulder dystocia is the strongest risk factor for a recurrent shoulder dystocia. Prior macrosomia, abnormal labor, and operative delivery dramatically increase the injury rate in subsequent pregnancies. Early induction of labor or cesarean section is indicated unless the infant is significantly smaller. Prediction of future outcomes is not a realistic endeavor in modern-day obstetric practice.

Keywords: prediction · prior knowledge · recurrence

Contents

12.1 Introduction 163
12.2 Defeatist Attitude 164
12.3 Mathematical Calculations 164
12.4 Prior Knowledge 165
12.5 Predictability 166
12.6 Conclusion 167

12.1 Introduction

It is well-known that many women who have previously been delivered of newborns with obstetric (traction) brachial plexus injuries at birth are at great risk for having a recurrent injury [1]. A history of shoulder dystocia, with or without an injury, is traditionally thought to identify a risk for recurrent dystocia, given a similar set of clinical findings [2].

J.A. O'Leary

Professor Obstetrics & Gynecology (retired), University of South Florida, Tampa, Florida, USA

J.A. O'Leary, *Shoulder Dystocia and Birth Injury*,
DOI 10.1007/978-1-59745-473-5_12, © Humana Press, a part of Springer
Science+Business Media, LLC 2009

12.2 Defeatist Attitude

More than 10 years ago [3], the problem of shoulder dystocia was summarized in a publication as follows: "Most of the traditional risk factors for shoulder dystocia have no predictive value for shoulder dystocia itself is an unpredictable event, and infants at risk of permanent injury are virtually impossible to predict." Thus, no protocol should serve to substitute for clinical judgment [3].

This defeatist philosophy has been repeated in some publications [3], often with the implication that the terms *prediction* and *prevention* are interchangeable. Actually, preventive medicine has seldom relied on prediction [3]. The elimination of devastating diseases, such as smallpox, tuberculosis, and puerperal fever, and the teratogenic effects of drugs did not hinge upon prospective identification of individuals who would contract a particular infection or would suffer from the untoward effect of a potentially teratogenic agent. Thus, the numerous publications that confirmed and reconfirmed the unpredictability of shoulder dystocia have not helped to decrease the number of fetal injuries. Instead, orthopedic centers specializing in the surgical repair of Erb palsy have mushroomed in the United States in recent years [3].

This fatalistic belief in the unpredictability of shoulder dystocia appears to have derived from two major considerations:

1. The perceived difficulty of detecting macrosomia reliably by sonography.
2. Mathematical calculations that claimed that an inordinate number of cesarean sections would be needed to reduce the rate of brachial plexus injuries.

Intrinsic to the first argument has been the concern that sonography may overestimate the fetal weight, coupled with lack of attention to the fact that, by an equal chance, it can underestimate it. The philosophy that sonographic assessment of fetal weight at term is unacceptably unreliable is not shared by many prominent experts. Apuzzio and associates [3] calculated that, using an estimated fetal weight threshold of 4,250 g as an indication for abdominal delivery for diabetic women, 76% of diabetes-related brachial plexus injuries could be prevented! It is interesting, furthermore, that with due recognition of its limitations, sonographic estimation of the fetal weight has been relied upon in many clinical situations, ranging from the determination of the expected date of confinement to detection of fetal growth retardation and the diagnosis of discordance between twins [3].

12.3 Mathematical Calculations

As for the mathematical calculation suggesting that 2,335 cesarean sections would be needed to prevent one brachial plexus injury [3], one need only remember that the generally quoted rate of arrest of the shoulders at birth is about 1% in the United States. Of these babies, approximately 7% die or suffer

Table 12.1 Algorithm for the Prevention of Recurrent Shoulder Dystocia

First encounter	Obtain prior delivery record. History about the mother's own birthweight, personal and family history of diabetes, past delivery of child large for gestational age, with or without birth injury. Glucola screening test for all patients.
Examination	Attention to maternal weight and weight gain. Detailed pelvic assessment: to be documented in detail.
Prenatal visits	Close attention to weight gain. Involve nutritionist if needed (in case of glucosuria: diabetic screening at any gestational length). Discuss cesarean delivery.
26–28 weeks	Repeat diabetic screening (glucola test). If 135 mg/dL or more at 1 hour, arrange 3-hour glucose tolerance test promptly. If the blood glucose level is 190 mg/dL after 1 hour, the patient is gestational diabetic. Ultrasound for abdominal circumference.
36–40 weeks	Estimate fetal weight clinically at every visit. If large for gestational age fetus at term is suspected, double-check fetal weight with ultrasound. Discuss cesarean delivery.
Term	If estimated fetal weight is the size of the prior birth or more, perform cesarean section.

permanent injury [3]. Thus, out of 1,500 infants delivered vaginally, one becomes damaged due to arrests of the shoulders. Accordingly, one does not have to be a statistician to recognize that the quoted calculation is grossly inaccurate. Besides, this and other estimations ignore the fact that what needs to be prevented is not the shoulder dystocia but the fetal injuries deriving from it.

The knowledge that most cases cannot be predicted should not stop physicians from preventing as many incapacitating fetal injuries, deriving from shoulder dystocia, as possible [4–10]. In most instances, this complication is not lightning out of the blue but the last stage of a process that can often be influenced by early recognition and careful elimination of factors conducive to this complication. Indeed, very little in obstetrics is truly predictable or for that matter in life itself. An algorithm designed to show a path that offers a chance for preventing shoulder dystocia-related birth injuries is shown [3] in Table 12.1.

12.4 Prior Knowledge

Knowledge of a prior shoulder dystocia clearly affects management and outcome of subsequent deliveries. The Johns Hopkins experience [11] demonstrated a scheduled cesarean delivery in 46% of the cases. There was a 28% brachial plexus palsy rate in cases delivered vaginally.

12.5 Predictability

When calculating the rise of shoulder dystocia in relation to birthweight in nondiabetic and diabetic women, various authors used a broad variety of approaches, end points, and interpretations. The most extensive and probably most reliable data were published by Nesbitt et al [12]. and were based on the combined material of more than 300 hospitals, involving more than one-half million deliveries in the year 1992 (Table 12.2) [3]. In this material, diabetic mothers giving birth to 4,000 g to 4,250 g babies experienced shoulder dystocia in about 8% of all instances. The rate increased to more than 20% when the birthweights exceeded 4,500 g. In nondiabetic patients, the fetal risks were comparable with those of infants of diabetic mothers who weighed 250 g less. The use of an extraction instrument increased the risk of arrest of the shoulders by approximately 40% [3].

Another study found that of those infants delivered under conditions of shoulder dystocia, 20% sustained injuries [3]. Among these, 30% suffered permanent neurologic or other deficits. These results are comparable with data deriving from other sources. They permit the calculation, therefore, that approximately 1 of 13 cases of shoulder dystocia entails permanent fetal sequelae [3].

Meier and Broste studied 28 women with a prior shoulder dystocia and a subsequent vaginal delivery and found a 14% recurrence rate [2]. Infants smaller than the prior birth had no recurrences. However, infants above 4,000 g and larger than the prior birth had a 50% recurrence rate! Among the larger infants, the likelihood of recurrent shoulder dystocia is 15.7% to 84.3% based on exact 95% confidence limits. All infants in this study weighing more than 4,000 g experienced a recurrence of shoulder dystocia [2].

Mehta et al., [4] in a 5-year study of 25,995 deliveries, observed a 10-fold increase in the incidence of shoulder dystocia but concluded that there was an inability to predict the complication. Moore and colleagues' study [5] of 26,208 deliveries demonstrated that infant birthweight in the index pregnancy and the use of a vacuum extractor were strong risk factors for recurrence.

Table 12.2 Recurrence of Shoulder Dystocia: 1,983 Dystocias with 377 Subsequent Births

Author	Previous Shoulder Dystocia (N)	Subsequent Vaginal Delivery (N)	Recurrent Shoulder Dystocia (N)	Percent (%)
Smith	201	42	5	9.8
Barker	254	93	1	1.1
Lewis	747	123	17	13.8
Flannnelly	114	36	5	13.9
Ginsberg	602	66	11	16.7
Wolfe	53	17	6	35.0
Total	1,983	377	39	12

In a report from Hutzel Hospital, Wolfe et al. [6] observed a massive 73-fold risk for shoulder dystocia. In addition, a Temple University [7] analysis of recurrent shoulder dystocia was associated with a 22.8% injury rate.

A similar study by Smith and Lane [8] analyzed 51 patients with a prior shoulder dystocia. They found a recurrence rate of 9.8%, which was 17 times greater than the background rate. Similar results from Louisiana State University included a 13.8% recurrence rate of which 82.4% were infants larger than the prior delivery [9]. They concluded that shoulder dystocia recurs at a rate seven times higher than the baseline risk. Significant risk factors were fetal macrosomia, maternal obesity, and infants larger than the previous delivery. They concluded that many cases can be anticipated by paying careful attention to the risk factors and clinical management.

There have been five series reviewing the risk of recurrent shoulder dystocia, and these ranged from 1.1% to 16.7% (Table 12.2) [10]. Interestingly, the review with the lowest proportion of subsequent vaginal deliveries had the highest recurrence rate (16.7%), and the one with the highest proportion of subsequent vaginal deliveries had the lowest recurrence (1.1%). Thus, whereas shoulder dystocia in a previous pregnancy greatly increases the risk of shoulder dystocia recurrence, it will not always happen in many cases because the next infant may be smaller and/or the decision to induce labor early is implemented.

However, the risk of recurrence in those women with brachial plexus injury in the previous pregnancy can be so much greater that delivery by repeat elective cesarean section is justified in all of these cases [8,11].

12.6 Conclusion

In the 21st century, it is well-known that the vast majority of women with a prior shoulder dystocia will request or decide on a primary cesarean section. Proper and full informed consent requires that the care providers clearly define the higher likelihood of recurrent shoulder dystocia delivery problems (10% to 85%).

References

1. Al-Quttan M, Al-Kharfy T. Obstetric brachial plexus injury in subsequent deliveries. *Ann Plast Surg* 1996;37:545–548.
2. Meier P, Broste S. Estimating the risk of recurrent shoulder dystocia. *Female Patient* 1992;17:27–91.
3. Apuzzio J, Ventzileos A, Iffy L. Shoulder dystocia (chapter 13). In: Ramieri J, Iffy L, eds. *Operative Obstetrics*. 3rd ed. London and New York: Taylor & Francis; 2006:253–63.
4. Mehta S, Blackwell S, Chadha R, Sokol R. Mode of delivery following shoulder dystocia and its recurrence rate. *Am J Obstet Gynecol* 2006;189:45, 117 (abstract).
5. Moore H, Reed S, Batra M, Schiff M. Risk factors for recurrent shoulder dystocia, Washington State 1987–2004. *Obstet Gynecol* 2007;109:79S.

6. Wolfe H, Dierker L, Gross T, Treadwell M, Sokol R. Recurrence of shoulder dystocia in a subsequent delivery. *Am J Obstet Gynecol* 1997;168:433–434.
7. Quintero C, Grotegut C, Lidicker J, Mulla W, Lingamaneni A, Dandolu V. How do deliveries complicated by shoulder dystocia differ from non index deliveries. *Obstet Gynecol* 2007;109:91S.
8. Smith R, Lane C. Shoulder dystocia: What happens at the next delivery? *Br J Obstet Gynecol* 1994;101:713–715.
9. Lewis D, Raymond R, Perkins M, Brooks G, Heymann A. Recurrence rate of shoulder dystocia. *Am J Obstet Gynecol* 1995;172:1369–1371.
10. Baskett T. Shoulder dystocia: Best practice & research. *Clin Obstet Gynecol* 2002:16:57–68.
11. Gurewitsch E, Landsberger E, Jain A, Cha S, Johnson T, Allen R. Does knowledge of prior shoulder dystocia affect management and outcome in subsequent deliveries. *Am J Obstet Gynecol* 2006;189:42, 103.
12. Nesbitt T, Gilbert W, Herrchen B. Shoulder dystocia and associated risk factors with macrosomic infants born in California. *Am J Obstet Gynecol* 179:476–480.

Chapter 13
Predisposing Factors for Shoulder Dystocia-Related Birth Injuries: Causation Analysis

Leslie Iffy, Joseph J. Apuzzio, and Vijaya Raju

Summary This chapter contradicts the claim that more than half of all brachial plexus injuries are associated with uncomplicated deliveries. Infants are injured much more frequently with macrosomia and operative delivery. Twenty-five percent of infants suffer injury, and 5% to 22% become permanent. Shoulder dystocia was recorded in 97% of 135 cases.

Keywords: birth injury · large babies · LGA · macrosomia

Contents

13.1   Clinical Background   169
13.2   Database   170
13.3   Data Analysis   173
13.4   Clinical Interpretation   173
13.5   Conclusion   175

13.1 Clinical Background

Contemporary medical publications cite a variety of predisposing factors leading to shoulder dystocia with the implication that their relative frequency in the background of this complication defines their respective roles in the causation of associated fetal injuries. In some of the authors' previous publications, it was pointed out that, when cases without coincidental damage are excluded, the relative importance of the various predisposing factors differs from that quoted in the obstetric literature [1,2]. It was found that, in cases of fetal injury, macrosomia and the use of extraction instruments were more prevalent than generally thought. In addition, injuries involving the central nervous system (CNS) were far more frequently associated with shoulder dystocia than the literature had acknowledged [3,4].

L. Iffy
Professor of Obstetrics & Gynecology, University of Medicine & Dentistry of New Jersey, New Jersey Medical School, Newark, New Jersey, USA

J.A. O'Leary (ed.), *Shoulder Dystocia and Birth Injury*,
DOI 10.1007/978-1-59745-473-5_13, © Humana Press, a part of Springer
Science+Business Media, LLC 2009

13.2 Database

Birth injuries often involve litigation in the United States. For this reason, our earlier mentioned reports were based on cases of shoulder dystocia that involved potential or actual litigation on account of irreversible injury sustained by the neonate. Those cases occurred between 1976 and 1991. Using the same source, the data presented herein rest upon a new series of similar incidents that took place in various parts of the United States between 1982 and 2003.

Some of these were not followed by legal action. As a selection criterion, the remaining ones were restricted to those cases where the litigation process had been concluded before the time of the development of this review. The above outlined data selection has provided 135 cases, collected on the grounds of the following criteria [2]:

1. Neonatal brachial plexus lesion persisting for 6 months or more after birth with or without documented diagnosis of shoulder dystocia.
2. Damage to the CNS of the neonate, still demonstrable 6 or more months after birth, against a background of reference to arrest of the shoulders in the medical records.
3. Perinatal death associated with the clinical diagnosis of shoulder dystocia.

Divided into 5-year categories, the times of the events are shown in Table 13.1. Also distributed into 5-year groups, the maternal ages at the times of the childbirth are displayed in Table 13.2. The parity of the mothers is indicated in Table 13.3.

Most but not all records provided information about the Apgar score. Distributed into three groups, the relevant data are listed in Table 13.4. The nature of the injuries found among these neonates is described in Table 13.5.

Whereas most records offered adequate details about the perinatal events, some others did not. Therefore, the frequency of diabetes and hypertension associated with shoulder dystocia–related injuries was probably underestimated (Table 13.6). The same comment is applicable to the documented protraction and arrest disorders

Table 13.1 Chronology

	Years				
	1981–1985	1986–1990	1991–1995	1996–2000	2001–
Number of cases	3	25	64	40	3

Time of occurrence in 135 cases of shoulder dystocia–associated permanent neonatal damage.

Table 13.2 Maternal Age

	Age Groups (y)						
	<15	15–19	20–24	25–29	30–34	35–39	40–44
No. of cases	2	12	29	51	28	12	1

Maternal age at the time of the accident in the cases included in "chronology."

Table 13.3 Maternal Parity

Number of	0	1	2	3	4	5	6
Previous births	50	53	24	4	2	0	2

Number of previous childbirths of mothers included in the study.

Table 13.4 The Apgar Scores of Neonates

	Scores Divided into Three Groups		
	0–3	4–6	7–10
1-minute score	56	38	39
5-minute score	19	22	86

Note that the numbers do not add up to 135 because in some records, the Apgar score was not documented.

Table 13.5 Types of Neonatal Injury Associated with 135 Cases of Shoulder Dystocia

Nature of Injury	Number of Cases
Brachial plexus lesion	121
Traumatic injury to the shoulder joint or clavicle	3
Cerebral palsy	12
Intracerebral hemorrhage	11
Head trauma	2
Developmental delay	1
Seizure disorder	2
Perinatal demise	3

The definition of types of injuries rests upon the interpretations stated in the medical records. Neonates who suffered cerebral palsy tended to have low Apgar scores.

Table 13.6 Antepartum and Intrapartum Complications Associated with Shoulder Dystocia–Related Birth Injuries

Nature of Complications	Number of Documented Cases
Diabetes mellitus	35 (27%)
Hypertension (pregnancy-induced or chronic)	29 (21%)
Protraction and arrest disorders:	
First stage of labor	38 (28%)
Second stage of labor	39 (29%)

The above numbers are probably underestimations. Many patients were not tested for diabetes. Some blood pressure elevations may have remained undocumented. The labor curve was not indicated in several cases, thus, some arrest or protraction disorders may have been overlooked or simply not mentioned in the records.

during labor. The relationships among the length of the gestation, the fetal weight, and the method of delivery are presented diagrammatically in Fig. 13.1.

The ethnicity of the mothers could not always be determined. Most likely, they were similar to the population of the United States at large. The professionals who conducted the deliveries included obstetricians, residents in training, family physicians, and nurse midwives, in accordance with the quoted sequence in terms of frequency.

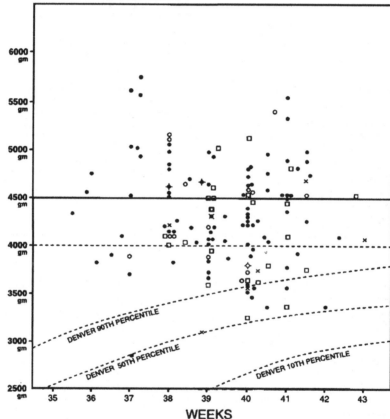

**METHOD OF DELIVERY IN 135 CASES
OF SHOULDER DYSTOCIA RESULTING
IN FETAL DAMAGE**

Fig. 13.1 The above presented cases of shoulder dystocia followed 90 instances of spontaneous vaginal delivery of the head, 23 vacuum extractions, 14 forceps procedures and 7 sequential use of vacuum and forceps instruments. One of the latter and 2 spontaneous deliveries of the caput were followed by the Zavaneli maneuver. One injury occurred in connection with a repeat cesarean section.

13.3 Data Analysis

In the current study, 70 neonates were male and 65 were female. The moderate male preponderance is consistent with that prevailing in the general population [5]. In four instances, the cord was cut deliberately after the delivery of the head but prior to the extraction of the body of the child. These unusual, catastrophic cases were described in detail in a recent publication [6].

In terms of maternal age and parity, there may have been a tendency for this complication to occur in the advanced reproductive years among women of low parity (Table 13.2 and Table 13.3). Low 1-minute Apgar score was frequent among the cases (Table 13.4). The number of CNS injuries was high (Table 13.5). Those infants who eventually developed such injury usually had low Apgar scores at birth. The demonstrated rates of diabetes (26%) and hypertension (21%) were high in this material, even if their numbers were probably underestimated (Table 13.6). The same applies to protraction and arrest disorders, based on Friedman's criteria [7], in the first (28%) and second stages (29%) of labor.

As shown in Fig. 13.1, a disproportionately high number of very large babies suffered damage in connection with shoulder dystocia. Fifty-seven of the 135 (42%) neonates weighed >4,500 g. Only 27% of them were <4,000 g. More than 90% of the newborns were large for gestational age (LGA) according to the Denver criteria [8]. As noted by other investigators in the past [9], instrumental deliveries (33%) were frequent in the background of shoulder dystocia–related injuries. The number of vacuum extractions exceeded forceps deliveries, reflecting the increasing popularity of the "ventouse" in the New World [10].

During the study years, cesarean sections outnumbered vaginal breech deliveries at least 10-fold. Nonetheless, in contrast with three breech-related Erb palsies, only one case of brachial plexus damage was associated with abdominal delivery [11].

It is a matter of considerable interest that only in four instances was the diagnosis of shoulder dystocia not mentioned in the records. Thus, in 97% of the cases, this complication was recognized by the health care personnel in charge.

13.4 Clinical Interpretation

It has been proposed that damage to the brachial plexus relatively often occurs spontaneously *in utero* before the time of the delivery [12–14]. In light of this hypothesis, the rarity in this material of irreversible brachial plexus injury in connection with cesarean section is striking, taking the fact into account that some 20% to 25% of all babies were born by the abdominal route in the United States during the study years. Consequently, the findings presented herein support those literature data that are in conflict with the concept that a significant proportion of brachial plexus injuries occur spontaneously *in utero* [1,2,9,11,15].

The previously published series of cases [2] and those here described show similarities in terms of maternal age, parity, and the high frequency of CNS damage with or without coincidental injury to the brachial plexus. They are also in agreement with regard to the frequency of low Apgar scores, the high rates of diabetes and hypertension, and the often observed arrest and protraction disorders during the preceding labor processes. Similarly consistent in the two studies was the high rate of very large newborns who suffered permanent damage in connection with arrest of the shoulders at delivery. More than 40% of these neonates weighed >4,500 g. Thus, a small group of very big babies suffered a disproportionately high number of injuries. Those weighing <4,000 g contributed little more than 25% of shoulder dystocia–related injuries in either of the two series. This fact invalidates the belief that most cases of shoulder dystocia–related injuries involve fetuses weighing <4,000 g [16].

The frequency of hypoxic and/or traumatic damage to the brain (23%) was comparable in this review to that previously reported. This trend had already been noted more than four decades ago [17] but was dismissed subsequently by authors whose end point of investigation was other than neonatal CNS damage. This study confirms the existence of a close association between arrest of the shoulders at birth on the one hand and permanent CNS injury of the neonate on the other.

The above summarized data show that investigations, based on analysis of factors that predispose for shoulder dystocia, do not provide accurate information about their relative importance with regard to the causation of fetal injuries associated with arrest of the shoulders. The data presented in Fig. 13.1 demonstrate convincingly that LGA fetal status and macrosomia play a more important role in the etiology of fetal injuries than generally recognized [3,4,16,18]. The same conclusion applies to extraction instruments, the use of which entails only a moderate predisposition for arrest of the shoulders [19] but a substantial risk of shoulder dystocia–related fetal damage [2].

According to data collected by the American College of Obstetricians and Gynecologists, arrest of the shoulders complicates about 1.4% of vaginal deliveries [20], of which close to 10% causes permanent neonatal damage [21]. In Sweden, the incidence of birth injury is almost twice as high [22], perhaps as a result of the relatively high birthweights in Scandinavian populations. On the other hand, much lower rates of shoulder dystocia and associated neonatal injuries have been reported from Great Britain [23]. This circumstance suggests that differing training patterns and management may offer at least a partial explanation for the wide discrepancies among the observed results. It deserves consideration that the definition of shoulder dystocia, as generally understood in the United States [24], differs from that recognized in some other countries [25,26]. As explained in another chapter of this volume, the same consideration applies to the routine management of the birthing process at various epochs in North America. Recent books of "perinatology" provide markedly different instructions than those contained in standard textbooks of "obstetrics," published in the middle of the past century [27,28]. So it happens that those were the days when shoulder dystocia was rare, and these are the times when arrest of the shoulders and its dire sequelae are frequent. The idea than the exploding rates of fetal injuries are attributable to better nutrition and increasing number of diabetics in the population and thus bigger babies, or an epidemic increase of spontaneous "*in utero*" injuries, may be consoling but is unconvincing in the light of the fact that, under comparable conditions, they have not changed during the past 40 years in the British Islands [23].

The contemporary literature leaves one under the impression that, rather than searching for solutions, the relevant publications offer unconvincing excuses for the state of affairs that surround the problem of shoulder dystocia both in the medical and legal arenas [18,29,30]. The data presented herein contradict the claim that "more than half of all brachial plexus injuries are associated with uncomplicated deliveries [13,31]." In this series, only in 3% of the cases was the diagnosis of arrest of the shoulders in the records ignored, overlooked, or interpreted in good faith as absent. A retrospective review of the authors' previously published 107 cases [2] revealed that only on nine occasions did the personnel in charge claim unawareness of the occurrence of this complication; a rate of 8%. Despite overwhelming evidence indicating the opposite [2,17], contemporary authorities prefer to believe that arrest of the shoulders at birth is not conducive to perinatal morbidity [32]. More observant authors [33], having reported a 10-fold increase in the rate of shoulder dystocia in the State of Maryland between 1979 and 2003, made no attempt to explain how such an inexplicable increase could conceivably occur, and cause a commensurate proportion of fetal damage, if most such injuries were spontaneous "*in utero*" events unrelated to the obstetric management. The alternative explanation, namely that this 21st century epidemic may have something to do with the obstetric management, is just as unpopular today as it was in the mid-1800s when Dr. Semmelweis searched for the cause of puerperal fever in the Vienna Lying-in-Hospital.

13.5 Conclusion

Claims contending that shoulder dystocia–related injuries are "exceedingly rare [31,34]" are contradicted by statistics indicating that, in case of shoulder dystocia, about 25% of the infants suffer brachial plexus injury [35] and of these 5% to 22% become permanent [36]. Actually, even the earlier quoted statistics circulated by the American College of Obstetricians and Gynecologists offer little basis for undue optimism.

When considering the current literature, one is bound to develop the impression that questions are many and answers are few [37]. Instead, fanciful ideas circulate in abundance. Until the questions are answered through further research aimed at "prevention" rather than "prediction [3,4,20,21,26]," it may be expedient to include contemporary routine management of labor and delivery, as described in standard textbooks and promoted by professional organizations, among the risk factors for shoulder dystocia and the associated fetal injuries.

In 97% of the cases of brachial plexus palsy, a shoulder dystocia was recorded. These findings support the literature that is in conflict with the concept that plexus injuries occur spontaneously *in utero* [1,2,9,11,15]. Macrosomia was present in 75% of the infants.

References

1. Iffy L. A vallak elekadasa szulesnel. *Magy Noorv Lap (Budapest)* 1993;56:13–16.
2. Iffy L, Varadi V, Jakobovits A. Common intrapartum denominators of shoulder dystocia related fetal injuries. *Zbl Gynak* 1994;116:33–37.
3. American College of Obstetricians and Gynecologists. Technical Bulletin. Fetal macrosomia. No. 159. Washington, DC: ACOG; 1991.
4. American College of Obstetricians and Gynecologists. Practice Bulletin. Fetal macrosomia. No. 22. Washington, DC: ACOG; 2000.
5. Jakobovits A, Jakobovits AA, Viski A. Sex ratio of the stillborn fetuses and neonates dying in the first week. *Early Human Development* 1987;15:131–135.
6. Iffy L, Varadi V, Papp E. Untoward neonatal sequelae deriving from cutting of the umbilical cord before delivery. *Med Law* 2001;20:627–634.
7. Friedman EA. *Labor: Clinical Evaluation and Management.* 2nd ed. New York: Appleton-Century-Crofts; 1978.
8. Lubchenco LO. *The High Risk Infant.* Philadelphia: W.B. Saunders; 1976:114.
9. Benedetti TJ, Gabbe SC. Shoulder dystocia. A complication of fetal macrosomia and prolonged second stage of labor with midpelvic delivery. *Obstet Gynecol* 1978;52:526–529.
10. Miksovsky P, Watson WJ. Obstetric vacuum extraction: State of the art in the new millennium. *Obstet Gynecol Survey* 2001;56:736–751.
11. Iffy L, Pantages P. Erb's palsy after delivery by cesarean section. *Med Law* 2005;24:955–962.
12. Gherman RB, Ouzounian JG, Miller DA, Kwok L, Goodwin M. Spontaneous vaginal delivery: A risk factor for Erb's palsy? *Am J Obstet Gynecol* 1998;178:423–427.
13. Gherman RB, Ouzonia JG, Goodwin TM. Brachial plexus palsy: An in utero injury? *Am J Obstet Gynecol* 1999;180:1303–1307.
14. Jennett RJ, Tarby TJ. Disuse osteoporosis as evidence of brachial plexus palsy due to intrauterine fetal maladaptation. *Am J Obstet Gynecol* 1998;178:423–437.
15. Allen RH, Bankoski BR, Butzin CA, Nagey DA. Comparing clinician-applied loads for routine, difficult and shoulder dystocia deliveries. *Am J Obstet Gynecol* 1994;171:1621–1627.
16. Walle T, Hartikainen-Sorri AL. Obstetric shoulder dystocia. Associated risk factor, prediction and prognosis. *Acta Obstet Gynecol Scand* 1993;72:450–454.
17. McCall JO Jr. Shoulder dystocia: A study of aftereffects. *Am J Obstet Gynecol* 1962;83:1486–1490.
18. Gross TL, Sokol RJ, Williams T, Thompson K. Shoulder dystocia: A fetophysician risk. *Am J Obstet Gynecol* 1987;156:1408–1418.
19. Nesbitt TS, Gilbert WM, Herrchen B. Shoulder dystocia and associated risk factors with macrosomic infants born in California. *Am J Obstet Gynecol* 1998;179:476–480.
20. Nocon JJ, McKenzie DK, Thomas LJ, Hansell RS. Shoulder dystocia: Analysis of risks and obstetric maneuvers. *Am J Obstet Gynecol* 1993;168:1732–1739.
21. American College of Obstetricians and Gynecologists. Practice Patterns. Shoulder dystocia. No. 7. Washington, DC: ACOG; 1997.

22. Mollberg M, Hagberg H, Bager B, Lilja H, Ladfors L. High birthweight and shoulder dystocia: The strongest risk factor for obstetric brachial plexus palsy in a Swedish population-based study. *Acta Obstet Gynecol Scand* 2005;84:654–669.
23. Evans-Jones G, Kay SPJ, Weindling AM, Cranny G, Ward A, Bradshaw A, Hermon C. Congenital brachial plexus palsy: Incidence, cause and outcome in the United Kingdom and Republic of Ireland. *Arch Dis Childhood Fetal and Neonatal* 2003;88:F185–189.
24. O'Leary JA. Shoulder dystocia: Prevention and treatment. In: Iffy L, Apuzzio JJ, Vintzileos AM, eds. *Operative Obstetrics*. 2 nd ed. New York: McGraw-Hill; 1992:234–243.
25. Roseveas S, Stirrat GM. *Handbook of Obstetric Management*. Oxford: Blackwell Science, Ltd.; 1996:251.
26. Papp Z. *A Szuleszet Nogyogyaszat Tankonyve*. Budapest: Semmelweis Publ; 1999:432.
27. Greenhill JP. *Obstetrics*. 11th ed. Philadelphia: W.B. Saunders; 1955:278.
28. Bryant RD, Danforth DN. Conduct of normal labor. In: Danforth DN, ed. *Textbook of Obstetrics and Gynecology*. 2 nd ed. New York: Harper & Row; 1971:561–584.
29. Medical Malpractice. Verdicts, Settlements & Experts. Vol. 18, No. 10, October 2000.
30. O'Leary JA. *Shoulder Dystocia and Birth Injury*. New York: McGraw-Hill; 1992.
31. Gherman RB. New insight to shoulder dystocia and brachial plexus injury. *Obstet Gynecol Survey* 2002;58:1–2.
32. Levy A, Sheiner E, Hammel RD, Hershkovitz R, Haliak M, Katz M. Shoulder dystocia: a comparison of patients with and without diabetes mellitus. *Arch Gynecol Obstet* 2006;273:203–206.
33. Dandolu V, Lawrance L, Gaughan JP, Grotegut C, Harmanil OH. Trends in the rate of shoulder dystocia over two decades. *J Mat Fetal Neonat Med* 2005;18:305–310.
34. Gherman RB. Shoulder dystocia: Prevention and management. *Obstet Gynecol Clin N Am* 2005;32:297–305.
35. Chrisoffersson M, Rydhstroem H. Shoulder dystocia and brachial plexus injury: A population-based study. *Gynecol Obstet Invest* 2002;53:42–47.
36. Jevitt CM. Shoulder dystocia: Etiology, common risk factors and management. *J Midwifery Women's Health* 2005;50:485–497.
37. Jakobovits A. Medico-legal aspects of brachial plexus injury: The obstetrician's point of view. *Med Law* 1996;15:175–182.

Chapter 14

Recognition, Classification, and Management of Shoulder Dystocia: The Relationship to Causation of Brachial Plexus Injury

Michael S. Kreitzer

Summary Using a classification for shoulder dystocia provides insight into a greater understanding of the mechanisms of injury. Failure of the shoulders to deliver spontaneously increases the risk of fetal injury, and traction on the head can injure the brachial plexus. Scientific evidence, based on birthing simulations, has demonstrated that brachial plexus stretch during shoulder dystocia does *not* exceed naturally occurring stretch in the absence of shoulder dystocia, indicating that permanent injury resulting from *over*-stretching (rupture or avulsion) does not occur unless external traction is applied.

Keywords: brachial plexus injury (BPI) · dystocia · restitution · traction

Contents

14.1 Introduction 179
14.2 Definition and Incidence 181
14.3 Modern-Day Classification 185
14.4 Management 190
14.5 Causation of Brachial Plexus Injury 202
14.6 Conclusion 205

14.1 Introduction

In the spontaneous delivery of an averaged sized or relatively small infant, the shoulders will usually deliver immediately after the head, during the same contraction. As fetal size increases relative to pelvic size and shape, the stepwise sequential cardinal movements of normal labor are more easily appreciated, with spontaneous delivery of the shoulders following external rotation of the head by the next contraction. As seen in Fig. 14.1 (cardinal movements of

M.S. Kreitzer
Attending Physician, Overlook Hospital, Summit, NJ, USA; Clin. Assoc. Prof,
OBIYN, University of Medicine and Dentistry of NJ, USA; Senior Risk Management
Consultant, Princeton Insurance Co, Princeton, NJ, USA

J.A. O'Leary (ed.), *Shoulder Dystocia and Birth Injury*,
DOI 10.1007/978-1-59745-473-5_14, © Humana Press, a part of Springer
Science+Business Media, LLC 2009

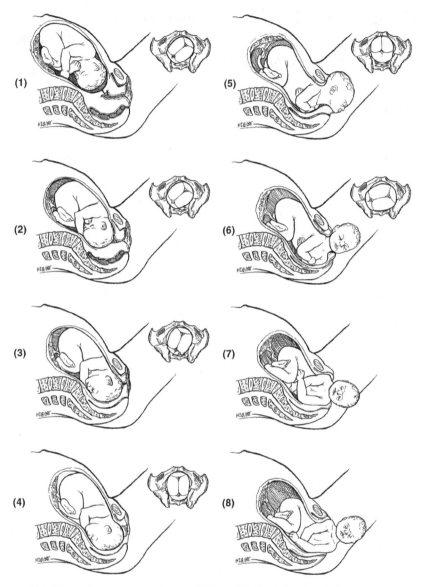

Fig. 14.1 Cardinal movements of normal labor. (1) Head floating, before engagement. (2) Engagement, flexion descent. (3) Further descent internal rotation. (4) Complete rotation, beginning extension. (5) Complete extension, head emerges. (6) Restitution (external rotation). (7) Anterior shoulder appears under pubic bone. (8) Posterior shoulder delivers

normal labor), the anterior shoulder appears under the pubic symphysis, which acts as a fulcrum, permitting delivery of the posterior shoulder (and arm) over the perineum, following the curve of the sacrum along the shape of the pelvic axis (Fig. 14.2). The anterior shoulder then emerges from beneath the pubis and in most cases the shoulders are born spontaneously [1,2], with no traction required. There is no need to hurry delivery of the shoulders during the same contraction [3], but if needed to aid delivery, or if immediate extraction is advisable, traction must be applied slowly, "gently" and "in-line," maintaining the alignment of the cervical and thoracic spine [1] (Fig. 14.3). Oblique traction bends the neck and risks excessive stretching of the brachial plexus [1] (Fig. 14.4).

When fetal size exceeds 4,000 g (8 lb 14 oz), obstruction of the various cardinal movements may occur resulting in an increased incidence of labor protraction/arrest, use of oxytocin, cesarean section, operative vaginal delivery, and shoulder dystocia [4–6]. In recent years, the term *macrosomia* has been redefined, first from 4,000 to 4,500 g, and then to 5,000 g in a nondiabetic gravida, and to 4,500 g in women with diabetes. However, this does not change the fact that beginning at 4,000 g in the nondiabetic and 3,500 g (7 lb 12 oz) in the diabetic gravida, an increased risk for shoulder dystocia exists, regardless of which definition of macrosomia is used [4,5].

14.2 Definition and Incidence

There is no single accepted definition of shoulder dystocia. As a result, it is reasonable to assume that the lack of uniformity in defining shoulder dystocia has resulted in underreporting of its incidence [4–9]. The simplest definition is a

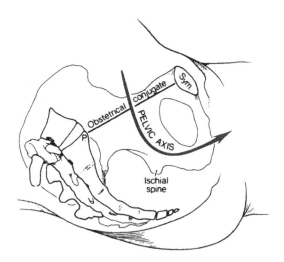

Fig. 14.2 Curvature of pelvic axis

Fig. 14.3 Use of "in-line" traction

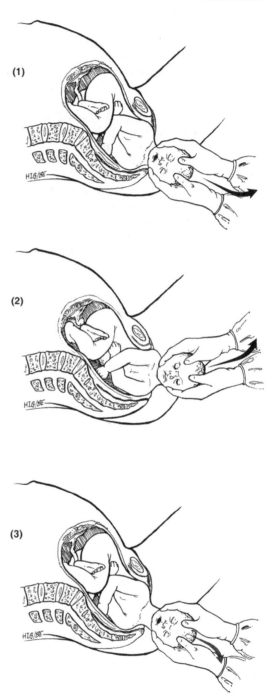

Fig. 14.4 Oblique downward traction

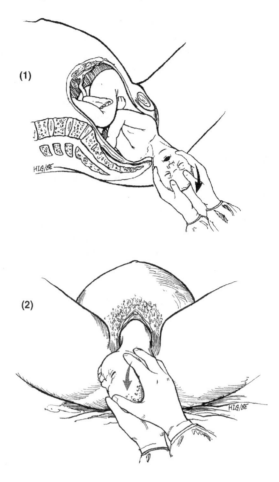

delay, or failure, of the shoulders to *spontaneously* deliver after the fetal head [4,10,11]. Other definitions require documentation of specific release maneuvers or other procedures to substantiate the diagnosis. Still another definition is the subjectivity of a clinician's judgment, noted in the chart, that shoulder dystocia occurred. The most widely used description of shoulder dystocia includes the failure of the shoulders to deliver despite the application of "gentle," "usual," or standard" traction; all subjective, imprecise, undefined terms. Recently, Lerner [12] has coined the term "minimum necessary" traction, claiming without any supporting evidence or references that "routine" or "moderate" traction is used in most deliveries. It is noteworthy that Smeltzer [10] has written that "fetal head traction in the delivery of the anterior shoulder is not helpful in normal delivery, and a harmful habit when shoulder dystocia is present", and Danforth [13] emphasized that "gentle traction should only be applied if the anterior shoulder is *already* beneath the symphysis, and approaching the subpubic arch."

With regard to brachial plexus injury (BPI), it has long been accepted [8,14–16], since the seminal work of Sever [17], that overstretching of the brachial plexus by lateral traction causes both transient and permanent injuries and occurs in either/both the anterior and posterior shoulder (Fig. 14.4 and Fig. 14.5). He also demonstrated that BPI can occur *in utero*, as a result of malpresentation. More recently, Allen et al. [18,19] found that increasing amounts of force tend to be applied as difficulty in delivering the shoulders increases, observing that men and women applied similar degrees of neck-bending forces in both a downward and upward direction. They also found that the rate of application of force was important; concluding that the faster force is applied to the fetal head, the more vulnerable the fetus is to injury.

Therefore, if the recognition of shoulder dystocia (SD) is not made prior to applying traction, and delivery is accomplished by that traction, BPI can and does occur prior to or without SD being recognized. This would explain why retrospective studies that do not define SD, or define SD as not having occurred

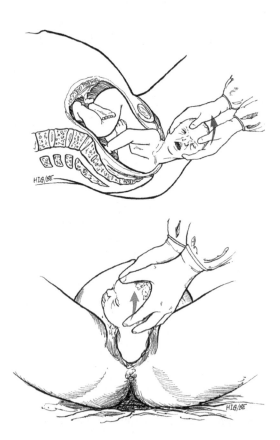

Fig. 14.5 Oblique upward traction

until after traction or maneuvers have been applied, could conclude that BPI occurs in the absence of SD in up to 50% of cases [8,20,21,22,26].

Use of maneuvers to define SD has been criticized by some authors [7,16], and others have suggested that a delay or failure of the shoulders to deliver spontaneously, within a specific interval or time frame, could more objectively define SD and improve reporting of its incidence. In this regard, Iffy [23] advocates a definition used in much of Europe and in some American obstetric services: that arrest of the shoulders is not deemed to have occurred until, and unless, the shoulders and body have not been expelled during the next contraction that follows delivery of the head. In support of this definition, he points to the work of Stallings [24], as well as 10,000 deliveries over a 30-year period at his own institution [25], showing that delivery in the course of two uterine contractions has no adverse fetal effects.

In contrast, Spong and Beall [7,16] propose that a head-to-delivery time exceeding 60 seconds be used to define shoulder dystocia, based on *prospective* evaluation of unselected deliveries. The incidence of SD, defined by the use of obstetric maneuvers, was 11%, with only half being documented [7], and based on head-to-body delivery time, the SD incidence was 14%, with only 3% being coded on the medical record [16]. These observations are much higher than the previously reported incidence of up to 4% [4] and suggest that the arbitrary use of a 60-second time interval to define SD may lead to premature intervention, as the physiology of labor is not considered in this definition. A two-step delivery occurs in up to 50% of primiparous and 25% of multiparous births, and standard American textbooks over the past 50 years describe spontaneous delivery during two separate uterine contractions as a physiologic phenomenon [1,3,25].

It is this author's opinion that the most functional definition of shoulder dystocia is also the simplest: a delay or failure of the shoulders to deliver spontaneously, *without* the aid of traction or specific maneuvers. Since the failure to deliver spontaneously increases the risk of injury [26], this definition would permit early recognition and the avoidance of traction prior to recognition, leading to prompt application of accepted shoulder dystocia maneuvers, and successful management, without injury in most cases [14]. Improved reporting of incidence could then be anticipated.

14.3 Modern-Day Classification

Though its occurrence is classically thought of as a disproportion between the fetal shoulders and the bony maternal pelvis, soft tissue obstruction has long been recognized as a cause of shoulder dystocia [3,17]. More recent texts, however, discount the fact that soft tissue obstruction at the vaginal outlet can and does result in a delay or failure of the shoulders to deliver spontaneously, and that it also occurs at cesarean section. (Table 14.1)

Table 14.1 Kreitzer Classification of Shoulder Dystocia Injuries

1. Shoulder dystocia at cesarean section
2. Shoulder dystocia at vaginal delivery
   • Soft tissue dystocia after restitution
   • Bony dystocia after restitution
   • Bony dystocia due to failure of restitution

14.3.1 Shoulder Dystocia at Cesarean Section

See Chapter 17.

14.3.2 Shoulder Dystocia at Vaginal Delivery

Though its occurrence cannot be reliably predicted, deliveries at increased risk for shoulder dystocia can often be identified by obstetric and medical history, evaluation of fetal weight and position, careful pelvic assessment, and the course of labor, thus permitting anticipation of and preparation for a potentially difficult delivery. Unexpected shoulder dystocia clearly creates an emergency atmosphere, and additional help must often be summoned. However, this does not preclude a calm approach and implementation of an appropriate well-rehearsed plan of management that reflects an understanding of how the different types of shoulder dystocia occur. O'Leary [27] warns that panic is likely to result in the "Three P's" pulling (traction), pushing (maternal and fundal pressure), and pivoting (twisting of the head), all increasing the likelihood of injury to the baby. While waiting for additional assistance from nursing, anesthesia, and pediatrics, the posterior pelvis should be examined [3,28], the infant's airway should be cleared, and a nuchal cord should be ruled out.

14.3.3 Soft Tissue Dystocia After Restitution

After external rotation (restitution), the anterior shoulder is usually visible, or easily palpable beneath the symphysis, and delivery should occur with the next contraction in a patient with gynecoid pelvis. Occasionally, particularly in an obese primipara, delivery of the posterior shoulder may be delayed by the soft tissue of the perineum if an episiotomy has not been done. Once recognized, an episiotomy will usually result in prompt delivery, with or without traction. If, for some reason, an episiotomy is not done, or does not result in delivery, and immediate extraction is indicated, genuinely "gentle" in-line traction in an upward direction (Fig. 14.3) will deliver the posterior shoulder (and arm) followed by the anterior shoulder, as in a spontaneous delivery. Oblique traction must be avoided [17]. An equally effective method may be to deliver the anterior shoulder first (Fig. 14.3), but care must be taken before applying traction, to make sure the anterior shoulder is already beneath the symphysis, approaching the subpubic arch [13]. Rapid, forceful or oblique traction angulating the neck more than 30 degrees is excessive and must be avoided [17,29] or brachial plexus injury may occur (Figs. 14.4 and 14.5).

In a patient with a narrow subpubic arch (android or anthropoid pelvis), delivery of the head and shoulders is directed more posteriorly, increasing the likelihood of perineal obstruction. Unless an episiotomy is made, downward traction in this circumstance is more likely to be obliquely applied, risking significant perineal laceration and anterior brachial plexus injury (Fig. 14.4).

Soft tissue shoulder dystocia is rarely, if ever, documented because an episiotomy or "standard" or "usual" or "gentle" traction most often results in delivery without injury. However, injury to either the anterior or posterior arm does occur as a result of obliquely applied lateral traction exceeding 30 degrees (excessive angulation). Though transient injury is more likely because the resistance to traction is less than from bony dystocia, this author is unaware of any data in this regard and has never seen soft tissue shoulder dystocia documented. Of note, neonatal injury in these cases would be reported as having occurred in the absence of shoulder dystocia, as the maternal record would not reflect any difficulty in delivery. Therefore, it would not be unreasonable to assume that rapid, other than "gentle" traction, and/or obliquely applied traction, to overcome soft tissue dystocia, may be responsible for some, or at least an occasional case of permanent brachial plexus injury.

In recent years, there has been an anti-"routine" episiotomy sentiment in much of the obstetric community that has led to the reluctance to use this procedure even when indicated. In supervising resident physicians, this author has observed a number of unnecessarily difficult deliveries in primiparous patients who did not have an episiotomy of any size. I am aware of one infant with a short-lived (4 hour) weakness of the posterior arm and another with a BPI of the anterior arm that resolved prior to discharge.

14.3.4 Bony Dystocia After Restitution

The most common type of bony shoulder dystocia also occurs after external rotation. Restitution indicates that the shoulders have rotated into the A-P = antero-posterior or oblique diameter, and that at least the posterior shoulder is in the pelvis [1]. In a gynecoid pelvis, the midpelvis and outlet seldom present a bony obstruction to delivery at this point [10], unless the fetus is large. If the pelvis is flat (platypelloid), even if the fetus is not macrosomic (<4,000 g), and the labor is normal or precipitous, the anterior shoulder may get stuck, neither visible nor palpable, behind the pubic bone (Fig. 14.6).

If spontaneous delivery does not occur with maternal pushing after the nose and mouth have been suctioned and a nuchal cord is found to be absent, bony

Fig. 14.6 Anterior shoulder
dystocia after restitution

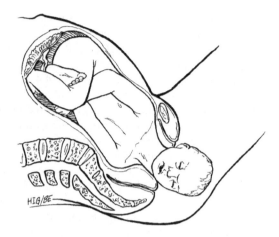

shoulder dystocia is present. Until this obstruction is relieved by use of appropriate maneuvers, as signaled by the appearance or palpation of the anterior
shoulder under the symphysis approaching the subpubic arch, there is no role
for traction of any kind and maternal pushing must cease.

14.3.5 Bony Dystocia Due to Failure of Restitution

In normal labor, the fetal head delivers by extension and the chin delivers over
the perineum. At this stage, the shoulders are oriented toward the transverse
diameter of the pelvis, not yet ready to pass through the midpelvis. External
rotation (restitution) signals alignment of the shoulders in the A-P or oblique
diameter as they negotiate the midpelvis, either during the same or subsequent
contraction that delivers the head. Shoulder dystocia most often occurs in
patients with a platypelloid (flat) or relatively small gynecoid pelvis after
restitution, but its occurrence in the absence of external rotation is heralded
by the "turtle sign," where the fetal chin retracts against the perineum (Fig. 14.7).

In patients with a narrow funnel type (anthropoid or android) pelvis, the
midpelvis and pubic arch are narrow, and the sidewalls are parallel or convergent. These pelvic types favor the OA = occiput anterior or OP = occiput posterior
position as the head descends through the midpelvis, as opposed to the transverse position common to the gynecoid pelvis. As the head delivers over the
perineum, the transversely oriented shoulders may become wedged in the
narrow midpelvis, unable to turn to the A-P or oblique diameter with maternal
pushing, resulting in a persistent turtle sign (Fig. 14.8). Though data is lacking,
it is likely that when shoulder dystocia occurs unexpectedly in infants of average
weight, a certain percentage will be associated with this pelvic type.

In patients with a flat pelvis, the A-P dimensions at all levels are decreased
and the transverse dimensions are wide. Shoulder dystocia will occur 8 to 10

Fig. 14.7 Turtle sign

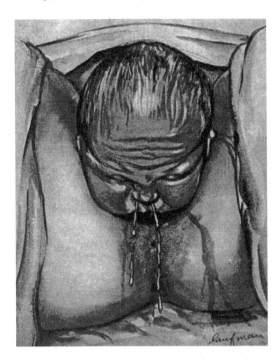

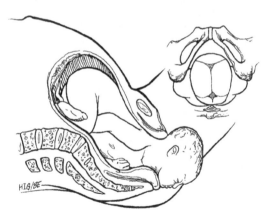

Fig. 14.8 Turtle sign in funnel pelvis (shoulders transversely oriented)

times more frequently in women with this pelvic type [27]. As the head descends through the midpelvis in the transverse position, the shoulders may become obstructed at the inlet in an A-P or oblique orientation. This situation will most often result in arrest of labor, with delivery by cesarean section. However, if the shoulders have molded at the inlet and the vertex has molded into the lower pelvis during a protracted labor, and the infant's neck is long enough to allow delivery of the head, often by forceps or vacuum extraction, the chin will retract

Fig. 14.9 Turtle sign in
bilateral shoulder dystocia

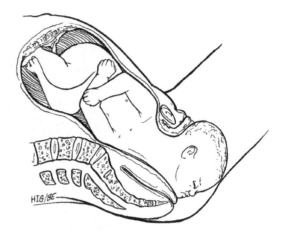

forcefully against the perineum in the turtle sign. With the shoulders stuck at
the inlet, this creates a "potentially undeliverable" bilateral shoulder dystocia
[10] (Fig. 14.9). Fortunately, this circumstance is uncommon, with most obstetricians never knowingly encountering this situation in their careers. Based on
the above descriptions, it should not be surprising that appropriate management of SD occurring without external rotation would differ from that after
restitution. When the turtle sign persists, even those who define SD as being
present when "gentle," "usual," or "standard" traction has not accomplished
delivery must recognize that as the shoulders are either transversely oriented or
stuck at the inlet and *any* application of traction cannot be justified [10]. In this
circumstance, the posterior pelvis must be examined first [28].

14.4 Management

Use of the following maneuvers or procedures to manage shoulder dystocia is
summarized in the algorithms (Figs. 14.10 and 14.11). The merits of each are
discussed below.

- *Episiotomy*
  If an episiotomy was not done prior to delivery of the head, there is no
  rational basis for avoiding cutting of the perineum after shoulder dystocia
  has been recognized. It will eliminate possible soft tissue interference and can
  only facilitate implementation of other maneuvers. An existing episiotomy
  should be enlarged when dealing with SD, but episio-proctotomy can be
  delayed pending the result of initial maneuvers.
- *McRoberts Position* (Hip and Thigh Hyperflexion)
  Hyperflexion of the patient's legs against the abdomen to facilitate delivery had
  been in use for many years [3] before its importance was re-emphasized by

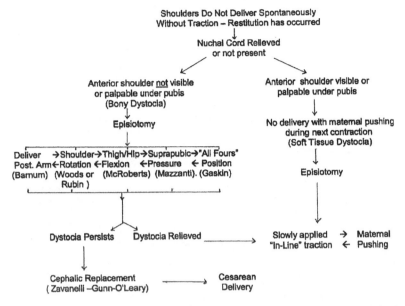

Fig. 14.10 Algorithm: Shoulders do not deliver spontaneously without traction—restitution has occurred

Gonik [30] and McRoberts. As stated by Smeltzer [10], the simplicity of application of this position (Fig 14.12) hides an elegant complexity of the physical and mechanical forces that it invokes, by simultaneously reversing all of the factors tending to cause shoulder dystocia, by the dorsal lithotomy position.

- *Effects of McRoberts Position*
  1. The anterior shoulder is elevated and moves cephalad, flexing the fetal spine toward the anterior shoulder. If bilateral SD is present, this elevation and flexion pushes the posterior shoulder over the sacrum and through the inlet. If the posterior shoulder is in the pelvis it will move toward the hollow of the sacrum.
  2. Straightens the maternal lumbar and lumbosacral lordosis, essentially removing the promontory as an obstruction to the inlet.
  3. Removes all weight-bearing forces from the sacrum, the main pressure point of the pelvis in the lithotomy position, permitting the inlet to open to its maximum dimension.
  4. The inlet is brought into the plane perpendicular to the maximum maternal expulsive force.

The success of this position is signaled by relaxation of the "turtle sign," if bilateral shoulder obstruction is present, followed by external rotation. If only the anterior shoulder is obstructed, movement of the posterior shoulder into the sacral hollow allows the anterior shoulder to drop under the pubic bone, permitting normal delivery.

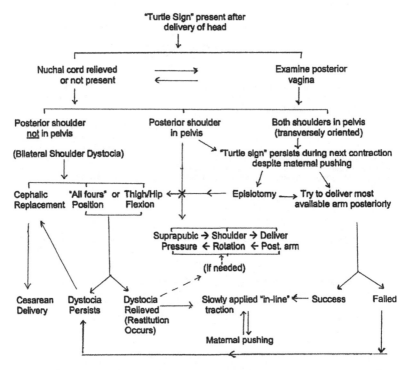

Fig. 14.11 Algorithm: Turtle sign present after delivery of head

Though Gonik et al [31] objectively documented that this position reduces shoulder extraction forces, brachial plexus stretching, and clavicular fracture, it has not clearly been shown to reduce the incidence of brachial plexus injury. When compared to patient groups not utilizing this position, however, the overall trauma rate was four times less in the "McRoberts" group. In Gonik's experience freeing of this obstruction seems to allow a spontaneous delivery. However, O'Leary [27] indicates that additional maneuvers are almost always required, while Poggi [32] points out that it is less effective in obese patients who may not be capable of achieving the desired hyperflexion.

It must be emphasized that traction is inappropriate while the shoulder is impacted behind the pubic bone, and should not be applied until the anterior shoulder appears under the symphysis or is easily palpable, signaling relief of the obstruction. Success in relieving shoulder dystocia by the McRoberts position merits its use in most cases as one of the initial maneuvers. However, its use prophylactically has been shown to be of no value [33].

- *Suprapubic Pressure*

Suprapubic pressure may be used as a primary maneuver, after McRoberts positioning and in association with efforts to rotate the shoulders. Effective SPP = suprapubic pressure is best applied by an assistant with pressure

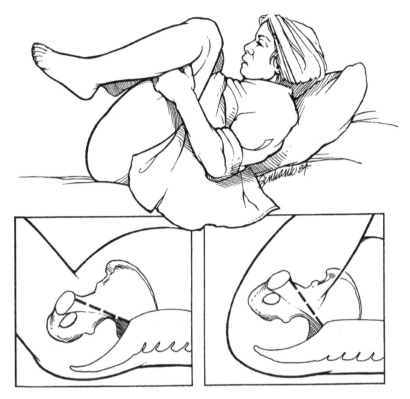

Fig. 14.12 The McRoberts position. (From Gabbe S, Niebyl J, and Simpson JL. *Obstetrics. Normal and Problem Pregnancies.* New York: Churchill Livingstone; 1986.)

directed posteriorly or from behind the anterior shoulder toward the baby's face [34]. This will adduct the shoulders forcing them into an oblique diameter of the pelvis. Use of the palm is preferable to using the fist and is most effective in conjunction with simultaneous vaginally applied pressure to the back of the anterior shoulder (Fig. 14.13). Anterior shoulder impaction will be relieved in 60% to 80% [8,29] of cases by the combination of hyperflexion of the thighs and suprapubic pressure, but neither maternal pushing nor traction should be implemented until it is clear that the shoulder dystocia is relieved.

- *Rotational Maneuvers*

  Using the principal of the screw, Woods [35] presented a wooden model to demonstrate that although the shoulders might be too large to be delivered through the pelvis directly (by maternal pushing or traction), it might be possible to effect delivery by a screwing motion. He recommended exerting pressure to the anterior (clavicular) surface of the posterior shoulder. If movement of the shoulder occurred, fundal pressure or maternal Valsalva was added until the posterior shoulder had rotated 180 degrees to the anterior (Fig. 14.14).

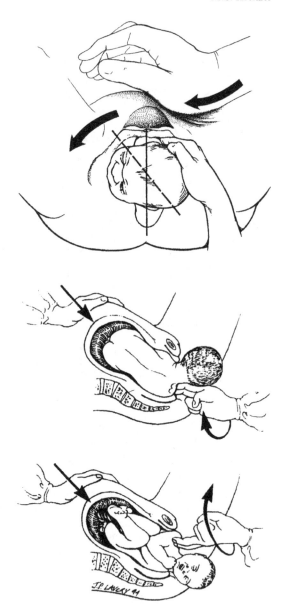

Fig. 14.13 Suprapubic pressure in association with Rubin rotation of the anterior shoulder. (Modified from Pauerstein C. *Clinical Obstetrics.* 1987; and Gabbe S, Niebyl J, and Simpson JL. *Obstetrics. Normal and Problem Pregnancies.* New York: Churchill Livingstone, New York; 1986.)

Fig. 14.14 The Woods screw maneuver. (From O'Grady JP, Gimovsky ML, McInhargie CJ, eds. *Operative Obstetrics.* Baltimore: Williams & Wilkins, 1995.)

- Rubin [36] emphasized the importance of having both the infant's shoulders brought forward toward the chest, and showed that this adduction of the shoulders resulted in a smaller circumference of the baby's body than the abducted shoulder position of the Woods rotation. He actually recommended two maneuvers:

1. Laterally applied pushing on the mother's abdomen to rock the shoulders from side to side.
2. Pushing the posterior (scapular) surface of the most available shoulder.

If the shoulders are at first directed anteroposteriorly, this would displace the shoulders into the longer oblique diameter. In addition, as in the Woods rotation the posterior shoulder could be rotated 180 degrees. The alliteration "shoving scapulas saves shoulders" is a useful reminder (Figs. 14.15 and 14.16).

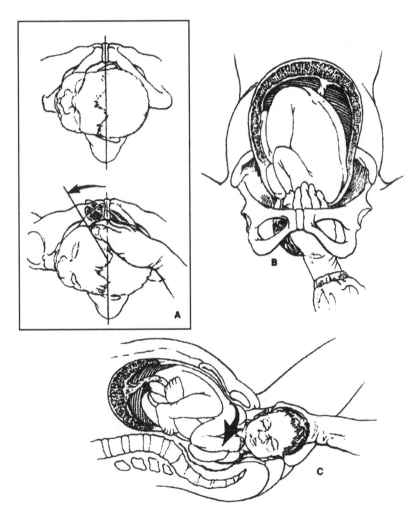

Fig. 14.15 Rubin rotation of anterior shoulder to the oblique pelvic diameter. (From Hankins GDV, Clark SL, Cunningham FG, et al., eds. *Operative Obstetrics*. Baltimore: Appleton & Lange, 1995.)

Fig. 14.16 Rubin rotation of posterior shoulder 180 degrees. (From Gabbe S, Niebyl J, and Simpson JL. *Obstetrics. Normal and Problem Pregnancies.* New York: Churchill Livingstone; 1986.)

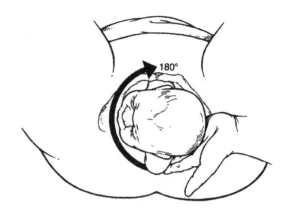

Rotation of the shoulders may be used a primary maneuver but should be abandoned quickly if the shoulders do not move. Both the Woods and Rubin maneuvers are more successful if combined with suprapubic pressure applied in a direction facilitating the vaginal rotation (Fig. 14.13). It must be strongly emphasized that all rotational forces must be applied to the clavicle or scapula and *never* to the baby's head.

- *Delivery of the Posterior Arm (Barnum Maneuver)*
  In the 1940s and 1950s, the Woods and Barnum [37] maneuvers were the prevailing standard of care, in place of traction, for shoulder dystocia management, and during that time period a 400% reduction in brachial plexus injury was noted [38]. As previously discussed, hip hyperflexion was reintroduced in the 1980s by Gonik and has become the primary maneuver for most practitioners, allowing for atraumatic delivery in many, but not all, cases [39]. Poggi et al. [32] have shown, by geometric analysis, that delivering the posterior arm reduces the obstruction by more than a factor of 2, relative to the McRoberts maneuver. She suggests that its use as a primary maneuver should not be considered unorthodox, particularly in obese patients, many of whom are unable to achieve maximum hyperflexion due to soft tissue obstruction. She also points out that delivery of the posterior arm has been assumed to be associated with a higher rate of birth injury because its use most often follows the failure of other maneuvers. In support of her position, she refers to Baskett and Allen [40], who reported no neonatal injuries when posterior arm delivery was used as the primary shoulder dystocia maneuver in nine cases. In addition to describing the dramatic benefit in reducing the shoulder diameter, she emphasizes the risk of downward traction to the anterior shoulder. In agreeing with Poggi, it is this author's opinion that once SD is recognized, the application of *any* downward traction in an effort to deliver the anterior shoulder first is unphysiologic, as the force applied is counter to the upward direction of pelvis axis (Fig. 14.2) and increases the likelihood of BPI. If the anterior shoulder is stuck, reaching for the posterior arm will *always* be a better early choice than applying downward traction (Fig 14.17).

Fig. 14.17 Delivery of posterior arm. (A) To bring the fetal wrist within reach, exert pressure with the index finger at the antecubital junction. (B) Sweep the fetal forearm down over the front of the chest. (From Sandberg E. *Am J Obstet Gynecol* 195;152:481.)

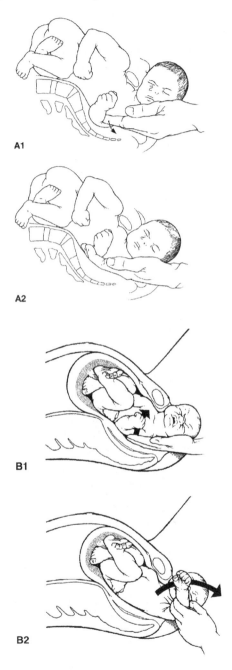

A1

A2

B1

B2

- *The All-Fours Maneuver (Gaskin)*

  The all-fours maneuver was introduced to the United States by Ina May Gaskin in 1976 and has found its greatest acceptance among midwives and family practitioners. In 1998, Bruner et al. [41] reported on 82 consecutive cases of shoulder dystocia in 4.452 births (1.8% incidence) over 20 years. All cases were managed primarily by the all-fours maneuver (Fig. 14.18), and midwives did most of the deliveries. In 83% (68 of 82), the fetus was delivered with the next contraction, *without* the need for any additional maneuvers. In 12 cases, rotation of the fetal shoulders to the oblique position was performed, and in two patients the posterior fetal arm was delivered with the patient in the all-fours position. The average recognition of shoulder dystocia to delivery time was 2 to 3 minutes (range, 1 to 6 minutes), and none of the patients had received anesthesia or were delivered by forceps or vacuum extraction.

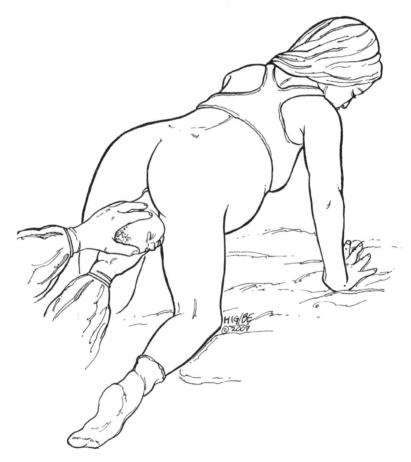

Fig. 14.18 Gaskin (all-fours) maneuver

The most significant observations of this study were the negative findings. Though 50% of the newborns weighed more than 4,000 g, and 21% weighed more than 4,500 g, there were *no* cases of brachial plexus injury; transient or permanent. In addition, no newborn experienced seizures, hemorrhage, hypoxic ischemic encephalopathy, cerebral palsy, or a fractured clavicle, and all maternal and neonatal morbidity occurred in cases with a birthweight more than 4,500 g (P = .0009), as described in Table 14.2.

The precise mechanism by which the Gaskin maneuver relieves shoulder impaction has not been studied, but the mere act of turning from the supine to the hands-and-knees, using gravity to relieve all weight-bearing forces on the sacrum, may be enough to provide relief of the obstruction. Of note, shoulder dystocia was defined as the inability to deliver the shoulders *without* the aid of specific maneuvers. Because nurse midwives did most of the deliveries, it is likely that shoulder dystocia was recognized when the shoulders failed to deliver during the contraction that followed delivery of the head. Though the use of traction and frequency of episiotomy was not mentioned, any application of downward traction in a patient in the all-fours position would have been applied to the posterior fetal shoulder, delivering the posterior shoulder (and arm) first; following the curve of the pelvic axis. In contrast, downward traction applied to a patient in the supine or McRoberts position would be applied to the anterior shoulder, counter to the pelvic axis. Because no BPI occurred in the study, it is reasonable to assume that the amount of traction applied along the pelvic axis, to effect delivery, was less than would be required with the patient in the supine position, and reduced the likelihood of injury. In addition, use of other established shoulder dystocia maneuvers was apparently facilitated by the all-fours position.

This author has no experience with the Gaskin maneuver, but the advantages and results stated by Bruner warrant its incorporation into general clinical practice. Even in patients with epidural anesthesia, moving the patient into the all-fours position should not be difficult, if adequate assistance is present.

- *Cephalic Replacement (Gunn-Zavanelli-O'Leary Maneuver; See Chapter 9)*
  Cephalic replacement was first performed by Gunn (1976) and Zavanelli (1978). In 1985, Sandberg [42] reported on the maneuver being used in desperation by Dr. Zavanelli when all other maneuvers had failed after restitution (Fig 14.19). Cesarean section delivery of a 12 lb 2 oz infant, in good condition (Apgar 7/10), was accomplished 67 minutes after reinsertion of the fetal head. Also in 1985, O'Leary and Gunn [43] reported on the use of cephalic replacement in anticipation of the undeliverable bilateral shoulder dystocia heralded by the turtle sign (Fig. 14.20).

Table 14.2 Four Cases of Shoulder Dystocia Managed Primarily with the All-Fours Maneuver and Associated with Maternal (1.2%) or Neonatal (4.9%) Morbidity

Estimated Gestational Age (wk)	Parity	Birth-weight (g)	Condition of perineum	Apgar score		Diagnosis delivery internal (min)	Morbidity
				1 min	5 min		
41	1	4,536	2° Laceration	6	8	3.5	Postpartum hemorrhage (no transfusion required)
40	2	4,984	1° Laceration	2	7	3.5	Humerus fracture, 1-min Apgar score <3
41	4	5,096	1°Episiotomy	2	9	5	1-min Apgar Score <3
36	5	4,536	Intact	5	6	2	5-min Apgar score <6

From Bruner JP, Drummond SB, Meenan AL, Gaskin IM. All-fours maneuver for reducing shoulder dystocia during labor. *J Reprod Med* 1998;43:439–443.

Fig. 14.19 Cephalic
replacement after restitution

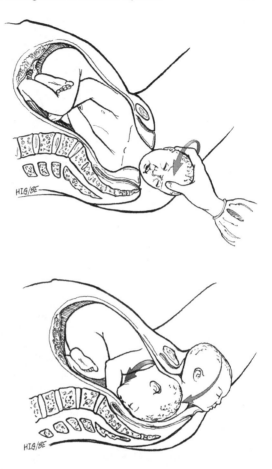

- *Other Techniques*
  Over the years, a number of other techniques have been described to facilitate delivery in cases of shoulder dystocia. Most obstetricians in the United
  States have no experience with these rarely used methods listed below, and
  for interested readers references are provided.

  Use of parallel forceps (1962) [44]
  Hibbard maneuver (1969) [30,45,46]
  Deliberate fracture of clavicle [1]
  Chavis instrument (1979) [1]
  Cleidotomy (1983) [1]
  Symphysiotomy (1986) [47]
  Abdominal rescue (1992) [48]

Fig. 14.20 Cephalic
replacement in bilateral
shoulder dystocia

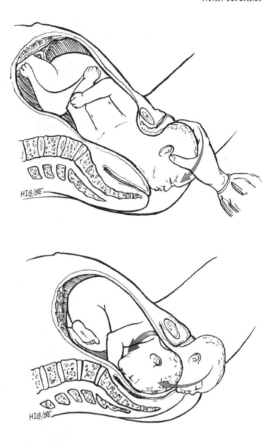

14.5 Causation of Brachial Plexus Injury

It is clear that "failure of the shoulders to deliver spontaneously places both the
pregnant women and fetus at risk for injury" [26], but if traction has not been
applied prior to the recognition of shoulder dystocia, delivery can be accomplished without injury to the fetus in most cases, if a well-rehearsed plan of
action is implemented [14]. However, BPI does occur as a result of traction
applied prior to recognition of SD even if subsequent relief of the obstruction
has been accomplished by appropriately executed maneuvers. Therefore, if *not*
recognized prior to the application of traction that results in both delivery *and*
injury, shoulder dystocia would not be recorded as having occurred. This would
explain why retrospective reviews that do not define shoulder dystocia, or
define it as having occurred only after traction has failed or maneuvers have
been applied, underreport its incidence, even in the presence of injury [20,22,49].
In addition, most of these same retrospective reviews do not distinguish
between transient and permanent injury, or separate compression injuries

from traction-related injuries. Even those studies that address permanent injury have inadequate follow-up, lacking information on imaging studies (MRI or CAT scan), electromyography (EMG) of injured neonates, or on the incidence of pediatric surgery done in an attempt to improve function. As a result, these articles also fail to separate compression injuries from the "stretch" injuries resulting in avulsion, rupture, or neuroma of the brachial plexus [50]. Gherman et al. [51] compared transient and permanent BPI retrospectively from national birth injury and shoulder dystocia databases. However, they defined SD as the need for ancillary maneuvers after initial attempts at traction were unsuccessful and also *excluded* cases of BPI that occurred in the absence of shoulder dystocia being coded: resulting in underreporting. In addition, they found 17 cases of transient injury, but no cases of permanent injury, associated with "spontaneous" (would include use of traction by their definition of SD) vaginal deliveries, as well as a high percentage (12%) of permanent injuries in cases where fundal pressure had been used.

Because lack of uniformity in defining SD has resulted in underreporting of its incidence, and underreporting has led to the lack of correlation between the occurrence of BPI and SD, it is not surprising that speculation has led to unsubstantiated theory suggesting that etiologies other than traction can cause permanent injury due to rupture or avulsion of the brachial plexus [52].

Although prolonged compression and immobility *in utero* can result in permanent injury, and a positive EMG can be demonstrated immediately after delivery [53], this injury is extremely rare. Because muscle atrophy is likely to be present as well, and osteoporosis of the affected arm may also be found [54–56], a traction-related etiology is easily excluded in these rare cases. If *in utero*-acquired BPI is a relatively frequent event, it should occur in a higher percentage of neonates born by cesarean section. Instead, existing studies show that the overwhelming majority of infants with BPI noted at cesarean section show no evidence of atrophy or osteoporosis, are otherwise neurologically normal, have not been tested by EMG [57], and lack information on imaging studies or incidence of surgery done to improve function. Because lateral traction is applied to either the anterior or posterior brachial plexus at cesarean section, during extraction of the head or delivery of the shoulders, there is no other mechanism, actual or theorized, that would explain a rupture or avulsion in an infant delivered abdominally without labor. Therefore, it is not reasonable to attribute these injuries to *in utero* causation preceding labor or delivery.

Transient BPI has occasionally been described in totally spontaneous deliveries where shoulder dystocia has not occurred and no traction has been applied [58,59]. These transient injuries may be due to compression, mild stretching resulting from asynclitism [59], or malpresentation [17], but the claim that avulsion or rupture might be due to "endogenous" factors (expulsive uterine forces and maternal pushing) capable of overstretching the brachial plexus [52] is unsubstantiated. This so-called tractor-trailer theory is actually more compatible with traction as a cause of injury, not the momentum of uterine forces that might occur after impaction behind the pubic bone. Because of the intermittent nature of contractions and the resistance of the pelvis, labor and delivery is simply not a high-momentum process, even when precipitous, and any stretching of the brachial plexus that might occur after impaction would be minimal and not considered capable of causing permanent injury [60] unless traction is applied [61,62]. Because the fetus is confined in a muscle-lined bony pelvis, marginally capable of permitting delivery, there is no similarity to the sustained speed of an unconfined tractor-trailer capable of the "jack-knife" position. In addition, if obstruction of the pubic bone were capable of causing injury by compressing the brachial plexus during labor, bruising of the soft tissue over the *shoulder*, not the arm, face, or neck, should be evident in *all* cases, and would be similar to the damage sustained by a trailer striking an overpass after the tractor passes underneath. This acute-type permanent compression injury has never been described or reported, and in any event would not be capable of "overstretching," resulting in rupture or avulsion.

Regarding causation, in 2007 Allen et al., [62] using a sophisticated birthing simulator and fetal model, demonstrated that "SD itself does not pose additional brachial plexus stretch" to the anterior shoulder, over naturally occurring deliveries unaffected by SD. They also found that the degree of stretch in the posterior brachial plexus was greater during routine deliveries than in SD deliveries and concluded that the degree of brachial plexus stretch demonstrated by their study "would be unlikely to cause injury in neonates independent of additional, externally applied force."

To this author's knowledge, there is not even a single case report of permanent injury due to rupture or avulsion, in an otherwise normal infant, in the absence of traction having been applied. In addition, our pediatric colleagues in neurology, orthopedics, and neurosurgery who evaluate and treat BPI recognize that avulsion or rupture results from excessive stretching of the brachial plexus by abduction (lateral traction). In a large series of surgically treated obstetric brachial plexus injuries, Ubachs et al. [63] noted that neuroma formation, rupture, or avulsion was found in all patients. The obstetric history of each patient also mentioned factors such as shoulder dystocia with extreme lateral traction of the fetal head or a difficult breech delivery, in most cases combined with asphyxia. Therefore, though it is evident that a transient injury may occur from compression or mild stretching during a completely spontaneous delivery, there is no direct evidence to support the assumption that the same forces can cause permanent injury due to rupture or avulsion.

Retrospective reviews dealing with the management of SD [8,39,64] indicate that no specific maneuver has been proved superior to others with the regard to the rate of neonatal injury. Nerve or bone injury has been observed in 25% of infants with SD regardless of the procedure used to disimpact the shoulder. All these studies either do not define SD or define it as having occurred after traction has failed and other maneuvers have been used. By itself, this lack of uniformity in defining SD could explain why McFarland et al. [39] concluded that neonatal and maternal morbidity increased as the number of maneuvers increased, whereas Gherman et al. [49] found that additional maneuvers did not increase the rate of neonatal bone fractures or brachial plexus injury.

In contrast, only the study by Bruner et al., [41] using the all-fours (Gaskin) maneuver primarily, was successful in achieving vaginal delivery with a much lower incidence of neonatal morbidity. In that study, shoulder dystocia was defined as the inability to deliver the shoulders *without* use of additional maneuvers. Noteworthy is the absence of *any* brachial plexus injury in this large group of patients delivered mainly by nurse midwives and family practitioners. This outcome strongly suggests that the all-fours position is superior to other accepted shoulder dystocia maneuvers, and/or that recognition of shoulder dystocia occurred prior to the application of traction capable of injury.

As noted by crofts, et al [65], the incidence of BPI in the United Kingdom has not changed despite the identification of "best practice" in the 1990s. In their recent study of forces applied during simulation of SD they demonstrated that excessive traction was common, and opined that their findings probably represented current practice. In acknowledging that "the amount of force applied during SD is an important factor in the development of BPI," they concluded:

- "Clearly, we need a better understanding of how to diagnose SD safely"
- "Clinicians must follow recommended maneuvers accurately," and must "abandon a maneuver quickly once it has failed, without resorting to increasing traction" to overcome the obstruction.

14.6 Conclusion

It is evident that lack of recognition and underreporting has prevented us from knowing the true incidence of shoulder dystocia. It is also clear that it is the use of traction in the management of shoulder dystocia, recognized or not, that most affects the incidence of neonatal injury. In addition, there is no scientific evidence to support the notion that shoulder dystocia, by itself, is capable of causing permanent brachial plexus injury.

A plea is made here to put aside divisive, litigation-motivated speculation related to causation of permanent BPI, as well as misleading emphasis on the predictability of shoulder dystocia or the definition of macrosomia. In the future, we must focus on how to reduce the persistently high incidence of neonatal injury. It is this author's opinion that this effort must begin with:

1. A uniform, functional definition of shoulder dystocia.
2. Identification of patients at increased risk of shoulder dystocia at delivery by paying closer attention to the obstetric and medical history; careful pelvic assessment; estimated fetal weight; and the course of labor.

If we can just agree on a simple definition that permits recognition *before* potentially injurious traction is applied, the next generation of obstetric practitioners may be able to initiate *prospective* studies that will determine the true incidence and optimal management of shoulder dystocia.

Acknowledgments The author greatly appreciates the contributions of Brice Karsh, President, and Brian Evans, C.M.I., of High Impact Graphics (Englewood, Colorado) and Gail Joyiens-Salam of JS Transcription Service (Rahway, New Jersey) for their invaluable dedication and effort in helping to complete this chapter.

References

1. *Williams Obstetrics* 16th ed. New York: Appleton Century Croft; 1980:421.
2. *Williams Obstetrics.*22 nd ed. New York: McGraw-Hill; 2005:430.
3. Greenhill JP, *Obstetrics*. 11th ed. Philadelphia: Saunders; 1965:373.
4. American College of Obstetricians and Gynecologists. Practice Patterns: Shoulder Dystocia. No. 7. Washington, DC: ACOG; 1997.
5. American College of Obstetricians and Gynecologists. Technical Bulletin: Fetal macrosomia. No. 159. Washington, DC: ACOG; 1991.
6. Rouse DJ, Owen J Goldenberg RI, Oliver SP. The effectiveness and costs of elective cesarean delivery for fetal macrosomia diagnosed by ultrasound. *JAMA* 1996;276:1480–1486.
7. Spong CY, Beall M, Rodrigues D, Ross MG. An objective definition of shoulder dystocia: Prolonged head to body delivery time and/or use of ancillary obstetrical maneuvers. *Obstet Gynecol* 1995;12:338–341.
8. Gonik B, Hollyer VL, Allen R. Shoulder dystocia recognition: Differences in neonatal risks for injury. *Am J Perinatol* 1991;8:31–34.
9. Romoff A. Shoulder dystocia: Lessons from the past and emerging concepts. *Clin Obstet Gynecol* 2000;43:226–235.
10. Smeltzer, JS. Prevention and management of shoulder dystocia. *Clin Obstet Gynecol* 1986;29:299–308.
11. Benedetti TJ. Added complications of shoulder dystocia. Contemp OB/GYN Special Issue *OB/GYN and the Law* 1989;33:150–161.
12. Lerner HM. Shoulder dystocia: What is the legal standard of care. *OBG Management* 2006;18:1–14.
13. Danforth's Principles and practice of obstetrics 15th edition Philadelphia Saunders 1965;714.
14. Zuspan F, Quillipan E, *Douglas-Stromme Operative Obstetrics*. 5th ed. Norwalk, CT: Appleton & Lange; 1988.
15. Gross SJ, Shime J, Farine D. Shoulder dystocia: Predictors and outcome. *Am J Obstet Gynecol* 1987;156:334–336.
16. Beall MH, Spong C, McKay J, Ross G. Objective definition of shoulder dystocia: A prospective evaluation. *Am J Obstet Gynecol* 1998;178:934–937.
17. Sever JW. Obstetric paralysis: Its etiology, pathology, clinical aspects and treatment, with a report of 470 cases. *Am J Dis Child* 1916;12:541–578.
18. Allen R, Sorab J, Gonik B. Risk factors for shoulder dystocia: An engineering study of clinician-applied forces. *Obstet Gynecol* 1991;77:352–355.
19. Allen RH, Bankoski BR, Butzin CA, Nagey DA. Comparing clinician-applied loads for routine difficult, and shoulder dystocia deliveries. *Am J Obstet Gynecol* 1994;171:1621–1627.

20. Gilbert WM, Nesbitt TS, Danielsen B. Associated factors in 1611 cases of Brachial Plexus injury. *Obstet Gynecol* 1999;93:536–540.
21. Allen RH. Associated factors in 1611 cases of brachial plexus injury [letter]. *Obstet Gynecol* 1999;94:482–483.
22. Gherman RB, Quzounian JG, Miller DA, Kwok L, Goodwin TM. Spontaneous vaginal delivery: A risk factor for Erb's palsy? *Am J Obstet Gynecol* 1998;178:423–427.
23. Iffy L. Shoulder dystocia. *Am J Obstet Gynecol* 1987;156:1416.
24. Stallings SP, Edwards RK, Johnson JWC. Correlation of head-to-body delivery intervals in shoulder dystocia and umbilical artery acidosis. *Am J Obstet Gynecol* 2001;185:268–274.
25. Iffy L, Apuzzio J, Ganesh V. A randomized control trial of prophyiactic maneuvers to reduce head-to-body delivery time in patients at risk for shoulder dystocia (letter). *Obstet Gynecol* 2003;102:1089–1090.
26. American College of Obstetricians and Gynecologists. Practice Bulletin: Shoulder Dystocia. No. 40. Washington, DC: ACOG; 2002.
27. O'Leary JA. *Shoulder Dystocia and Birth Injury: Prevention and Treatment.* 2 nd ed. New York: McGraw-Hill; 2000;8:107.
28. Harris BA. The Zavanelli maneuver: 12 years of recorded experience [letter]. *Obstet Gynecol* 1999;1:159.
29. Benedetti TJ. Shoulder dystocia. *Contemp Ob/Gyn* 1995;March:39–43.
30. Gonik B, Stringer C, Held B. An alternative maneuver for management of shoulder dystocia. *Am J Obstet Gynecol* 1983;145:882–884.
31. Gonik B, Allen R, Sorab J. Objective evaluation of the shoulder dystocia phenomenon: Effect of maternal pelvic orientation on force reduction. *Obstet Gynecol* 1989;74:44–48.
32. Poggi SH, Spong CY, Allen RH. Prioritizing posterior arm delivery during severe shoulder dystocia. *Obstet Gynecol* 2003;101:1068–1072.
33. Beall MH, Spong CY, Ross MG. A randomized controlled trial of prophylactic maneuvers to reduce head-to-body delivery time in patients at risk for shoulder dystocia. *Obstet Gynecol* 2003;102:31–35.
34. Mazzanti GA. Delivery of the anterior shoulder. *Obstet Gynecol* 1959;13:606–609.
35. Woods CE. A principle of physics as applicable to shoulder delivery. *Am J Obstet Gynecol* 1943;45:796–812.
36. Rubin A. Management of shoulder dystocia. *JAMA* 1964;189:835–844.
37. Barnum CG. Dystocia due to the shoulders. *Am J Obstet Gynecol* 1945;50:439–442.
38. Adler J, Patterson RL. Erb's palsy: Long term results of treatment in 88 cases. *J Bone Joint Surg* 1967;49A:1052–1074.
39. McFarland MB, Langer O, Piper JM, Berkus MD. Perinatal outcome and the type and number of maneuvers in shoulder dystocia. *Int J Obstet Gynecol* 1996;55:219–224.
40. Baskett TF, Allen AC. Perinatal implications of shoulder dystocia. *Obstet Gynecol* 1995;86:14–17.
41. Bruner JP, Drummond SB, Meenan AL, Gaskin IM. All-fours maneuver for reducing shoulder dystocia during labor. *J Reprod Med* 1998;43:439–443.
42. Sandberg E. The Zavanelli maneuver: A potentially revolutionary method for the resolution of shoulder dystocia. *Am J Obstet Gynecol* 1985;153:592–595.
43. O'Leary J, Gunn D. Cephalic replacement for shoulder dystocia. *Am J Obstet Gynecol* 1985;153:592–596.
44. Shute WB. Management of shoulder dystocia with the Shute parallel forceps. *Am J Obstet Gynecol* 1962;84:936–9.
45. Hibbard L. Shoulder dystocia. Obstet Gynecol 169;34:424–429.
46. Hibbard LT. Coping with shoulder dystocia. *OB/GYN* 1982;20:229–233.
47. Hartfield VJ. Symphysiotomy for shoulder dystocia. *Am J Obstet Gynecol* 1986;155:22 K.
48. O'Leary JA, Cuva A. Abdominal rescue after failed cephalic replacement. *Obstet Gynecol* 1992;80:514–516.

49. Gherman RB, Quzounian JG, Goodwin TM. Obstetric maneuvers for shoulder dystocia and associated fetal morbidity. *Am J Obstet Gynecol* 1998;178:1126–1130.
50. Kreitzer MS. Brachial plexus injury: The role of shoulder dystocia [letter]. The *Female Patient* 2005;30:7.
51. Gherman RB, Quzounian JG, Satin AJ, Goodwin TM, Phelan JP. A comparison of shoulder dystocia associated transient and permanent brachial plexus palsies. *Obstet Gynecol* 2003;102:544–548.
52. Sandmire HF, Demott RK. Erb's palsy: Concepts of causation. *Obstet Gynecol* 2000;95:940–942.
53. Dunn DW, Engle WA. Brachial plexus palsy: Intrauterine onset. *Pediatr Neurol* 1985;1:367–369.
54. Jennett RJ, Taby TJ. Disuse osteoporosis as evidence of brachial plexus palsy due to intrauterine fetal maladaption. *Am J Obstet Gynecol* 2001;185:276–277.
55. Eng GE. Neuromuscular disease. In: Avery GB, Fletcher MA, MacDonald MG, eds. *Neonatology*. 4th ed. Philadelphia: J.B. Lipincott; 1994:1164–1116.
56. Alfonso I, Alfonso DT, Papazian O. Focal upper extremity neuropathy in neonates. *Semin Pediatr Neurol* 2000;7:4–14.
57. Gherman RB, Goodwin TM, Quzounian JG, Miller DA, Paul RH. Brachial plexus injury associated with cesarean section: An in-utero injury? *Am J Obstet Gynecol* 1997;177:11162–11164.
58. Jennett RJ, Tarby TJ, Kreinick CJ. Brachial plexus palsy: An old problem revisited. *Am J Obstet Gynecol* 1992;166:1673–1677.
59. Allen RH, Gurewitsh ED. Temporary Erb-Duchenne palsy without shoulder dystocia or traction to the fetal head. *Obstet Gynecol* 2005;105:1210–1212.
60. Antonucci MC, Pitman MC, Eid T, et al. Simultaneous monitoring of head-to-cervix forces, intrauterine pressure and cervical dilation during labor. *Med Eng Phys* 1997;19:317–326.
61. Allen RH, Edelberg S. Brachial plexus palsy causation (published erratum in Birth 2003;30:210) *Birth* 2003;30:141–143.
62. Allen RH, Cha SL, Kronker LM, Johnson TL, Gurewitsch ED. Comparing mechanical fetal response during descent, crowning, and restitution among deliveries with and without shoulder dystocia. *Am J Obstet Gynecol* 2007;196:539–541.
63. Ubachs JMH, Sloof ACI, Peeters LLH. Obstetric antecedents of surgically treated obstetric brachial plexus injuries. *Br J Obstet Gynecol* 1995;102:813–817.
64. Nocon JJ, McKenzie DK, Thomas LJ, Hansall RS. Shoulder dystocia: An analysis of risks and obstetric maneuvers. *Am J Obstet Gynecol* 1993;168:1732–1739.
65. Crofts J, Ellis D, James M, et al. Pattern and degree of forces applied during simulation of shoulder dystocia. *Am J Obstet Gynecol* 2007;197:156.e1.

Chapter 15
Minimizing the Risks of Shoulder Dystocia-Related Fetal Injuries

Leslie Iffy

Summary The rate of injury can be reduced. Prediction of the complication is not the solution. Prevention does not require prediction. The foundations of the science of medicine were laid down by Hippocrates not Nostradamus!

Keywords: injury · prediction · prevention · risk factors

Contents

15.1   Introduction   209
15.2   Preconceptual Risk Factors   211
15.3   Antenatal Risk Factors   212
15.4   Intrapartum Risk Factors   213
15.5   Diagnosis of Shoulder Dystocia   214
15.6   Childbirth in America and Abroad   217
15.7   Etiology and Prevention   219
15.8   Considerations Pertaining to Method of Delivery   219
15.9   Conclusion   221

15.1 Introduction

As its title indicates, this chapter does not try to reiterate the "party line" about the inevitability of Erb and Klumpke palsies. Instead, it reflects the author's learning and experience, gained during five decades of practice in four countries of two continents. The admission of this "bias" may save precious time for readers who embrace the dogma that "most traditional risk factors of shoulder dystocia have no predictive value, shoulder dystocia itself is an unpredictable event, and infants at risk of permanent injury are virtually impossible to predict [1]." This section intends to challenge this comfortable philosophy [2–4], using

L. Iffy
Professor of Obstetrics & Gynecology, University of Medicine & Dentistry of New Jersey, New Jersey Medical School, Newark, New Jersey, USA

J.A. O'Leary (ed.), *Shoulder Dystocia and Birth Injury*,
DOI 10.1007/978-1-59745-473-5_15, © Humana Press, a part of Springer
Science+Business Media, LLC 2009

209

the argument spelled out in a recent textbook [5]: "Preventive medicine seldom relied on prediction. The elimination of devastating diseases . . . did not hinge upon prospective identification of individuals who would contract a particular infection or would suffer from the untoward effect of a potentially teratogenic agent."

Prevention does not require prediction. However, shoulder dystocia is one of those entities that allows evidence-based risk assessment with a reasonable degree of accuracy [5,6]. The fatalistic acceptance of the inevitability of certain birth injuries is a new phenomenon in modern medicine, probably specific to obstetrics.

Despite declining maternal and perinatal mortality rates, birth-related fetal injuries increased in North America during the past 50 years (Table 15.1) [7–13]. A report documenting a more than fivefold increase in one institution in the course of 15 years outlines an emerging problem of epidemic proportions (9).

The prominent place of large fetal size in the causation of shoulder dystocia has gained general recognition [5,14–16]. Therefore, numerous articles have discussed the question of whether or not fetal macrosomia can be detected prospectively. A variety of other predisposing factors have also been recognized [5,9,10,14–19] (Table 15.2). These have been identified in the background of injuries associated with arrest of the shoulders at delivery with disturbing frequency [23]. Most of them, and, in fact, even macrosomia itself, can be modified by appropriate antenatal and/or intrapartum management. These factors can be logically distributed into three groups.

Table 15.1 Chronology of the Changing Incidence of Shoulder Dystocia in North America

Author(s)	Year of Publication or Years of Data Collection	Reported Rate of Incidence in Terms of Percentage of All Childbirths (%)
Schwartz and McClelland [7]	1960	0.15
Seigworth [8]	1966	0.38
Hopwood [9]	1966–1976	0.2
Benedetti and Gabbe [10]	1978	0.34
Parks and Zeil [11]	1978	1.9
Hopwood [9]	1976–1981	1.1
S.J. Gross et al. [12]	1980–1985	0.85*
T.L. Gross et al. [13]	1982–1983	1.6
Nocon et al. [1]	1966–1990	1.4
ACOG Bulletin [2]	2000	1.4

Note the increasing incidence of arrest of the shoulders at birth during the five decades since the late 1950s.
*Percentage of all vaginal deliveries.

Table 15.2 Risk Factors Predisposing for Shoulder Dystocia*

Preconceptual	Antenatal	Intrapartum
Inadequate pelvis (platypelloid)	Impaired glucose tolerance	Fetal malpresentation or malrotation
Small maternal stature	Gestational diabetes	Dysfunctional labor
History of large birth-weight for the mother	Excessive maternal weight gain in pregnancy (>35 lb)	Induction of labor
History of LGA baby	LGA fetal status	Augmentation of labor with oxytocin
Previous shoulder dystocia	A-P trunk diameter exceeding BPD by >1.4 cm	Conduction anesthesia
Maternal obesity	Postdated pregnancy	Protraction or arrest disorder in the first and/or second stages of the labor
Long birth interval (>10 years)	Floating fetal head at term in primigravidas	Midcavity or low forceps or vacuum extraction and sequential use of the instruments
Family history of diabetes		Cutting umbilical cord before delivery of the shoulders
Personal history of (gestational) diabetes		

A-P, antero-posterior; BPD, biparietal diameter.
*Although mentioned as a predisposing factor for shoulder dystocia in some textbooks and articles [16,20–22], for reasons explained elsewhere, short umbilical cord is not included in the list.

15.2 Preconceptual Risk Factors

The mother's historical data are useful indicators of possible future problems. The birth of a previous LGA baby is a red flag for another, even larger child. Personal or family history of diabetes requires immediate attention. Fetal macrosomia can be avoided or limited in severity by timely provision of diabetic diet and medication [24].

Inadequate pelvic capacity is often associated with small maternal stature (≤5 feet 2 inches), although it may occur even among well-developed women [25]. Therefore, detailed antenatal pelvic assessment is of outstanding importance [26]. It is to be remembered that it was the recognition of the crucial role of the female pelvic configuration in the birthing process that turned traditional midwifery, practiced by granny midwifes, into a branch of the science of medicine. The fact that opinions questioning the value of pelvic assessment still find their way into medical journals [27] is a bizarre phenomenon that, beyond the constitutionally protected right to free speech, has no rational explanation.

15.3 Antenatal Risk Factors

Routine prenatal testing for diabetes has been a standard procedure in teaching institutions for decades both in America and Europe. This being the case, selective screening, based on certain risk factors, is an anachronism in the 21st century, conducive to the trend shown in Table 15.1 [5,23,28,29]. Early treatment of glucose intolerance is protective against fetal macrosomia [24]. Omission of routine glucose screening invites, therefore, complications with grave dangers both for the unborn child and for the obstetrician [13].

Excessive maternal weight gain should and, in most instances, can be controlled. Assessment of the fetal weight at term gestation is another obligatory routine. Suspicion of LGA fetal status, or inability to assess the fetal weight clinically, is a compelling reason for sonographic evaluation. Unfortunately, the belief that "ultrasonography is an inaccurate predictor of macrosomia [30]" has been inoculated into the minds of obstetricians so deeply that no evidence to the contrary is likely to remove it soon. Actually, the range of error of sonographic estimation of the fetal weight and size is unchanged throughout the pregnancy [31–33]. Thus, it is just as reliable for assessing LGA status as it is for detecting growth restriction or discordance between twin pairs.

The reservations about diagnosing "macrosomia" with ultrasound (interpreted as $\geq$4,500 g in America and $\geq$4,000 g elsewhere) has been motivated by fear that overestimation of the fetal weight could lead to unnecessary cesarean sections. This argument ignores the fact that, above the 4,000 g weight range, current sonographic growth standards tend to underestimate the fetal weight [5,34,35]. In the $\geq$4,500 g weight group, the probability of underestimation is 80% [15,34,36]. Therefore, the real problem is the frequent underestimation of the weights of some grossly macrosomic fetuses rather than the less ominous consequences of occasional overestimations.

Several studies have demonstrated that, above certain weight limits, elective abdominal deliveries can eliminate many birth-related injuries [38,39]. In response, some biostatistical analyses were published, claiming that ultrasound is not able to confirm or exclude macrosomia with acceptable accuracy [2,40]. Intrinsic to the twisted logic of the voodoo mathematics involved in these studies is the premise that, if "Sonographer A" estimated a fetus actually weighing 4,475 g as 3,800 g, but "Sonographer B" reported a calculated weight of 4,510 g, then "A" correctly excluded macrosomia, whereas "B" falsely diagnosed macrosomia.

The dictum "The most ignorant teacher can ask questions that the wisest of students cannot answer" highlights the above-mentioned statistical formulas. In response to a wrong question, sonography gives a wrong answer. Ultrasound cannot determine whether, by a couple of grams, a fetus is more or less than 650 g at 24 weeks, or 2,500 g at 35 weeks, or 4,000 g at 42 weeks gestation. This naive "yes or no" question serves as a fig leaf for those who prefer to ignore rather than address the problem. What sonography can do is to define fetal weight within a standard error of $\pm$10%. The suggestion that practicing obstetricians should ignore this information removes one leg of the stool on which they sit at times of critical decision making.

Sonographic techniques have been described for comparative head, trunk, shoulder girdle, and abdominal circumference measurements [41,42]. These data provide valuable clues for assessing shoulder dystocia related risks. Their use in borderline cases, instead of blindly relying on one's "judgment [1]," makes a difference comparable with investing in stocks and bonds versus trying to become prosperous by playing blackjack in Las Vegas.

15.4 Intrapartum Risk Factors

Many risk factors that emerge during labor are the sequelae of those previously described. Dysfunctional labor often derives from relative feto-pelvic dispro-portion, secondary to large fetal size, borderline pelvic capacity, nonmalleable caput due to postdated gestation, or a combination of some of them.

Malrotation, deflexion, or asynclitism of the head, detectable clinically at ≥5 cm cervical dilation, can create or exaggerate disproportion. In such circum-stances, oxytocin may exacerbate already prevailing uterine exhaustion [25] and lead to further complications, shoulder dystocia included [10,28]. Arrest or protraction disorder in the second stage of labor carries similar implications and often invites the use of an extraction instrument. Whereas a relatively safe choice when the pelvis is adequate and the fetal size is average, forceps or vacuum extraction can be a shortcut to catastrophe when the opposite is the case [5,6,18,28].

A bizarre recommendation, stating that pelvic assessment is unnecessary for the conduct of labor but is required before instrumental extraction [43], lures physicians into a territory where disaster looms high on the horizon. Some critical pelvic dimensions no longer can be assessed by manual pelvimetry after the fetal head has already engaged in the pelvis. Misconceptions such as this may well explain why catastrophic shoulder dystocia so frequently is associated with extraction procedures [10,28].

The idea that a large object, such as a big head, cannot be squeezed through a small opening is not difficult to conceptualize. Builders of jails have taken this expediency into account for centuries, as have manufacturers of men's hats and, in more recent times, jury members at malpractice trials. Why some physicians think that this simple fact is irrelevant to childbirth is a puzzle. The same applies to the never substantiated belief that women with inadequate pelvis are rare in modern times [43]. Actually, pelvic inadequacy is frequent in high-risk popula-tions and is more a rule than an exception among women who are ≤5 feet tall. It is thought provoking that the loss of interest of obstetricians in the female pelvis that followed the disappearance of x-ray pelvimetry from clinical practice coincided with the rapid increase of arrests of the shoulders at delivery and of the ensuing litigations [44].

Whether conduction anesthesia diminishes myometrial activity has been disputed for decades. Eventually, the acknowledgment of this phenomenon had to be smuggled into the obstetric literature, not unlike the soldiers of Greece into the city of Troy. The horse was a Solomonic decision, declaring that under epidural anesthesia, the second stage of labor is "normal" for primigravidas even if it lasts 3 hours, versus a 2-hour limit without anesthesia. Because conduction anesthesia is perceived as a "right" by contemporary women facing labor, its routine use is not disputed in this chapter. Nor is the fact ignored, however, that it tends to reduce both voluntary and nonvoluntary expulsive efforts. This effect increases the need for forceps, vacuum-assisted, and cesarean deliveries. For the same reason, conduction anesthesia is also counterproductive for breech delivery, where good expulsive efforts are needed for the safe delivery of the aftercoming head [45] and to avoid the occurrence of nuchal arms; another complication conductive to brachial plexus injury. The same is true for vacuum extractions, where the maternal forces are critically important [46] and, by logical deduction, for shoulder dystocia as well. It is important, therefore, to minimize the effect of conduction anesthesia at the time of the contemplated delivery, whenever predisposing factors for arrest of the shoulders are present. It is worth remembering that the increasing use of conduction anesthesia during labor also coincided with the exponential increase of shoulder dystocia incidents.

The risks of sequential use of extraction instruments has been documented extensively [10,18,28]. Thus, few situations can justify this approach. Probably the only circumstance that may provide an explanation for this practice is well-documented malfunctioning of a vacuum instrument. Although the nature of the ensuing fetal injuries varies, brachial plexus damage is frequent among them [28]. Therefore, avoiding the application of one instrument after another serves best the interests of both patient and obstetrician.

15.5 Diagnosis of Shoulder Dystocia

Shoulder dystocia has no generally accepted definition. The forthcoming one probably fairly reflects the prevailing perception of American obstetricians: "Most investigators agree that (shoulder dystocia) has occurred when, in the absence of spontaneous expulsion of the fetus, the standard delivery procedure of gentle downward traction of the fetal head has failed to accomplish delivery [14]."

A different interpretation has been prevalent, although also disputed, in some European countries [47,48], based on the knowledge that the delivery of the head and the rest of the fetal body during two different uterine contractions is a physiologic phenomenon [21,49,50]. Part and parcel of this concept is the understanding that the retraction of the delivered head toward the perineum after the cessation of the contraction is not "ipso facto" evidence of shoulder dystocia but a natural consequence of uterine relaxation. It is a disquieting experience for the uninitiated that the face of the child gradually turns blue before the next contraction builds up. However, babies are born in good condition after such "two-step deliveries [51]," indicating that the change in color reflected reduced skin and not impaired brain circulation. Clinical experience [5,52] and relevant research [53] both prove that, in the absence of extraction attempts, unassisted delivery of the head and the body during two separate contractions entails no adverse effect. Another advantage of two-step deliveries is the expression of fluid inhaled by the fetus during the process of labor [5,49,50] (Fig. 15.1). In case of meconium aspiration, this

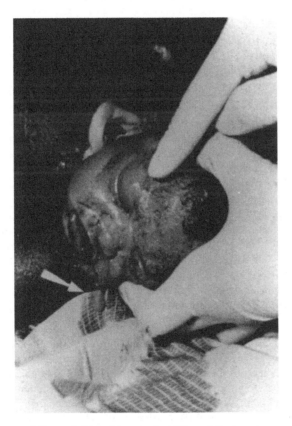

Fig. 15.1 Two-step delivery of a high-risk parturient. The umbilical cord was wrapped around the neck of the fetus twice. This complication was suspected on account of recurrent variable fetal heart rate decelerations during the second stage of labor. No attempt was made to extract the body of the child after the emergence of the head. The umbilical cord was loosened slightly around the neck. With the occurrence of the next uterine contraction, mucus was squeezed out of the lungs of the baby (see arrow). The contraction expelled the body spontaneously. The child was born in vigorous condition. (Courtesy of Dr. Vivic Johnson.)

protective mechanism is forfeited if the body is extracted from the birth canal immediately.

To comprehend the effects of the delayed expulsion of the body, one must understand the mechanism of a spontaneous delivery process [51]. During its progress in the pelvic cavity, the fetal head passes through the inlet in occipito-transverse rotation. In the midpelvis, the ischial spines reduce the transverse diameter. Thus, during its descent, the head must rotate 90 degrees to bring the biparietal diameter to the narrowest available space. The passage of the shoulders, positioned in the transverse diameter, through the inlet coincides with that of the anteroposteriorly rotated head across the midpelvis, as nature designed them in such a manner that the distance between the shoulders and the greatest circumference of the head is the same as that between the planes of the inlet and the midpelvis. Thus, both can optimally accommodate the corresponding pelvic structures at the same time.

Still in the transverse diameter, as the uterus contracts, the shoulders descend into the true pelvis while the contraction delivers the caput in occipito-anterior rotation. At this point, one of two things can happen:

1. The contraction continues and rotates the shoulders into the anteroposterior diameter, thus bringing the shortest diameter of the chest between the ischial spines. In this process, the head, maintaining its normal relationship with the shoulders, passively rotates 90 degrees; a phenomenon described as *external rotation*. The contraction then expels the rest of the body seconds after the head. This mechanism occurs during the unassisted deliveries of most multiparous and about one-half of nulliparous women.
2. Having expelled the caput, the contraction stops and the uterus relaxes. As a result, the head, still in occipito-anterior rotation, retracts against the perineum. Often referred to as the "turtle sign," this event is frequently interpreted as diagnostic of shoulder dystocia. Actually, when the next contraction develops 2 to 3 minutes later, the shoulders inside and (passively) the head outside rotate 90 degrees and, almost invariably, the body is expelled spontaneously without need for intervention.

The method of two-step delivery takes the fact into account that, before turning into the anteroposterior diameter, the shoulders cannot pass through the midpelvis. Thus, prior to the external rotation of the head, attempts at extraction are futile and dangerous. Intervention is both undesirable and unnecessary, as the period of rest between the contractions allows the reestablishment of the uterine and chorionic circulations and, thus feto-maternal gas exchange [54].

It has been reported that the majority of shoulder dystocia–associated fetal injuries involve manipulative delivery of the body within 3 minutes of the emergence of the head [23]. Apparently, some injuries derive from the erroneous assumption that extraction of the body shortly after the emergence of the head is necessary to avoid fetal damage. Experience shows that the opposite is true. In the course of more than 30 years, though about 10,000 two-step deliveries were conducted in the author's service, no hypoxic fetal injury, conceivably attributable to the delivery technique, has been observed. Initiating oxytocin infusion at the moment of the delivery of the head, or increasing its rate of flow, is conducive to the development of a strong enough subsequent contraction to ensure the timely expulsion of the shoulders and the rest of the body.

The two-step delivery method is effective for reducing the risk of arrest of the shoulders at birth and its consequences [5,52]. The acceptance of this approach for managing the birthing process requires the dismissal of misconceptions about the dangers that supposedly threaten the child between the time of the delivery of the head and the expulsion of the rest of the body. Actually, prior to the occurrence of the next uterine contraction, these perils are virtually nonexistent.

It deserves mention, furthermore, that the application of a scalp electrode to the head permits the monitoring of the fetal condition during this uterine resting phase just as effectively as at any other time during the labor. Thus, with regard to the risks that the method involves, the overanxious doctor does not need to rely on experiments on lambs or unsubstantiated hypotheses.

15.6 Childbirth in America and Abroad

Childbirth is a phenomenon that human beings have experienced throughout the ages. In this process, a variety of beliefs developed about its conduct. Fascinating though the insights and rituals of primitive cultures may be, this section deals with ideas that are pertinent to contemporary obstetric practices. Prevailing concepts about the proper conduct of delivery have limited scientific foundation. This is understandable if one considers that, whereas it is easy to set up experimental models for antepartum and even intrapartum events, the dramatic moments of the birthing process offer limited scope for research. This fact is well-mirrored in obstetric textbooks, if one cares to compare their contents from edition to edition. Whereas other aspects of perinatal physiology and pathology have undergone significant changes, the description of the process of delivery was passed on for decades from one volume to the next, and often also from one author to another, with little change.

The belief that the child's body needs to be removed from the birth canal by manual extraction after the delivery of the head has been stated in several textbooks printed in Western, Central, and Eastern Europe [20,55–61]. Some others, while discussing the mechanism of labor at length, bypass the question of how finally the neonate enters the world [62–64]. The suggestion that after the emergence of the head, manipulation involving traction is the desirable delivery method, is even more prevalent in standard textbooks on this continent [65–68]. Nonetheless, some American [69] and Canadian [70] authors have pointed out with emphasis that refraining from intervention until the occurrence of the next uterine contraction is the safest conduct of childbirth. Prominent in this regard was the textbook of Danforth, where the relevant chapter warned physicians strongly against intervening during the time between the delivery of the head and the development of the next uterine contraction [71]:

> Most patients deliver spontaneously if simply let alone . . . after the head is born. In a completely unaided delivery there may be a pause . . . temporarily the patient has no urge to bear down. . . . Shortly, as the uterus resumes effective contraction, the shoulders are forced into and down through the pelvis, at the same time rotating so that one shoulder is behind the pubis and the other in the hollow of the sacrum. This rotation of the shoulders into the anteroposterior diameter of the pelvis causes the baby's head to rotate the back of the head toward the side of the mother where the fetal back was during labor. This is the external restitution phase of the mechanism of labor. The anterior shoulder stems or pivots underneath the symphysis, and the posterior shoulder is forced outward. As the posterior shoulder emerges over the perineum, both shoulders advance together, and the rest of the baby follows without delay or particular mechanism.

The above described two-step delivery method [51] is favored by many English, Scottish, and Irish obstetricians. Surprisingly, this fact does not always transpire in the medical literature of the United Kingdom. It is interesting that textbooks written for British midwives place more emphasis upon the importance of refraining from extracting the body after the delivery of the head [72,73] than do those addressed to physicians. Nonetheless, some European obstetric textbooks unequivocally state that the critical criterion for the diagnosis of shoulder dystocia is continued retention of the fetal body after the end of the contraction that followed the one that had delivered the head [47,48].

The old routine that recommended the cutting of the umbilical cord wrapped around the fetal neck, before the delivery of the body [21], was reiterated uncritically in modem obstetric texts up to the early years of the 21st century [50,66,67,69]. Refreshing exceptions are the previously cited British books for midwives. These warned against [72] or even forbade [73] such intervention.

The never substantiated idea that the delivery of the shoulders may be prevented by a short umbilical cord or by one wrapped tightly around the neck of the fetus still emerges at times in the literature [22]. This hypothesis ignores the fact that the cord can be pulled out of its insertion at the navel with relatively little force. This happened in a well-documented case, as the doctor tried to ease the nuchal cord around the head of a child [74]. Besides, the force of the uterus can tear the placenta off its implantation site as happens occasionally when fetus and placenta are expelled together. Thus, it is obvious that the cord cannot stop the delivery of the shoulders by overriding the expulsive force of the contracting uterus. The strength of the latter not only exceeds any accoucheur's but even tops that of the much admired biceps muscles of boxing champion Muhammad Ali.

Ignored for decades, this dangerous practice only received attention recently in this century [53,75–77], after the publication of case reports describing incidents of catastrophic neurologic damage deriving from severing the cord before the delivery of the shoulders [74,78]. Having been spelled out in one new textbook [79], the condemnation of this practice still awaits reiteration in others.

Meanwhile, relevant catastrophes continue to occur. The author has first-hand knowledge of two, as yet unpublished, incidents where the occurrence of shoulder dystocia, associated with severance of umbilical cord, resulted in serious neurologic damage in the neonates. One of these followed the cutting of the cord by the physician in order to resolve shoulder dystocia.

15.7 Etiology and Prevention

Undoubtedly, the increasing incidence of shoulder dystocia in obstetric practice is related to changes in our society in general and in the practice of obstetrics in particular. Obvious predisposing factors are the increasing prevalence of obesity [14], escalating incidence of diabetes among gravidas [5], women's demand for conduction anesthesia during labor, widespread use of oxytocin for the induction or augmentation of labor [10], frequent use of extraction instruments [10,28], and decreased understanding even among specialists of the role of the female pelvic structure in the birthing process. The task of quantitating the roles of the various recognized or suspected contributory factors is difficult. One theory that obviously cannot explain this trend is that up to 50% of all brachial plexus injuries are spontaneous *in utero* events, unrelated to the delivery process and its management [80].

Discouraged physicians may extract solace from the reassurance that many if not most Erb palsies have nothing to do with the birthing events [81]. However, those obstetricians who, in the course of a long career, have seen no case of Erb palsy without difficulty having been encountered at the time of the delivery of the shoulders, will remain skeptic [5]. Rare exceptions may exist, but the idea that the exceptions are the rule is too far-fetched to be credible.

15.8 Considerations Pertaining to Method of Delivery

In 2002, Hanna et al. published a multicenter study showing that vaginal deliveries carried a 3% risk of fetal death or injury [82]. The protocols of their investigation permitted vaginal deliveries up to 4,000 g estimated body weight. Besides, labor was "augmented" with oxytocin in more than one half of all instances. Because this practice pattern was far more liberal than those prevailing in America, the deriving danger was about threefold higher than what comparable gravidas in the United States had to face [83]. Nonetheless, after prompt acceptance of the validity of the cited study by British authorities [84], the American College of Obstetricians and Gynecologists quickly followed suit and warned obstetricians to avoid the dangers of vaginal breech deliveries [85].

For reasons mentioned, this decision has been disputed subsequently. None-theless, it established an important principle, namely that there must be a limit to the risks that physicians, anxious to maintain their technical skills, can expose their patients to. Indeed, if the actual risk is even only 1%, elective abdominal delivery may well be a reasonable choice, noting that the child predestined to be injured cannot be "predicted" with certainty.

Based on more than 500,000 childbirths, in 1998 Nesbitt and his associates [6] calculated the risk of shoulder dystocia based on three major factors: (1) maternal glucose tolerance; (2) fetal weight; (3) use of extraction instrument (Table 15.3). Noting that the risk of permanent brachial plexus damage associated with shoulder dystocia has been close to 10% in this country [86], the chance of significant fetal injury can be calculated with reasonable accuracy on the ground of the cited authors' data (Table 15.4).

Table 15.3 Correlations Between Birthweights and the Incidence of Shoulder Dystocia

| Birthweight (g) | Nondiabetic Women | | Diabetic Women | |
| | | Method of Delivery | | |
	Spontaneous (%)	Instrumental (%)	Spontaneous (%)	Instrumental (%)
3,500–3,749	0.5	1.5	2.5	4
3,750–3,999	2.5	3.5	5	8
4,000–4,249	5	7.5	8	12
4,250–4,499	8	12	13	18
4,500–4,749	13	20	23	27
4,750–5,000	21	23	29	35

Simplified tabulation of the data published by Nesbitt et al., [6] based on more than 500,000 childbirths in the State of California.

Table 15.4 Risk of Shoulder Dystocia–Related Fetal Injury According to Fetal Weight, Maternal Glucose Tolerance, and Method of Delivery

| Birthweight (g) | Nondiabetic Women | | Diabetic Women | |
| | | Method of Delivery | | |
	Spontaneous	Instrumental	Spontaneous	Instrumental
3,500–3,749	1/2,000	1/666	1/400	1/250
3,750–3,999	1/400	1/285	1/200	1/125
4,000–4,249	1/200	1/135	1/125	1/83
4,250–4,499	1/125	1/83	1/77	1/62
4,500–4,749	1/77	1/50	1/44	1/37
4,749–5,000	1/48	1/43	1/35	1/28

The calculation has been based on the statistics of Nesbitt et al. [6] as shown in Table 15.3. It rests upon the premise that about 1 out of 10 incidents of shoulder dystocia is associated with permanent injury of the child. Because the reported frequency of injury in connection with arrest of the shoulders at birth varies on a broad scale in the practices of obstetricians [86], the actual risk for any individual physician may be lower or higher than the above estimates indicate.

The premise used for the presented calculation, namely that 1 out of 10 cases of shoulder dystocia entails long-range damage to the child, is supported by certain considerations:

(A)   Whereas the widely referred to statistics use brachial plexus injury as an end point [86], actually more than 10% of all fetal injuries involve the central nervous system exclusively without any Erb or Klumpke palsy [28].
(B)   The fact that most shoulder dystocias occur in less than 4,000 g babies [1,87], whereas close to 75% of those who sustain damage weigh more than 4,000 g [28], indicates clearly that the risk of injury is markedly higher than average in the $\geq$4,000 g groups.

Analysis of the here presented information leads to the conclusion that currently prevailing guidelines instruct physicians to tolerate risk of fetal damage as high as 3%; a higher degree of danger than what has been ruled to be unacceptable in connection with vaginal breech deliveries.

The argument that reliance on sonographic assessment of the fetal size could lead to unnecessary cesarean sections has little validity in light of the knowledge that current growth standards tend to underestimate fetal weight at term gestation and that at the 5,000 g range, the weights of 80% of all fetuses are underestimated [15,34]. Because the danger of underestimation (fetal injury) far exceeds that of overestimation (unnecessary cesarean section), the widely quoted warnings about avoidable cesarean sections are clearly misguided.

For this author, a 1% risk of fetal injury appears to be the uppermost limit of acceptability. However, the perception of any particular mother may be different. The task of the physician is to determine the magnitude of the fetal and maternal risks with a reasonable degree of accuracy, rather than to be the final arbiter about the method of delivery. Duly conceding that no calculation can claim absolute validity, it is the contention of the writers that the direction of the tipping of the balance is obvious in most instances. It needs to be remembered, of course, that the pros and cons can shift during the labor process with the development of protraction and arrest disorders, deterioration in the condition of the fetus, and the emergence of situations where instrumental extraction may be needed for vaginal delivery [5,14,16].

15.9 Conclusion

Neither in obstetrics nor in other fields of medicine are the doctor's decisions infallible. The above suggestions do not claim, therefore, absolute validity. However, this fact does not justify blind acceptance of blatantly dangerous practice patterns. There is reason to believe that, based on the above outlined principles, the rate of shoulder dystocia–related fetal injuries can be reduced drastically and immediately. Further improvement requires continued search for prevention [88] and the abandonment of the idea that the key to the solution is "prediction." The foundations of the science of medicine were laid down by Hippocrates not Nostradamus.

References

1. Nocon JJ, McKensie DK, Thomas LJ, Hansell RS. Shoulder dystocia: An analysis of risks and obstetric maneuvers. *Am J Obstet Gynecol* 1992;168:1732–1737.
2. American College of Obstetricians and Gynecologists. Practice Bulletin. Fetal macrosomia. No. 22. Washington, DC: ACOG; 2000.
3. Bryant DR, Leonardi MR, Landwehr JR, Bottoms SE. Limited usefulness of fetal weight in predicting neonatal brachial plexus injury. *Am J Obstet Gynecol* 1998;179:686–689
4. Donelly V, Foran A, Murphy J, McFarland P, Keane D, O'Herlihy C. Neonatal brachial plexus palsy: An unpredictable injury. *Am J Obstet Gynecol* 2002;187:1209–1212.
5. Ramieri J, Iffy L. Shoulder dystocia. In: Apuzzio JJ, Vintzileos MA, Iffy L, eds. *Operative Obstetrics.* 3rd ed. London: Taylor & Francis: 2006:253–263.
6. Nesbitt TS, Gilbert WM, Herrchen B. Shoulder dystocia and associated risk factors with macrosomic infants born in California. *Am J Obstet Gynecol* 1998;179:476–480.
7. Schwartz RC, McClelland D. Shoulder dystocia. *Obstet Gynecol* 1958;11:468–471.
8. Seigworth GI. Shoulder dystocia: Review of five years experience. *Obstet Gynecol* 1966;28:764–767.
9. Hopwood HG Jr. Shoulder dystocia: Fifteen years' experience in a community hospital. *Am J Obstet Gynecol* 1982;144:162–164.
10. Benedetti TJ, Gabbe SC. Shoulder dystocia: A complication of fetal macrosomia and prolonged second stage of labor with midpelvic delivery. *Obstet Gynecol* 1978;52:526–529.
11. Parks GD, Zeil HK. Macrosomia: A proposed indication for primary cesarean section. *Obstet Gynecol* 1978;52:407–409.
12. Gross SJ, Shime J, Farine D. Shoulder dystocia: Predictors and outcome. *Am J Obstet Gynecol* 1987;156:334–336.
13. Gross TL, Sokol RJ, Williams T. Shoulder dystocia: A fetal-physician risk. *Am J Obstet Gynecol* 1987;156:1408–1414.
14. O'Leary JA. *Shoulder Dystocia and Birth Injury.* New York: McGraw-Hill; 1992.
15. Mollberg M, Hagberg H, Bager B, Lilja H, Ladorfs L. High birthweight and shoulder dystocia: The strongest risk factor for obstetric brachial plexus palsy in Swedish population-based study. *Acta Obstet Gynecol Scand* 2005;84:654–659.
16. Beer E, Mangiante G, Pecorari D. Distocia delle Spalles. Rome, Italy: CIC Edizioni Internazionali ; 2006.
17. O'Leary JA. Shoulder dystocia. In: Iffy L, Apuzzio JJ, Vintzileos AM, eds. *Operative Obstetrics.* 2 nd ed. New York: McGraw-Hill; 1992:234–243.
18. Benedetti TJ. Shoulder dystocia. In: Pauerstein CJ, ed. *Clinical Obstetrics.* New York: John Wiley & Sons; 1987:871–882.
19. Hernandez C, Wendel GD. Shoulder dystocia. *Clin Obstet Gynecol* 1990;33:526–534.
20. Tawler J, Butler-Manual R. *Modern Obstetrics for Student Midwifes.* London: Lloyd - Luke Ltd.; 1973:371.
21. Greenhill JP. *Obstetrics.* 11th ed. Philadelphia: W.B. Saunders; 1955:983.
22. Ogueh O, Al-Tarkait A, Vallerand D, Rouah F, Morin L, Benjamin A, Usher RH. Obstetrical factors related to nuchal cord. *Acta Obstet Gynecol Scand* 2006;85:810–814.
23. Iffy L, Varadi V. A vallak elakadasaval kapcsolatos magzati serulesek korocki tenyezoi. *Magy Noorv Lap (Budapest)* 2001;64:365–371.

24. Chin-Chu L, River J, River P, Blix PM, Moawad AH. Good diabetic control in pregnancy and favorable fetal outcome. *Obstet Gynecol* 1986;67:51–56.
25. Schulman H. Uterine dystocia. In: Iffy L, Kaminetzky HA, ed. *Principles and Practice of Obstetrics & Perinatology*. New York: Wiley; 1981:933–939.
26. Diegmann EK, Nichols R. Clinical pelvimetry. In: Apuzzio JJ, Vintzileos MA, Iffy L, eds. *Operative Obstetrics*. 3rd ed. London: Taylor & Francis; 2006:33–40.
27. Martel MJ, MacKinnon CJ. Guidelines for vaginal birth after previous cesarean birth. *J Obstet Gynecol Canada* 2004;26:660–663.
28. Iffy L, Varadi V, Jakobovits A. Common intrapartum denominators of shoulder dystocia related birth injuries. *Zbl Gynak* 1994;116:33–37.
29. Gabbe SC, Graves CR. Management of diabetes mellitus complicating pregnancy. *Obstet Gynecol* 2003;102;857–868.
30. American College of Obstetricians and Gynecologists. Practice Patterns. Shoulder dystocia. No 7. Washington, DC: ACOG; 1997.
31. Manning FA, Romero R. *Sonography in Obstetrics and Gynecology*. 5th ed. Stanford, CT: Appleton & Lange; 1991:517–536.
32. Deter RH, Hadlock FP. Use of ultrasound in detection of macrosomia: A review. *J Clin Ultrasound* 1985;13:519–524.
33. DuBose TJ. Assessment of fetal age and size: Techniques and criteria. In: Berman MC, Cohen HL, eds. *Diagnostic Medical Sonography. Obstetrics and Gynecology*. 2 nd ed. Philadelphia: Lippincott; 1997:359–398.
34. American College of Obstetricians and Gynecologists. Technical Bulletin. Fetal macrosomia. No. 159. Washington, DC: ACOG; 1991.
35. Chien PFW, Owen P, Kahn KS. Validity of ultrasound estimation of fetal weight. *Obstet Gynecol* 2000;95:856–860.
36. Loeffler FE. Clinical fetal weight. *J Obstet Gynaecol Br Commonw* 1967;74:675–677.
37. Best G, Pressman EK. Ultrasonographic prediction of birth weight in diabetic pregnancies. *Obstet Gynecol* 2002;99:740–744.
38. McFarland LV, Raskin M, Daling JR, Benedetti TJ. Erb/Duchene's palsy: A consequence of fetal macrosomia and method of delivery. *Obstet Gynecol* 1986;68:784–788.
39. Langer O, Berkus MD, Huff RW. Shoulder dystocia: Should the fetus weighing ≥ 4,000 grams be delivered by cesarean section? *Am J Obstet Gynecol* 1991;165:831–837.
40. Rouse DJ, Owen J, Goldenberg RL, Oliver SP. The effectiveness and costs of elective cesarean delivery for fetal macrosomia diagnosed by ultrasound. *JAMA* 1996;276:1480–1488.
41. Cohen B, Penning S, Major C, Ansley D, Porto M, Gante T. Sonographic prediction of shoulder dystocia in infants of diabetic mothers. *Obstet Gynecol* 1996;88:10–13.
42. Jazayeri A, Heffron JA, Phillips R, Spellacy WN. Macrosomia prediction using ultrasound fetal abdominal circumference of 35 centimeters or more. *Obstet Gynecol* 1999;93:3–526.
43. O'Grady JP, Gimovsky ML, Mollhargie CJ. *Vacuum Extraction in Modern Obstetric Practice*. New York: The Parthenon Publ. Group; 1995:43.
44. Medical Malpractice, Verdicts, Settlements & Experts, Vol. 18, No 10, October 2000.
45. Weingold AP. The management of breech presentation. In: Iffy L, Charles D, eds. *Operative Perinatology*. New York: Macmillan; 1984:537–553.
46. Dhanraj DN, Baggish MS. The vacuum extractor (ventouse) for obstetric delivery. In: Apuzzio JJ, Vintzileos MA, Iffy L, eds. *Operative Obstetrics*. 3rd ed. London: Taylor & Francis; 2006:299–310.
47. Roseveas SK, Stirrat GM. *Handbook of Obstetric Management*. Oxford: Blackwell Science; 1996:251.
48. Szabo I. Koros vajudas es szules. In: Papp Z, ed. *A Szuleszet-Nogyogyaszat Tankonyve*. Budapest: Semmelweis Konyvklado; 1999:397–490.

49. Bryant RD, Danforth DN. Conduct of normal labor. In: Danforth DN, ed. *Textbook of Obstetrics and Gynecology*. 2 nd ed. New York: Harper & Row; 1971:581–584.
50. Bottoms SF, Sokol RJ. Mechanisms and conduct of labor. In: Iffy L, Kaminetzky HA, eds. *Principles and Practice of Obstetrics & Perinatology*. New York: Wiley; 1981:815–838.
51. Iffy L, Apuzzio J, Ganesh V. A randomized controlled trial of prophylactic maneuvers to reduce head-to-body delivery time in patients at risk of shoulder dystocia. *Obstet Gynecol* 2003;102:1089–1090.
52. Iffy L. Shoulder dystocia. *Am J Obstet Gynecol* 1987;156:1416.
53. Stallings SP, Edwards RK, Johnson JWC. Correlation of head-to-body delivery intervals in shoulder dystocia and umbilical artery acidosis. *Am J Obstet Gynecol* 2001;185: 268–274.
54. Ramsey EM. Anatomy and pathology of uteroplacental circulation. In: Kaminetzky HA, Iffy L, eds. *New Techniques and Concepts in Maternal and Fetal Medicine*. New York: Van Nostrand Reinhold;1979:5–18.
55. Garrey MM, Govan ADT, Hodge C, Callander R. *Obstetrics Illustrated*. 2 nd ed. Edinburgh: Churchill Livingstone;1974:209–210.
56. Friedberg V, Heirsche HD. *Geburtshilfe*. Stuttgart: Georg Thieme Verlag; 1975:125–127.
57. Walker J, MacGillivray I, MacNaughton MC. *Obstetrics and Gynecology*. 9th ed. Edinburgh: Churchill Livingstone; 1976:318–397.
58. von Martius G. *Lehrbuch der Geburtshilfe*. Stuttgart: Georg Thieme Vertag; 1977:272–274.
59. Lampe L. *Szuleszet Nogyogyaszat*. Vol. 2. Budapest: Medicina;1981:418–419.
60. Munteanu I, Karadja V. Nasterea normala. In: Munteanu, ed. *Tratat de Obstetrica*. Bucuresti: Editura Academiei Romane; 2000:355–415.
61. Gaal J. Elettani vajudas es szules. In: Papp Z, ed. *Szuleszet-Nogyogyaszati Protokoll*. Budapest: Golden Book Publ;1999:291–299.
62. Moir JC. *Munro Kerr's Operative Obstetrics*. 7th ed. London: Bailliere, Tindall and Cox; 1964.
63. Merger R, Levy J, Melchior J. *Precis d'Obstetrique*. Paris: Masson; 1977.
64. Myerscough PR. *Munro Kerr's Operative Obstetrics*. 9th ed. London: Bailliere Tindall; 1977.
65. Eastman NJ, Hellman LM. *Williams Obstetrics*. 12th ed. New York: Appleton-Century-Crofts; 1961:448–449.
66. Ledger WJ. Labor and delivery. In: Willson RJ, Carrington ER, Ledter WJ, eds. *Obstetrics and Gynecology*. 7th ed. St. Louis: CV Mosby; 1983:381–414.
67. Cunningham FG, MacDonald PC, Gant NF, Leveno KJ, Gilstrap III LC. *Williams Obstetrics*. 19th ed. Norwalk, CT: Appleton & Lange; 1993:381–383.
68. Russell KP. The course and conduct of normal labor and delivery. In: Pernoll ML, Benson RC, eds. *Current Obstetric & Gynecologic Diagnosis & Treatment*. 6th ed. Norwalk, CT: Appleton & Lange; 1987:178–203.
69. Norwitz ER, Robinson JN, Repke JT. Labor and delivery. In: Gabbe SG, Niebyl JR, Simpson JL, eds. *Obstetrics*. 4th ed. New York: Churchill Livingstone; 2002:353–394.
70. Oxorn H. *Human Labor & Birth*. Norwalk, CT: Appleton-Century-Croft; 1986:140–141.
71. Bryant RD, Danforth DN. Conduct of normal labor. In: Danforth DN, ed. *Textbook of Obstetrics and Gynecology*. 2 nd ed. New York: Harper & Row; 1971:561–584.
72. Bennet VR, Brown LK. *Myles Textbook for Midwives*. 12th ed. Edinburgh: Churchill Livingstone; 1993:208–209.
73. Myles M. *Textbook for Midwives*. 10th ed. Edinburgh: Churchill Livingstone; 1985:313–314.
74. Iffy L, Varadi V. Cerebral palsy following cutting of the nuchal cord before delivery. *Med Law* 1994;13:323–330.
75. Flamm BL. Tight nuchal cord and shoulder dystocia: A potentially catastrophic combination. *Obstet Gynecol* 1999;94:853.

76. Mercer JS, Skovgaard RL, Peareara-Eaves J, Bowman TA. Nuchal cord management and nurse-midwifery practice. *J Midwifery Women's Health* 2005;50:373–379.
77. Iffy L, Gittens-Williams LN. Shoulder dystocia and nuchal cord [letter]. *Acta Obstet Gynecol Scand* 2007;86:523.
78. Iffy L, Varadi V, Papp E. Untoward neonatal sequelae deriving from cutting of the umbilical cord before delivery. *Med Law* 2001;20:627–634.
79. Stenchever MA, Gittens-Williams LN. Normal vaginal delivery. In: Apuzzio JJ, Vintzileos MA, Iffy L, eds. *Operative Obstetrics*. 3rd ed. London: Taylor & Francis; 2006:241–252.
80. Gherman RB, Ouzounian JG, Goodwin TM. Brachial plexus palsy: An in utero injury? *Am J Obstet Gynecol* 1999;180:1303–1307.
81. Sandmire HF, DeMott RK. Erb's palsy: Concepts of causation. *Obstet Gynecol* 2000;85:940–942.
82. Hanna ME, Hanna J, Dawson SA, Hodnett Ed, Saigal S, William AR. Planned cesarean section versus planned vaginal birth for breech presentation at term: A randomized multicentre trial. *Lancet* 2000; 356:1375–1383.
83. O'Leary JA. Vaginal delivery of the term breech. *Obstet Gynecol* 1979;53:341–343.
84. Lumley J. Any room left for disagreement about assisting breech birth at term? *Lancet* 2000;356:1368–1369.
85. American College of Obstetricians and Gynecologists. Mode of term singleton breech delivery. ACOG Committee Opinion No. 265. Washington, DC: ACOG; 2001.
86. American College of Obstetricians and Gynecologists. Practice Bulletin. Shoulder dystocia. No. 40. Washington, DC: ACOG; 2002.
87. Chien PFW, Owen P, Khan KS. Validity of ultrasound estimation of fetal weight. *Obstet Gynecol* 2000;1995:856–860.
88. O'Leary J, Leonetti H. Shoulder dystocia: Prevention and treatment. *Am J Obstet Gynecol* 1990;162:5–9.

Chapter 16
The Maternal Fetal Medicine Viewpoint: Causation and Litigation

Barry S. Schifrin and Wayne R. Cohen

Summary Identification of risk factors and discussion of these with the patient is critical to satisfactory outcomes.

Keywords: dystocia · legal · palsy · traction

Contents

16.1	Definition	227
16.2	Incidence and Etiology	229
16.3	Mechanism of Shoulder Dystocia	231
16.4	Fetal Risk Factors	232
16.5	Labor Risk Factors	232
16.6	Prediction Models	233
16.7	Clinical Management	234
16.8	Documentation	237
16.9	Defining the Standard of Care	238
16.10	Pitfalls in Diagnosis and Management	240
16.11	Legal Implications	241
16.12	Conclusion	244

16.1 Definition

Shoulder dystocia has been defined as "any non-spontaneous birth requiring extensive traction and specific maneuvers to disimpact the infant's shoulder girdle [1]." Others have defined it as a "...delivery requiring maneuvers in addition to gentle downward traction on the fetal head to effect delivery" or "...the tight approximation of the fetal head to the maternal perineum after the head is delivered [2]." Still others have simply relied on the delivering clinician's attestation that difficulty was encountered [3,4]. These definitions will depend on the

B.S. Schifrin

Consulting Obstetrician, Department of Obstetrics & Gynecology, Kaiser Permanente, Los Angeles Medical Center, Los Angeles, California, USA

J.A. O'Leary (ed.), *Shoulder Dystocia and Birth Injury*,
DOI 10.1007/978-1-59745-473-5_16, © Humana Press, a part of Springer
Science+Business Media, LLC 2009

amount of effort and sense of urgency, which varies considerably in these cases, as well as the objectivity and judgment of the clinician delivering the fetus [3–6].

In an effort to reduce some of the subjectivity in the diagnosis, others have used a definition of more than 60 seconds elapsing between delivery of the head and delivery of the shoulders [7]. The normal interval is about 24 seconds, and shoulder dystocia appears in about 75% of those in whom this interval is greater than 60 seconds. There is likely a rough correlation between the head-to-shoulder time interval and the number of maneuvers used before delivery of the shoulders with the degree of difficulty encountered in the delivery; but these are not always reliable indicators nor do they give credit for patience and gentleness.

As explained elsewhere in this volume, cases of shoulder dystocia that also involve brachial plexus injury (BPI) in the newborn account for a significant proportion of malpractice suits. The response to this spate of allegations of negligence surrounding BPI has engendered some novel explanations of provenance of shoulder dystocia and BPI all of which conspire to exculpate the obstetrician from any role in the causation of BPI. Both the dread of allegations of negligence and these theories have certainly modified that which is recorded in the (obstetric medical record). For example, recent literature has suggested a different provenance of brachial plexus injury depending upon whether "shoulder dystocia" is recorded in the medical record [8–12].

Similarly, conventional explanations of injury may be offered depending upon whether it is the "posterior" or "anterior" shoulder that is injured. Beyond this in the current foment about malpractice, physicians may be reluctant to commit the term *shoulder dystocia* to the chart, especially if the newborn demonstrates weakness or overt brachial plexus injury or other stigmata of mechanical injury. On numerous occasions, we have found "shoulder dystocia," or "difficult delivery" or "traumatic delivery" recorded in the neonatal record when it is absent from the obstetric record. In other situations, the mother may indicate that fundal pressure was used either before or after the delivery of the head. In any of these situations, it should be assumed that shoulder dystocia was encountered. From a neonatal standpoint, we have found institutions in which the diagnosis of brachial plexus injury is euphemistically designated as "weakness of the shoulder" (an entity for which there is no ICD-9 code).

As a practical matter, therefore, we consider the diagnosis of shoulder dystocia when special maneuvers, beyond the degree of gentle traction used commonly in normal deliveries, are necessary to effect the emergence of the shoulders. Further, this diagnosis should receive an ICD-9 code for shoulder dystocia in the medical record if the term appears anywhere in the mother or neonatal record or if any special maneuvers, including the McRoberts maneuver, fundal or suprapubic pressure are mentioned as part of the delivery process.

Other factors that may make the delivery more or less difficult are the vector and the degree of angulation of the neck during traction and the use of fundal pressure or maternal pushing that is used concurrently with attempts at delivery. The sequence of maneuvers may also play a role. Although there is no agreed upon sequence for management, it has been suggested that the delivery of the posterior arm should be the first maneuver [7,8]. Checking for and eliminating the compound presentation (the sacral hand wedge) may quickly resolve any difficulty in delivery or shoulder dystocia [13]. These various factors confound the ability to estimate the amount of force to which the nerve roots are exposed over time during the various obstetric maneuvers. Ultimately, the clinician appears to be an unreliable judge of the amount of force that he uses during these sessions [14], and whereas obstetricians may categorize the effort involved in managing shoulder dystocia as mild, moderate, or severe, there is no objective means to verify or validate such assessments. Irrespective, there is credible data to suggest that experience reduces both the incidence and risks of shoulder dystocia.

Believing that permanent BPI complicates only 1 case in 4,553 deliveries, Chauhan et al. [15] calculated that the average American College of Obstetricians and Gynecologists (ACOG) obstetrician performing 140 deliveries per year would encounter one such event in every 33 years of practice. This approach to the evaluation of brachial plexus injuries, even if the statistics were true, and without the evaluation of a single case, permits the authors to refer to these events as maloccurrences (i.e., an adverse event in which no negligence can be imputed). They also forward this approach to explain why the prevalence of injury has not decreased and may indeed be increasing [15].

16.2 Incidence and Etiology

The range of incidences of shoulder dystocia and its complications are presented in Table 16.1. Those clinical risk factors associated with an increased risk of shoulder dystocia and its consequences are listed in Table 16.2. Notwithstanding the numerous factors that increase the risk, shoulder dystocia is a complication that is not always foreseeable or reasonably preventable (other than by timely cesarean). It is certainly *not predictable* in the individual case, in the sense of predicting the future [1,16,20]. Even if one takes patients with the highest risk of shoulder dystocia (i.e., a repeat shoulder dystocia), it only occurs about 50% of the time.

The cause of neonatal brachial plexus injury has traditionally been assumed to be traction injury, not to the plexus, but to the affected nerve roots during delivery. This would seem to be the explanation in the majority of cases [21–23]. Whether sufficient traction to injure the plexus is necessarily the consequence of overly energetic maneuvers by the obstetrician or obstetric ineptness is less certain. Indeed, there is credible evidence that some cases of neonatal BPI occur prior to delivery or occur during delivery despite minimal or absent interference by the attendant [24–27]. or even at the time of cesarean section. As a minimum, at least some BPI occurs unrelated to excessive or misdirected efforts to extract impacted shoulders or the presence of shoulder dystocia. It has been estimated that BPI occurs in the absence of documented shoulder dystocia 15% to 50% of the time [8–10].

Table 16.1   Incidence Figures and References

	References	Incidence (%)
Shoulder dystocia	8–12	0.13–2.0
Brachial plexus injury	11, 13	5–25 of SD
All births	9, 15–24	0.5–5.4
With shoulder dystocia	—	50–85
Not preceded by shoulder dystocia	—	15–50
Permanent injury	16, 19,25, 26	20–50

SD, shoulder dystocia.

Given the limited ability to forecast the appearance of shoulder dystocia and the understanding that adverse fetal or maternal outcome may occur despite expert obstetric management, optimal outcome in an individual case is possible only if the attendant anticipates the problem when it is reasonable to do so, understands the nature of the disorder, and has a systematic approach to

Table 16.2   Risk Factors for Shoulder Dystocia/Erb Palsy

Demographic	
Prior shoulder dystocia	(OR 76.1, 95% CI 69, 84)*
Previous macrosomia	
Obesity	
Multiparity	
Advanced maternal age	
Short stature	
Maternal body weight	
Abnormal pelvic size/shape	
Antepartum	
Gestational diabetes	(OR 1.9, 95% CI 1.7, 2.1)*
Excessive weight gain	
Postdates pregnancy	
Male gender	
Intrapartum	
Malpresentation (nonbreech)	(OR 73.6, 95% CI 66, 83)*
Severe birth asphyxia	(OR 13.6, 95% CI 8.3, 22.5)*
Mild birth asphyxia	(OR 6.3, 95% CI 3.9, 10.1)*
Molding of the fetal head	
Precipitous labor	
Arrest of labor, abnormalities of descent	
Delivery	
Forceps delivery	(OR 3.4, 95% CI 2.7, 4.3)*
Vacuum extraction	(OR 2.7, 95% CI 2.4, 3.1)*
Physician experience	

OR, odds ratio; CI, confidence interval. *Data from Nesbitt, et al (Ref. 47).

management involving anticipation, preparation, and implementation that has been rehearsed and ready to employ without delay. Indeed, the problems of shoulder dystocia and its accompanying complications may be increasing in frequency [23]. perhaps related to the recent trends to increasing birthweight in turn related to improved maternal nutrition and obesity.

Although there always remains a degree of uncertainty about the inevitable appearance of shoulder dystocia, anticipation comes from a proper sequential analysis of the various prenatal, intrapartum, and delivery risk factors associated with shoulder dystocia. Several risk factors that make the problem at least foreseeable, the legal issue, are enumerated in Table 16.2.

The vast majority of cases of shoulder dystocia and its attendant serious complications are avoidable by performing cesarean delivery. More pertinent, perhaps, is the question of how much serious injury will be avoided when these labors are managed ideally by experienced accoucheurs including proper timing of cesarean delivery. Given the infrequency of occurrence, the multiplicity of factors contributing to shoulder dystocia, and/or brachial palsy, a controlled trial is unreasonable. More reasonably, some estimate of optimal outcome will come from the implementation of a comprehensive program of care beginning in the prenatal period based on logistic regression analysis of large data sets reflecting well-annotated clinical experience.

One approach to developing a value-based approach to management is to ask how many unnecessary cesarean deliveries would be required to prevent each case managed more or less conventionally. This approach, however, may not be totally satisfying from the perspective of setting clinical policy, because it is essentially an economic analysis that cannot readily incorporate the short-term and long-term indirect costs of more cesarean deliveries. It also fails to assess the value of an uninjured life. Notwithstanding the limitations of such a calculus, most of the available evidence does not support a policy of routine cesarean section for the fetus with suspected macrosomia [27,28], although this approach has more appeal in pregnancies complicated by diabetes [29].

16.3 Mechanism of Shoulder Dystocia

During normal labor in a gynecoid pelvis, the fetal head engages and descends to the midcavity in a transverse position. As internal rotation and delivery of the head proceed, the shoulders engage in the inlet, generally in an oblique diameter (although this is quite variable).

As the fetus descends through the birth canal and the head undergoes the cardinal movements of labor, the shoulders and the trunk accommodate to the birth canal serving to ensure proper engagement of the shoulders. This process has been termed *shoulder molding* [30]. This maneuver allows the posterior shoulder to negotiate the sacral promontory. With the shoulder girdle oriented obliquely, the anterior shoulder then stems beneath the symphysis and emerges under the subpubic arch. Several factors may, individually or in combination, confound the normal accommodation and descent of the shoulder girdle. These may relate to the fetus, to the pelvis, or to the rate of descent.

16.4 Fetal Risk Factors

Virtually all studies indicate that the most important risk factor is fetal size. Thus, fetal macrosomia (variously defined) has a very strong association with shoulder dystocia and its complications. There is, in fact, a direct relation between birthweight and the likelihood of shoulder dystocia. It is therefore not surprising that various factors associated with high birthweight (maternal diabetes, obesity, and excessive weight gain during pregnancy, and a history of large babies) are also associated with shoulder dystocia [18,31].

When the fetus is very large, the shoulders may be too broad to engage normally, and one or both shoulders may remain trapped at the inlet as the head delivers. More commonly, the posterior shoulder transverses the promontory, but the anterior shoulder becomes impacted behind the symphysis pubis. In the fetus of a diabetic mother, the bisacromial diameter is disproportionately large in relation to head size [32,33]. A similar phenomenon of disproportionate growth appears to be present in fetuses of nondiabetic mothers who encounter shoulder dystocia [31,33]. Thus, large fetal size and (perhaps more importantly) disproportionate growth of the trunk predispose to shoulder dystocia and, in turn, brachial plexus injury. This may occur in any fetus and may have some relationship to maternal obesity [34]. It must, however, be borne in mind that 20% to 50% of cases of brachial plexus injury occur in fetuses of average weight [35], and some are related to obstetric factors (e.g., compound presentation [13]) that are not associated with fetal macrosomia (i.e., birthweight greater than 4000 g).

16.5 Labor Risk Factors

It would be logical to assume that if shoulder dystocia and newborn brachial plexus palsy are strongly associated with large fetal weight, abnormalities of labor should share a similar association. The literature, however, is inconsistent in this regard. Several studies failed to demonstrate that dysfunctional labor patterns were precursors to difficult shoulder delivery [17,36–39]. Unfortunately, many of these studies did not use standardized definitions for labor dysfunctions or failed to control for parity. In fact, few studies have addressed thoroughly the relationships among labor disorders, shoulder dystocia, and brachial plexus injury. Most have confined their observations to descent in the second stage of labor, without objective, detailed analysis of patterns of dilatation or descent [36–38]. Better designed studies strongly suggest that first- and second-stage (arrest and protraction) disorders often precede brachial plexus injury [19,20,31,35,40,41]. Thus, properly evaluated, as many as three fourths of brachial plexus injuries are preceded by abnormal labor. Nevertheless, most labor abnormalities do not individually have high sensitivity for the confident prediction of shoulder dystocia or brachial plexus palsy [31]. Those labor abnormalities most commonly associated with difficult shoulder delivery are characterized by either sluggish dilatation and descent or (seemingly paradoxically) by exceptionally rapid descent [31].

One type of abnormal labor, the prolonged deceleration phase, appears to be a particularly strong independent predictor of Erb palsy [20,30,31]. It is a harbinger of second-stage labor abnormalities and difficulty with shoulder delivery [42]. When a prolonged deceleration phase occurs in the context of suspected macrosomia and other first-stage abnormalities, a cesarean section should be strongly considered. This relationship emphasizes the view that a prolonged deceleration phase actually is a problem of descent more than of dilatation, inasmuch as some descent of the presenting part is normally required for the last portion of dilatation to be accomplished as the cervix retracts around the presenting part.

Many cases of shoulder dystocia follow precipitate descent [4]. In these situations, one may presume inadequate time for normal shoulder accommodation results in the bisacromial diameter remaining in the anteroposterior diameter of the inlet when the head has delivered. The same process may explain the frequent association of instrumental delivery, vacuum or forceps, and shoulder impaction [18,41,43–47]. By accelerating the rate of descent artificially, insufficient time for the shoulders to conform to the pelvis results in their being in an abnormal position at the time of the expected engagement.

Many studies confirm that instrumental delivery, by vacuum or forceps, is an independent, strong risk factor for shoulder dystocia and brachial plexus injury, particularly when undertaken from the midpelvis [41,44–48]. Whether this is a consequence of the artificially rapid descent produced by instrumented traction or is simply a reflection of the fact that forceps or vacuum are more likely to be used and labor progress compromised when the fetus is very large is unclear. Certainly, the data strongly suggest that instrumental delivery should be avoided whenever there has been a preceding dysfunctional labor. Obviously, the risks and benefits of this kind of delivery must be weighed in individual situations, but as a generalization, it should be recognized that its use, particularly in association with other risk factors (suspected macrosomia, dysfunctional labor), carries a strong association with shoulder dystocia and subsequent injury.

16.6 Prediction Models

There are several approaches to identifying risk factors for adverse medical events. Most studies regarding risk factors for shoulder dystocia and Erb palsy have used univariate approaches; some have used multivariate modeling or discriminate analysis designed to estimate the individual contribution of specific factors to risk. In this regard, it is important to remember that only a minority of shoulder dystocia cases result in brachial plexus injury; and that

20% to 40% of brachial plexus palsies identified in the immediate newborn period were not preceded by documented shoulder dystocia.

A published prediction model [49]. incorporating birthweight and maternal size as major predictors had a high sensitivity for the prediction of shoulder dystocia. The shortcomings of this model are that it used only information available at the onset of labor and after delivery (birthweight). As such, it ignored the influence of intrapartum events on the predictability of injury in an individual case and used a parameter (birthweight) we have difficulty predicting.

A risk score for BPI (not shoulder dystocia!) has been recently developed based on the multiple logistic regression coefficients for various demographic and clinical observations including maternal body mass index, glucose intolerance, the deceleration phase and the second stage of labor, estimated fetal weight, and race [50]. Most of these variables were found to be independently associated with brachial plexus injury in a prior analysis [31]. The application of such prediction models will allow us to more broadly estimate how many additional cesarean sections would be required to prevent a case of neonatal BPI, assuming that the experience and skill of the obstetrician along with the philosophy of dealing with perceived macrosamia at term and management of aberrations of labor were held constant. It is important to recognize that such models will be population-specific, but not necessarily physician-specific. The relevance of the algorithm will depend on the baseline prevalence of fetal macrosomia and Erb palsy in the population, the racial and morphometric characteristics of the patients, and the prevalence of obesity and glucose intolerance. In theory, an optimal predictive model would need to be developed for each population (and for each physician!). A robust electronic database would make this possible, at least on a regional, if not a hospital-specific, basis. Alternatively, hospitals could match their own demographics to an existing model in order to enhance its sensitivity.

There are difficulties with interpreting risk factor information and using it clinically. For example, whereas macrosomia and its associated factors confer high risk, a substantial proportion (many studies suggest about half) of lower brachial plexus injuries occur in average-size babies. Some even occur in pre-term infants, albeit rarely. Multivariate analyses tend to support the importance of the factors mentioned above and explain their interaction. In one study, for example, gestational diabetes was not a significant risk factor in a multivariate model because its effects were explained by its association with maternal obesity and large fetal size [31]. New predictive models [50], which still require testing, may bring us closer to an understanding of how to use risk factor analysis to create guidelines for intervention.

16.7 Clinical Management

The obstetrician should have a logical strategy to confront shoulder dystocia, recognizing that each circumstance may require modifications. Many approaches have been suggested in the literature [16,51,52]. There exist no data clearly demonstrating the superiority of any particular maneuver or series of maneuvers. Clinical judgment (i.e., taking into account all the information [risk factors]. that are or should be known and making a reasonable plan) and skill are vital if successful atraumatic delivery is to occur. It is important that whatever efforts are made to effect delivery be done with slow, steady application of force. This may be less likely to result in injury than more robust forces applied over a short period of time [53]. Use of maneuvers prophylactically does not appear to be beneficial [54].

When the diagnosis of shoulder dystocia is made, pushing should cease and a vaginal examination should assess the position of the shoulders and the degree of descent of the posterior shoulder. In addition, the presence of a compound presentation (with the hand) should be sought (see later). Under most circumstances, the posterior shoulder will be found below the sacral promontory, near the ischial spines in the hollow of the sacrum, and the bisacromial diameter of the fetus will be in the direct anteroposterior diameter of the pelvis. If this is the case, the first maneuver should be directed toward rotating the shoulders into an oblique diameter of the pelvis [55,56].

This is generally most easily accomplished by rotating the posterior shoulder ventrally by pressure behind the scapula (i.e., clockwise from an left occiput transverse [LOT] position). To facilitate rotation, there may be pressure in the opposite direction applied to the ventral surface of the anterior shoulder through the abdominal wall. To accomplish this maneuver, the obstetrician inserts at least two fingers of the appropriate hand against the appropriate surface of the shoulders. The maneuver may also be used in either direction, and there is no evidence that forward or backward rotation is preferable. In either case, some complementary suprapubic pressure should be provided by an assistant. This pressure is to be directed posterolaterally on the mother's abdomen and is designed to push the anterior shoulder in the desired (i.e., opposite) direction. This maneuver requires clear communication between the obstetrician and assistant. Often, these maneuvers are sufficient to effect delivery.

Some obstetricians advocate awaiting the next uterine contraction before attempting to release the impacted shoulders. This may, in fact, be beneficial even in cases when shoulder complications are not anticipated. The extra time may allow gradual accommodation of the shoulder girdle to the birth canal and spontaneous assumption of an oblique position. Above all, when shoulder dystocia is diagnosed, it is important not to panic, not to rush, and not to place any traction on the fetal head and neck.

The McRoberts maneuver is widely recommended to be used early in the course of management [16]. It involves flexing the mother's thighs against her abdomen. This approach appears to be helpful in many instances [52,54,57–59], but questions have been raised as to the appropriateness of this maneuver as the primary response to shoulder dystocia because it may worsen the situation or cause maternal complications including gluteal pain, dysesthesia, symphyseal separation, sacroiliac joint dislocation, and transient lateral femoral cutaneous neuropathy [55,60,61]. Maintaining the patient in an exaggerated lithotomy position while actively pushing during the second stage of labor and the use of excessive force should be avoided. Experience with simulator models of shoulder dystocia suggests that attempts to rotate the shoulders place less force on the brachial plexus than does the McRoberts approach [55].

The Woods maneuver, described in 1943 [62], involves rotating the posterior shoulder 180 degrees to the anterior position. This will often result in its delivery beneath the pubic arch and does not require or induce any traction on the neck.

Another tactic that can be beneficial is delivery of the posterior arm [12]. With the anterior shoulder impacted against the pubic symphysis, the operator inserts a hand along the ventral surface of the fetus and locates the posterior arm, which is often extended. The operator flexes the arm gently at the elbow and draws it across the fetal chest, taking care not to force the arm into an unphysiologic position. Fracture of the humerus may result if the arm is extracted without first flexing the elbow and placing traction on the hand. Once the arm is extracted, the posterior then the anterior shoulder usually deliver easily. If not, application of the Woods maneuver is almost always effective.

When the initial examination after diagnosis reveals a compound presentation, extraction of the arm can be used as an initial maneuver, particularly if the posterior hand/arm is present. Whereas delivery of the presenting arm in a compound presentation generally requires little force, its extraction can be exceptionally difficult when the fetus is quite large. This affords little space for manipulation and flexion of the elbow, and fractures are not uncommon, despite the best efforts of the operator.

More aggressive approaches to shoulder dystocia have been advocated for situations that do not resolve with traditional methods. Symphysiotomy has been used effectively in some parts of the world but has never achieved acceptance in the United States or Europe [63–67]. It can have serious complications, and its success rate is unknown. The Zavanelli maneuver involves pushing the head back into the vagina, reversing the prior mechanism of labor, and delivering the fetus by cesarean section. A number of reports of success with this maneuver have been described, as have serious complications including death and subsequent neurologic injury [68–75]. The benefits of this procedure of last resort are not fully understood.

Intentional fracture of the clavicle is often mentioned as a technique for managing arrested shoulders. In theory, this approach may be helpful, but it is practiced rarely and in our experience is more easily said than done. Injury to the subclavian vessels or entry into the pleural space may occur, and some have suggested that its use be restricted to dead fetuses. Instrumental cleidotomy in a live fetus should be avoided because of the great risk of laceration of the subclavian vessels.

Maternal positions other than the traditional modified lithotomy position may be beneficial in alleviating shoulder impaction. Although controlled data are lacking, advocates of alternative positions for delivery say that hindrance of shoulder delivery is encountered rarely when women deliver in upright postures.

Squatting for delivery has several potential advantages in this regard. Delivery with the mother in the lateral position may also have some benefits, and good clinical success has been reported with the "all fours" position (i.e., with the patient on her hands and knees) [76,77]. McRoberts maneuver may be considered as an alternative posture for delivery. Almost no attention has been paid to the position of the accoucheur. At least theoretically, the sitting position at or below the level of fetal head provides a better estimation of the vector of traction than does the standing position.

Whatever maneuvers are used to treat shoulder dystocia, several principles should be paramount. Remain calm and give clear logical instructions to assistants and the patient; do not rush; and use a logical sequence of maneuvers to resolve the dystocia. Avoid the temptation to use intense fundal pressure or suprapubic pressure directed posteriorly. The primary purpose of this maneuver is to assist in rotation and perhaps secondarily to narrow the shoulder girdle. These maneuvers are not especially helpful and may result in fetal injury or even uterine rupture [78,79]. Once the anterior shoulder begins to stem beneath the symphysis, the force may be relaxed somewhat. Some experts sanction the use of fundal pressure at this point, but this is controversial [80]. Forsake attempts to deliver the anterior shoulder by traction on the neck and head. The only part of the fetus that should be manipulated is the shoulders, not the head or the neck. It is remarkable how little force is sometimes necessary to produce BPI, especially if applied in the wrong direction. Sometimes, a large episiotomy may be useful to eliminate soft tissue resistance to delivery and, most importantly, to allow sufficient room for intravaginal or intrauterine manipulation [81]. Its use is a matter of clinical judgment.

16.8 Documentation

Appropriate recording of the events associated with a shoulder dystocia in the medical record is vital. Such documentation serves an important function in allowing detailed and accurate interpretation of the delivery by those evaluating it in retrospect and indeed for reviewing one's own experience. This may be important from the points of view of education, billing, and risk management.

Although most annotations in the medical record in cases of shoulder dystocia begin with details of the delivery itself, this is insufficient. In fact, the delivery note should begin by summarizing the prenatal course up to the point of hospitalization. It should scrupulously record any demographic, obstetric, and prenatal factors that are associated with an increased risk of shoulder dystocia. If risks arise during labor, the record should include an itemization and an assessment of them and how they influenced the plans for managing labor and delivery. The record should demonstrate consideration was given to the likely risk of difficulties at delivery, the thoughtful preparation for them, and a discussion about these risks with the mother.

Table 16.3 Documenting the delivery complicated by shoulder dystocia

Times
  Delivery of the head
  Delivery completed
Risk factors
  Previous pregnancy
  Present pregnancy, especially diabetes
  Intrapartum
  Estimated fetal weight (EFW)
  Course of labor dilatation pattern, descent pattern
  Type of anesthesia used during labor and delivery
Delivery
  Use and type of episiotomy
    1. Maneuvers used, sequence, estimated amount of effort.
    2. Identification of anterior and posterior shoulders and their position at the outset of maneuvers.
    3. Presence of a compound presentation.
    4. An indication that throughout the maneuvers the fetal spine was maintained in the axial plane of the body.
    5. Maternal trauma
    6. Any difficulties with patient compliance potentially affect outcome.
    7. Personnel present at time of delivery.
    8. Examination of the infant in the delivery room.
Notification of personnel
  The neonatologist with specific recommendation to examine the fetal shoulders, spine, and extremities is helpful.
  Patient counseling for the next pregnancy. The note must reflect a reasonable estimate of the feasibility of safe vaginal delivery in a subsequent delivery. If the physician believes that a subsequent delivery should be done by cesarean section, this should be stated unequivocally in the chart and said directly to the mother.

A detailed delivery note should always be created (preferably dictated within a reasonable period of time after the delivery) and contain, at a minimum, the information contained in Table 16.3.

The neonatal record, in addition to a physical examination pertinent to identifying possible injuries, should include birthweight and head circumference, thoracic circumference, and abdominal circumference measurements of the newborn. The mother must be informed about the shoulder dystocia and the implications for the next delivery.

16.9 Defining the Standard of Care

If we define the standard of care in the anticipation and management of shoulder dystocia and brachial plexus birth injury to include that which a reasonably trained physician would do in extant circumstances, it is clear that a broad range of approaches to the problem, properly and timely executed (and annotated), would be acceptable.

All obstetric units should have a protocol for the anticipation and management of shoulder dystocia. Because it is often an unexpected event, it is necessary to call upon all of the necessary interdisciplinary resources and to have them available promptly. Each member of the team (obstetricians, nurses, anesthesiologists, neonatologists, neonatal resuscitation team, etc.) should be familiar with his or her role in the event a shoulder dystocia supervenes. Optimally, practice drills to ensure smooth operation of the protocol should be done periodically. Some obstetric units now require satisfactory participation in these drills for reappointment to the hospital staff.

16.9.1 Responsibilities of the Physician

The physician must identify and document risk factors from historical, prenatal, and intrapartum periods. He/she must document the discussion with the patient about these risks and the alternative options. In our opinion, these discussions of the risks and the stakes with the patient must occur during the labor when the risk calculus is modified on the basis of progress in labor and any new pertinent events—without coercion. There should be a discussion with the patient about what may occur in the event a shoulder dystocia occurs, preferably with a witness present. This should be annotated in the record. It may sometimes occur that the patient may refuse the recommendation of performing cesarean section. This also must be witnessed and annotated.

When a strong risk factor(s) exists and vaginal delivery is contemplated, it is necessary to alert the appropriate personnel and have them immediately available in anticipation of encountering a shoulder dystocia. Discuss the risks and plans, including the fact that no difficulties may be encountered, preferably with a witness present, and record in the chart that this discussion took place.

Shoulder dystocia must be immediately recognized and the emergency situation declared and assistance summoned: another obstetrician, nurse, anesthesiologist, and pediatrician. The time should be recorded and, as mentioned above, some time may be taken to elaborate everyone's role (including the patient's) before beginning any maneuver. The physician must avoid *any* lateral (downward) traction on the fetal head or neck beyond the minimum necessary to confirm the diagnosis. In all maneuvers, the fetal spine should be maintained erect! Fundal pressure and energetic pushing, especially while the anterior shoulder is trapped behind the pubic symphysis, must be scrupulously avoided as they only increase the amount of force necessary to overcome the impaction of the shoulders. The physician should perform the maneuvers in a logical sequence in a competent fashion to free the shoulders.

1. Explaining to the patient what is going on during the crisis to the extent possible.
2. Thoroughly examine the birth canal after delivery for injuries.
3. Thoroughly document the events of management in the medical record.
4. After the delivery, explain to the patient what happened, document this discussion, and provide emotional support to her and her family.
5. At some point, the physician must discuss with the patient his or her recommendations about the route of delivery for the next pregnancy! This must be documented in the chart and efforts taken to make sure that the patient indeed understands the recommendation.

16.9.2 Responsibilities of the Nursing Staff

1. Familiarity with hospital protocol for dealing with shoulder dystocia.
2. Participation in "shoulder dystocia drills" if available.
3. Discussing potential prenatal and intrapartum risk factors with the responsible physician.
4. Discussing with the patient what may occur in the event a shoulder dystocia occurs.
5. Assisting the physician with management of the dystocia (e.g., suprapubic pressure to rotate the shoulders; changing the patient's position to McRoberts, the lateral position, and the hands and knees position).
6. Calling for assistance from nurses and other personnel according to hospital protocol.
7. Recording time of delivery of the head, and delivery of the body, and which shoulder (anterior/posterior/right/left) delivered first.
8. Recording other significant events that occurred during delivery.
9. Providing emotional support to the patient and her family.

16.10 Pitfalls in Diagnosis and Management

The major pitfalls encountered by the obstetrician relate to the failure to be prepared for and to optimally manage shoulder dystocia. Preparation is obviously important when risk factors exist, although it must be borne in mind that shoulder dystocia may develop unexpectedly in the absence of any demonstrable risk factors. The potential for shoulder dystocia should be presumed to exist in any delivery. The likelihood of a good outcome when shoulder dystocia occurs is enhanced if appropriate anticipatory action has been taken to address it or to avoid it if an insurmountable situation is likely. Specifically, this involves being sure that timely observations are made before and during labor, that emerging risk factors are identified, including the course of labor, and that adequate help is promptly available in the delivery room from obstetricians, nurses, anesthesiologists, and pediatricians.

The failure to identify risk factors for shoulder dystocia most commonly resides in one or more of the following areas:

1. Failure to identify relevant aspects of the patient's previous obstetric history (prior large babies, shoulder dystocia, Gestational diabetes mellitus (GDM), instrumental delivery, dysfunctional labor).
2. Failure to identify pertinent factors that arise during prenatal care (relative glucose intolerance; frank diabetes, obesity, excessive weight gain, large estimated fetal weight, adverse pelvic architecture).
3. Failure to recognize the presence of intrapartum risk factors (development of dysfunctional labor, especially long deceleration phase and long second stage; anatomic features of the pelvis that predispose; large fetal weight).
4. Unfamiliarity with the proper way to perform maneuvers to relieve the shoulder impaction.
5. Failure to properly document all of the events of the labor and delivery.
6. Failure to properly estimate the likely success of safe vaginal delivery when forceps or vacuum are used.

If shoulder dystocia occurs, a retrospective analysis of the record should reveal the following documentation.

1. Documentation of a discussion of shoulder dystocia during prenatal care.
2. Estimated fetal weight prior to labor and during labor.
3. Results of the prenatal glucose challenge test and oral glucose tolerance tests.
4. Presence of maternal obesity or excessive weight gain.
5. Prior birthweights if the patient is a multipara.
6. Presence of prior shoulder dystocia if the patient is a multipara.
7. A history of instrumented vaginal delivery.
8. Clinical pelvimetry done during labor.
9. Recognition of labor abnormalities.
10. Documentation of fetal position and the mechanism of labor.
11. A specific tabulation of those factors influencing the decision to proceed with a trial of labor and vaginal delivery (i.e., a serial reevaluation of the probability of safe vaginal delivery when appropriate).

Shortcomings in documentation of the delivery are common. The dictated delivery note must contain a complete description of all the events that occurred once the diagnosis of shoulder dystocia was made. This should include a comment regarding the fact that every effort was made to keep the fetal neck in the axial plane during the delivery.

16.11 Legal Implications

Newborn brachial plexus palsy is one of the most common sources of obstetric malpractice litigation. The average settlement cost for cases of this sort is substantially higher than that of obstetric medical negligence suits in general, averaging nearly $500,000 in New York State (personal communication from Medical Liability Mutual Insurance Corporation, 2006).

Medical and legal attitudes about this disorder have changed in recent decades, resulting in more defense verdicts and a change in strategy on the part of plaintiff and defendant. It had been previously assumed that the presence of a neonatal brachial plexus abnormality was *prima facie* evidence of medical negligence, inasmuch as all such problems were assumed to be birth injuries resulting from excessive traction applied by the obstetrician abetted by fundal pressure. As a consequence, successful defense of such cases was quite uncommon, and plaintiff verdicts were common.

More recent evidence, noted above, has established clearly that not all cases are the consequence of the obstetrician's excesses, in part related to the awareness that fundal pressure is an inappropriate response to shoulder dystocia. Some transient neonatal Erb palsies occur in the absence of any difficulties at the time of delivery and have been documented in deliveries after perfectly normal labors and with essentially no more than superficial contact by the obstetrician at delivery. Some data suggest that there are cases in which the injury is an *in utero* event, unrelated to the delivery itself. As a consequence of these observations, the focus of litigation has shifted somewhat from the assumption that the presence of an injury is incontrovertible evidence of negligence to the notion that either the complication should have been anticipated (not predicted) based on preexisting risk factors (and the baby therefore delivered by cesarean) or that the maneuvers used to overcome shoulder dystocia at the time of delivery were employed inappropriately or negligently. The change in the frequency of plaintiff verdicts has not been accompanied by a diminution in the incidence of shoulder dystocia or BPI [82].

The ability to foresee the development of shoulder dystocia is quite limited at present, as detailed previously. Many of the allegations relating to these issues aver that the obstetrician failed to identify appropriately obesity, weight gain, or postdates, or failed to test for or appropriately diagnose gestational diabetes. There are often allegations that the obstetrician failed to determine the estimated fetal weight accurately. This may extend to criticism of the ultrasound technique and cast doubt on the individual's clinical acumen when the actual birthweight far exceeds the estimate. The failure to perform serial ultrasounds in high-risk patients or estimate the fetal weight can also be criticized.

The plaintiff may claim that the physician failed to offer elective cesarean delivery prior to labor in patients with multiple risk factors. Given sufficient risk factors, the patient must be informed and informed consent obtained (informed consent is *not* given). Allegations that, during labor, the obstetrician failed to recognize abnormal labor patterns that predispose to shoulder dystocia and nerve plexus injury or that the decision to perform operative vaginal delivery was inappropriate are common. Finally, mismanagement of shoulder dystocia when it occurs is often charged. This failure may include the use of inappropriate maneuvers to remove the impacted shoulder, the failure to use accepted maneuvers in these efforts, or the failure to have appropriately trained and experienced personnel at the time of delivery. In fact, the greater the severity of the nerve impairment, the more compelling will be the argument that excessive traction or traction applied in the wrong direction was used.

The keys to a successful defense of these cases include the presence of thorough and comprehensive prenatal and intrapartum records. The record should document the physician's concerns if there have been identified risk factors. In addition, it is vital the events of labor and delivery are documented in detail, including the rationale for any interventions during labor (use of oxytocin, vacuum, or forceps). If a shoulder dystocia is encountered, there must be clear documentation of maneuvers to relieve the problem and of other events at the delivery. Finally, it is important that the obstetrician be familiar with the details of the case and of both the theoretical and practical aspects of its management. Documentation of care should include the patient's participation in decision making.

In short, the record should show that the obstetrician exercised reasonable care in anticipating shoulder dystocia; advised the patient appropriately, and took all reasonable measures to manage it if it occurred. This would include the following minimum requirements:

Prenatal

1. Obtain and record a full obstetric history, with all available details of previous deliveries and their complications, birthweights and outcomes, especially with regard to prior shoulder dystocia, macrosomic infant, labor dysfunction, and instrumental delivery.
2. Obtain and document risk factors for macrosomia and perform and record tests for gestational diabetes, as appropriate.
3. Estimate the fetal weight near term and document this estimate.
4. Discuss shoulder dystocia and brachial plexus injury with all patients, just as the possibility of cesarean is discussed. Document that these discussions occurred.
5. Determine based on history and prenatal events whether there are risk factors for shoulder injury present.

Intrapartum

1. Estimate and document fetal weight.
2. Use labor curves to assess and document labor progress in dilatation and descent.
3. Reassess periodically during labor the likelihood of difficult shoulder delivery.
4. Adjust plans for delivery as new information emerges. Document all plans and observations and discuss with patient.
5. If shoulder dystocia is reasonably foreseeable and vaginal delivery is planned, be sure appropriate personnel are readily available at delivery.
6. If shoulder dystocia occurs, manage according to the principles outlined above and document all aspects of care.

16.12 Conclusion

It should be emphasized that if, after discussing the potential for shoulder dystocia with a patient, she desires cesarean section, either this wish must be granted or an agreement to pursue a trial of labor must be renegotiated! The physician may not decide on his or her own the benefits to the patient (the stakes) in this exercise in informed consent, which, in the final analysis, is obtained *from* the patient, not given to her.

After the fact, the defense is assisted materially by apology when appropriate; truthful discussions with the parents that are scheduled separately! not part of routine rounds.

References

1. Cunningham F. Dystocia Abnormal Presentation, Position, and Development of the Fetus In: *Williams Obstetrics*. 21st ed. New York: McGraw-Hill; 2001:459–464.
2. Cohen W, Friedman E. The pelvic division of labor. In: *Management of Labor*. Rockville: Aspen Publishers; 1989:19–60.
3. Acker D, Sachs B, Friedman E. Risk factors for shoulder dystocia. *Obstet Gynecol* 1985;55:762–768.
4. Acker D, Gregory K, Sachs B, Friedman E. Risk factors for Erb-Duchenne palsy. *Obstet Gynecol* 1988;71:389–392.
5. Spong C, Beall M, Rodrigues D, Ross M. An objective definition of shoulder dystocia: Prolonged head-to-body delivery intervals and/or the use of ancillary obstetric maneuvers. *Obstet Gynecol* 1995;86:433–436.
6. Beall M, Spong C, Ross M. A randomized controlled trial of prophylactic maneuvers to reduce head-to-body delivery time in patients at risk for shoulder dystocia. *Obstet Gynecol* 2003;102:31–35.
7. Gherman R, Ouzounian J, Goodwin T. Obstetric maneuvers for shoulder dystocia and associated fetal morbidity. *Am J Obstet Gynecol* 1998;178:1126–1130.
8. Jennett R, Tarby T, Kreinick C. Brachial plexus palsy: An old problem revisited. *Am J Obstet Gynecol* 1992;166:1673–1676.
9. Sandmire H, DeMott R. Erb's palsy without shoulder dystocia. *Int J Gynaecol Obstet* 2002;78:253–256.
10. Jennett R, Tarby T. Brachial plexus palsy: An old problem revisited again. II. Cases in point. *Am J Obstet Gynecol* 1997;176:1354–1356.
11. Beall M, Spong C, McKay J, Ross M. Objective definition of shoulder dystocia: A prospective evaluation. *Am J Obstet Gynecol* 1998;179:934–937.
12. Poggi S, Spong C, Allen R. Prioritizing posterior arm delivery during severe shoulder dystocia. *Obstet Gynecol* 2003;101:1068–1072.
13. Vacca A. The 'sacral hand wedge': A cause of arrest of descent of the fetal head during vacuum assisted delivery. *BJOG* 2002;109:1063–1065.
14. Allen R, Bankoski B, Butzin C, Nagey D. Comparing clinician-applied leads for routine, difficult, and shoulder dystocia deliveries. *Am J Obstet Gynecol* 1994;171:1621–1627.
15. Chauhan S, Magann E, McAninch C, Gherman R, Morrison J. Application of learning theory to obstetric maloccurrence. *J Matern Fetal Neonatal Med* 2003;12:203–207.
16. Shoulder Dystocia. Practice Bulletin. No. 40. Washington, DC: ACOG; 2002.
17. Donnelly V, Foran A, Murphy J, McParland P, Keane D, O'Herlihy C. Neonatal brachial plexus palsy: An unpredictable injury. *Am J Obstet Gynecol* 2002;187:1209–1212.

18. Nocon J, McKenzie D, Thomas L, Hansell R. Shoulder dystocia: An analysis of risks and obstetric maneuvers. *Am J Obstet Gynecol* 1993;168:1732–1737.
19. Gross S, Shime J, Farine D. Shoulder dystocia: Predictors and outcome. A five-year review. *Am J Obstet Gynecol* 1987;156:334–336.
20. Gross T, Sokol R, Williams T, Thompson K. Shoulder dystocia: A fetal-physician risk. *Am J Obstet Gynecol* 1987;156:1408–1418.
21. Kay S. Obstetricial brachial palsy. *Br J Plast Surg* 1998;51:43–50.
22. Dawodu A, Sankaran-Kutty M, Rajan T. Risk factors and prognosis for brachial plexus injury and clavicular fracture in neonates: A prospective analysis from the United Arab Emirates. *Ann Trop Paediatr* 1997;17:195–200.
23. Bager B. Perinatally acquired brachial plexus palsy—a persisting challenge. *Acta Paediatr* 1997;86:1214–1219.
24. Gurewitsch E, Johnson E, Hamzehzadeh S, Allen R. Risk factors for brachial plexus injury with and without shoulder dystocia. *Am J Obstet Gynecol* 2006;194:486–492.
25. Ouzounian J, Korst L, Phelan J. Permanent Erb palsy: A traction-related injury? *Obstet Gynecol* 1997;89:139–141.
26. Gherman R, Ouzounian J, Goodwin T. Brachial plexus palsy: An in-utero injury? *Am J Obstet Gynecol* 1999;180:1303–1307.
27. Keller J, Lopez-Zeno J, Dooley S, Socol M. Shoulder dystocia and birth trauma in gestational diabetes: A five-year experience. *Am J Obstet Gynecol* 191;165:928–930.
28. Ecker J, Greenberg J, Norwitz E, Nadel A, Repke J. Birth weight as a predictor of brachial plexus injury. *Obstet Gynecol* 1997;89:643–647.
29. Langer O, Berkus M, Huff R, Samueloff A. Shoulder dystocia: Should the fetus weighing greater than or equal to 4000 grams be delivered by cesarean section? *Am J Obstet Gynecol* 1991;165:831–837.
30. Hopwood H Jr. Shoulder dystocia: fifteen years' experience in a community hospital. *Am J Obstet Gynecol* 1982;144:162–166.
31. Welzsaeeker K, Deaver J, Cohen W. Labor characteristics and neonatal Erb palsy. *BJOG* 2007;114(8):1003–1009. Epub 2007 Jun 12.
32. Cohen B, Penning S, Ansley D, Porto M, Garite T. The incidence and severity of shoulder dystocia correlates with a sonographic measurement of asymmetry in patients with diabetes. *Am J Perinatol* 1999;16:197–201.
33. Modanlou H, Komatsu G, Dorchester W, Freeman R, Bosou S. Large-for-gestational-age neonates: Anthropometric reasons for shoulder dystocia. *Obstet Gynecol* 1982;60:417–423.
34. Ehrenberg H, Durnwald C, Catalano P, Mercer B. The influence of obesity and diabetes on the rislk of cesarean delivery. *Am J Obstet Gynecol* 2004;191:969–974.
35. Acker D, Sachs B, Friedman E. Risk factors for shoulder dystocia in the average-weight infant. *Obstet Gynecol* 1986;67:614–618.
36. Seigworth G. Shoulder dystocia. Review of 5 years' experience. *Obstet Gynecol* 1966;28:764–767.
37. Mehta S, Bujold E, Blackwell S, Sorokin Y, Sokol R. Is abnormal labor associated with shoulder dystocia in nulliparous women? *Am J Obstet Gynecol* 2004;190:1604–1607.
38. Lurie S, Levy R, Ben-Arie A, Hagay Z. Shoulder dystocia: Could it be deduced from the labor partogram? *Am J Perinatol* 1995;12:61–62.
39. McFarland M, Hod M, Piper J, Xenakis E, Langer O. Are labor abnormalities more common in shoulder dystocia? *Am J Obstet Gynecol* 1995;173:1211–1214.
40. Ouzounian J, Korst L, Phelan J. Permanent Erb's palsy: A lack of a relationship with obstetrical risk factors. *Am J Perinatol* 1998;15:221–223.
41. Benedetti T, Gabbe S. Shoulder dystocia. A complication of fetal macrosomia and prolonged second stage of labor with midpelvic delivery. *Obstet Gynecol* 1978;52:526–529.
42. Garrett K, Butler A, Cohen W. Cesarean delivery during second stage labor: Characteristic and diagnostic accuracy. *J Matern Fetal Neonatal Med* 2005;17:49–53.

43. Mehta S, Blackwell S, Bujold E, Sokol R. What factors are associated with neonatal injury following shoulder dystocia? *J Perinatol* 2006;26:85–88.
44. Baskett T, Allen A. Perinatal implications of shoulder dystocia. *Obstet Gynecol* 1995;86:14–17.
45. Peleg D, Hasnin J, Shalev E. Fractured clavicle and Erb's palsy unrelated to birth trauma. *Am J Obstet Gynecol* 1997;177:1038–1040.
46. McFarland L, Raskin M, Daling J, Benedetti T. Erb/Duchenne's palsy: A consequence of fetal macrosomia and method of delivery. *Obstet Gynecol* 1986;68:784–788.
47. Nesbitt T, Gilbert W, Herrchen B. Shoulder dystocia and associated risk factors with macrosomic infants born in California. *Am J Obstet Gynecol* 1998;179:476–480.
48. Mollberg M, Hagberg H, Bager B, Lilja H, Ladfors L. Risk factors for obstetric brachial plexus palsy among neonates delivered by vacuum extraction. *Obstet Gynecol* 2005;106:913–918.
49. Hamilton E, Wright E. Labor pains: Unraveling the complexity of OB decision making. *Crit Care Nurs Q* 2006;29:342–353.
50. Dyachenko A, Ciampi A, Fahey J, Mighty H, Oppenheimer L, Hamilton E. Prediction of risk for shoulder dystocia with neonatal injury. *Am J Obstet Gynecol* 2006;195:1544–1549.
51. Mazzanti G. Delivery of the anterior shoulder: A neglected art. *Obstet Gynecol* 1959;13:603–607.
52. Naef R III, Morrison J. Guidelines for management of shoulder dystocia. *J Perinatol* 1994;14:435–441.
53. Allen R, Sorab J, Gonik B. Risk factors for shoulder dystocia: An engineering study of clinician-applied forces. *Obstet Gynecol* 1991;77:352–355.
54. Poggi S, Allen R, Patel C, Ghidini A, Pezzullo J, Spong C. Randomized trial of McRoberts versus lithotomy positioning to decrease the force that is applied to the fetus during delivery. *Am J Obstet Gynecol* 2004;191:874–878.
55. Gurewitsch E, Kim E, Yang J, Outland K, McDonald M, Allen R. Comparing McRoberts' and Rubin's maneuvers for initial management of shoulder dystocia: An objective evaluation. *Am J Obstet Gynecol* 2005;192:153–160.
56. Rubin A. Management of shoulder dystocia. *JAMA* 1964;189:835–837.
57. Gonik B, Stringer C, Held B. An alternate maneuver for management of shoulder dystocia. *Am J Obstet Gynecol* 1983;145:882–884.
58. Gonik B, Allen R, Sorab J. Objective evaluation of the shoulder dystocia phenomenon: Effect of maternal pelvic orientation on force reduction. *Obstet Gynecol* 1989;74:44–48.
59. Gherman R, Goodwin T, Souter I, Neumann K, Ouzounian J, Paul R. The McRoberts' maneuver for the alleviation of shoulder dystocia: How successful is it? *Am J Obstet Gynecol* 1997;176:656–661.
60. Heath T, Gherman R. Symphyseal separation, sacroiliac joint dislocation and transient lateral femoral cutaneous neuropathy associated with mcRoberts' maneuver. A case report. *J Reprod Med* 1999;44:902–904.
61. Gherman R, Goodwin T. Shoulder dystocia. *Curr Opin Obstet Gynecol* 1998;10:459–463.
62. Woods C. A principle of physics as applicable to shoulder delivery. *Am J Obstet Gynecol* 1943;45:796–804.
63. Goodwin T, Banks E, Millar L, Phelan J. Catastrophic shoulder dystocia and emergency symphysiotomy. *Am J Obstet Gynecol* 1997;177:463–464.
64. Bergstrom S, Lublin H, Molin A. Value of symphysiotomy in obstructed labour management and follow-up of 31 cases. *Gynecol Obstet Invest* 1994;38:31–35.
65. Hartfield V. Subcutaneous symphysiotomy-time for a reappraisal? *Aust N Z J Obstet Gynaecol* 1973;13:147–152.
66. Gabbe D. Symphysiotomy. *Clin Obstet Gynaecol* 1982;9:663–683.
67. Lasbrey A. The symptomatic sequellae of symphysiotomy. *S Afr Med J* 1963;37:231–234.
68. Zelig C, Gherman R. Modified Zavanelli maneuver for the alleviation of shoulder dystocia. *Obstet Gynecol* 2002;100:1112–1114.

69. Kenaan J, Gonzalez-Quintero V, Gilles J. The Zavanelli maneuver in two cases of shoulder dystocia. *J Matern Fetal Neonatal Med* 2003;13:135–138.
70. Sandberg E. The Zavanelli maneuver: 12 years of recorded experience. *Obstet Gynecol* 1999;93:312–317.
71. Ross M, Beall M. Cervical neck dislocation associated with the Zavanelli maneuver. *Obstet Gynecol* 2006;108:737–738.
72. Graham J, Blanco J, Wen T, Magee K. The Zavanelli maneuver: A different perspective. *Obstet Gynecol* 1992;79:883–884.
73. Sandberg E. The Zavanelli maneuver extended: Progression of a revolutionary concept. *Am J Obstet Gynecol* 1988;158:1347–1353.
74. Spellacy W, Miller S, Winegar A, Peterson P. Macrosomia–maternal characteristics and infant complications. *Obstet Gynecol* 1985;66:158–161.
75. O'Leary J. Cephalic replacement for shoulder dystocia: Present status and future role of the Zavanelli maneuver. *Obstet Gynecol* 1993;82:847–850.
76. Bruner J, Drummond S, Meenan A, Gaskin I. All-fours maneuver for reducing shoulder dystocia during labor. *J Reprod Med* 1998;43:439–443.
77. Meenan A, Gaskin I, Hunt P, Ball C. A new (old) maneuver for the management of shoulder dystocia. *J Fam Pract* 1991;32:625–629.
78. Merhi Z, Awonuga A. The role of uterine fundal pressure in the management of the second stage of labor: A reappraisal. *Obstet Gynecol Surv* 2005;60:599–603.
79. Simpson K, Knox G. Fundal pressure during the second stage of labor. *MCN Am J Matern Child Nurs* 2001;26:64–70.
80. Flamm B. Shoulder dystocia and fundal pressure: A medical legal dilemma. *J Health Risk Manag* 2002;22:9–14.
81. Gurewitsch E, Donithan M, Stallings S, et al. Episiotomy versus fetal manipulation in managing severe shoulder dystocia: A comparison of outcomes. *Am J Obstet Gynecol* 2004;191:911–916.
82. Hankins G, Clark S, Munn M. Cesarean section on request at 39 weeks: Impact on shoulder dystocia, fetal trauma, neonatal encephalopathy, and intrauterine fetal demise. *Semin Perinatol* 2006;30:276–287.

Chapter 17
Brachial Plexus Injury at Cesarean Section

Michael S. Kreitzer and James A. O'Leary

Summary Brachial plexus traction injury can occur at the time of cesarean section delivery. This results from the operator's failure to recognize soft tissue incisional dystocia. Avoiding traction on the infant's head and enlarging the incision in the uterus and/or abdominal wall will prevent infant and maternal injury.

Keywords: incision · traction

Contents

17.1 Introduction 249
17.2 Incidence 250
17.3 Mechanism 250
17.4 Discussion 253
17.5 Clinical Experience 255
17.6 Conclusion 255

17.1 Introduction

It must be emphasized that cesarean delivery is no guarantee against birth trauma associated with extraction of the fetus, even at the time of a cephalic presentation. Gentle and appropriate techniques for delivery of the arms and head remain essential. Undue traction and hyperextension or lateral flexion of the head must be avoided. Fetal injury may occur with the use of improper traction or attempted delivery of the head through too small an incision, even with a smaller infant. This soft tissue dystocia is rarely, if ever, recorded in the patient's medical records.

M.S. Kreitzer
Attending Physician, Overlook Hospital, Summit, NJ, USA; Clin. Assoc. Prof,
OBIYN, University of Medicine and Dentistry of NJ, USA; Senior Risk Management
Consultant, Princeton Insurance Co, Princeton, NJ, USA

J.A. O'Leary (ed.), *Shoulder Dystocia and Birth Injury*,
DOI 10.1007/978-1-59745-473-5_17, © Humana Press, a part of Springer
Science+Business Media, LLC 2009

17.2 Incidence

The incidence and type of fetal injury identified at cesarean delivery is well characterized and well understood (Table 17.1). The most commonly identified injury at cesarean delivery is fetal laceration, and its incidence has been reported to be as high as 3%. One might hypothesize that the risk of fetal injury at cesarean delivery is low, especially considering that the cesarean delivery is purported to limit birth trauma in certain cases (i.e., breech presentation). This supposition is supported by the observation that major birth trauma has decreased over the past several decades in response to rising cesarean rates [1]. Certain injuries such as clavicular fracture appear to be unrelated to the mode of delivery and can be seen with cesarean as well as vaginal delivery, making the point that fetal injuries commonly attributed to vaginal delivery can be seen with cesarean delivery as well [1].

17.3 Mechanism

A uterine, fascial, and/or skin incision that barely permits delivery of the head, or requires the use of vacuum or forceps assistance, can result in a delay or failure to deliver the shoulders, necessitating enlargement of the incision. If the inadequacy of the incision is not appreciated early, and corrected, strong lateral traction applied to either the anterior or posterior brachial plexus can result in injury to the infant's brachial plexus (Figs 17.1 and 17.2).

In a recent study of fetal injury associated with cesarean delivery, Alexander et al. [1] found that injury occurred in 3.4% of infants where a "T" or "J" uterine incision was required for delivery, indicating inadequacy of the initial low transverse incision. Nine cases of brachial plexus injury occurred in this series

Table 17.1 Type and Incidence of Fetal Injury Identified in 37,110 Cesarean Deliveries

Type	Number (Incidence per 1,000)
Total number of injuries*	418 (11.3)
Skin laceration	272 (7.3)
Cephalohematoma	88 (2.4)
Clavicle fracture	11 (0.3)
Facial nerve palsy	11 (0.3)
Brachial plexus injury	9 (0.2)
Skull fracture	6 (0.2)
Long bone fracture	8 (0.2)
Intracranial hemorrhage	2 (0.1)
Other†	20 (0.5)

*Nine patients had two fetal injuries.
†Includes abnormal bruising, subconjunctival hemorrhage, abrasion, and minor injuries not able to be classified.

Fig. 17.1 Upward traction
at cesarean section

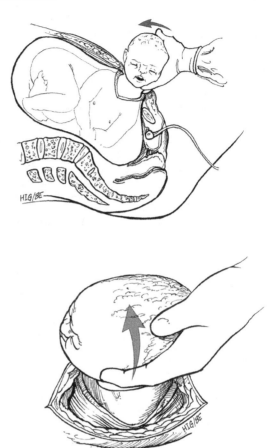

of 418 deliveries associated with various fetal injuries. Four of the nine cases of brachial plexus injury occurred in patients who did not experience labor. The data did not specifically analyze any of these nine cases regarding permanent versus transient injury, type of incision ("T" or "J"), infant birth weight >4,000 g, or difficulty in delivery of either the head or body.

In 1997, Gherman et al. [2] retrospectively reported on six cases of Erbs palsy in infants born by "atraumatic" cesarean section. Four palsies occurred in the anterior and two in the posterior arm, and all persisted at 1 year of age. Though acknowledging that a difficult cesarean delivery and "failure to rotate the fetal vertex to the OA position before delivery" can cause brachial plexus injury, they *excluded* "cases with reported difficulty in delivering the fetal vertex." In concluding that brachial plexus palsies associated with cesarean delivery "appear to be of intrauterine origin and are more likely to persist," they speculated that "long-standing in utero stretching may account for the

Fig. 17.2 Downward
traction at cesarean section

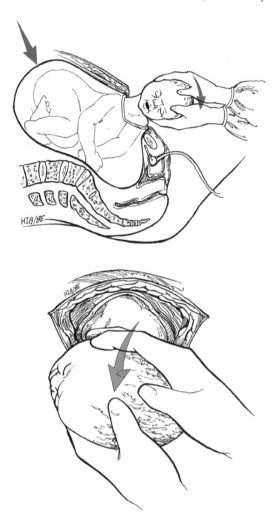

permanence of these injuries." Close analysis strongly indicates that these
conclusions are erroneous, for the following reasons:

- "All infants were otherwise neurologically normal," with none exhibiting
  muscle atrophy at birth. The absence of atrophy is not consistent with the
  theorized "long-standing in utero stretching" or "events antedating the
  delivery," such as prolonged compression or immobility. Because none of
  the infants were tested by electromyography (EMG) soon after delivery, the
  absence of muscle atrophy in the affected limb indicates that injury occurred
  at the time of delivery, and was not "long-standing [2]."

- Lack of reported difficulty in delivering the vertex was accepted as conclusive evidence that no difficulty occurred. Underreporting was not even considered a possibility. In addition, there was no consideration of the fact that delivery of the vertex may be atraumatic, whereas delivery of the shoulders can be obstructed despite the common use of both anteriorly and posteriorly directed traction and fundal pressure (Figs 17.1 and 17.2). Though the injured infants were followed for 1 year, no imaging studies or information regarding neonatal surgery was presented. The additional conclusion, that it is "virtually certain that traction at delivery played no role" cannot be supported, since these is no other mechanism, actual or theorized, that would explain BPI without atrophy at birth, in an infant delivered abdominally prior to labor.

17.4 Discussion

In 1999, the National Institutes of Health established a Cesarean Registry to prospectively address several contemporary issues related to cesarean delivery [1]. This registry included all patients undergoing cesarean delivery at network centers during the study period, providing the opportunity to explore uncommon complications of cesarean delivery, including fetal injury. Using data obtained from this registry, the author reported the incidence of fetal injury at cesarean delivery and classified the types of injury [1] (Table 17.1).

It is interesting to find that five of the cases of brachial plexus injury identified in this study were seen in cesarean delivery for dystocia, and that four of the nine cases occurred in women who did not labor at all (Table 17.2).

Table 17.2 Demographic Characteristics and Delivery Outcome of Women Undergoing Cesarean Delivery Complicated by Fetal Injuries Compared with Cesarean Births without Such Injuries*

Characteristic	Cesarean Delivery with Fetal Injury (N = 418)	Cesarean elivery without Fetal Injury (N = 36,692)	P Value
Maternal age by mean ± SD	27.0 ± 6.2	27.8 ± 6.4	.03
Nulliparity	223 (54)	14,888 (41)	<.001
Race			<.001
White	240 (51)	14,451 (41)	
Black	100 (24)	11,192 (32)	
Hispanic	93 (23)	9,139 (26)	
Other	7 (2)	672 (2)	
Body mass index (mean ± SD)	27.2 ± 6.9	27.2 ± 7.0	1.0
Birthweight more than 4,000 g	61 (15)	4,493 (12)	.14
Gestational age (mean weeks ± SD)	38.3 ± 3.5	38.2 ± 3.3	.02
Less than 37 weeks	85 (20)	7,332 (20)	.84

SD, standard deviation.
*Data are presented as n (%), except where otherwise indicated.

In fact, several types of fetal injury commonly associated with difficult vaginal delivery occurred in women who did not labor and underwent an elective repeat cesarean delivery (Table 17.3). In addition to brachial plexus injury, these include cephalohematoma, clavicular fracture, and long bone fracture. The key surgical factors appear in Table 17.4. This observation suggests that cesarean delivery does not in and of itself preclude major birth trauma [1].

Table 17.3. Indication for Cesarean Delivery and the Risk of Fetal Injury*

Indication for Cesarean Delivery	Cesarean Delivery with Fetal Injury	Cesarean Deliveries (N)	P Value
Primary	318 (1.5)	21,798	
Dystocia	111 (1.4)	8,122	<.001
Nonreassuring fetal heart rate	79 (1.5)	5,404	
Abnormal presentation	61 (1.4)	4,321	
Other	24 (0.7)	3,329	
Unsuccessful trail of forceps or vacuum	43 (6.9)	628	
Repeat	100 (0.7)	15,312	
No VBAC attempt	66 (0.5)	12,565	<.001
Failed VBAC	33 (1.2)	2,687	
Unsuccessful trail of forceps or vacuum	1 (1.7)	60	

VBAC, vaginal birth after cesarean delivery.
*Data are reported as n (%) or number. Chi-square analysis was used t o determine whether the incidence of fetal injury varied by indication for cesarean delivery in both primary and repeat cesarean delivery.

Table 17.4. Selected Surgical Factors at Cesarean Delivery in Relation to Fetal Injury*

Factors	Cesarean Delivery with Fetal Injury (N = 418)	Number of Cesarean Deliveries (N = 37,110)	P Value
Incision to delivery time, min			.002[†]
3 or less	61 (19)	3,266	
4–5	56 (14)	4,037	
6–10	146 (10)	14,405	
11–15	84 (9)	8,902	
More than 15	64 (10)	6,214	
Skin incision type			1.0
Pfannenstiel	328 (11)	29,072	
Midline	88 (11)	7,795	
Uterine incision type			.003
Transverse	385 (11)	35,040	
Vertical	24 (14)	1,779	
T or J	8 (34)	237	

*Data are shown as n (per 1,000) or number.
[†]A test of trend was used to determine whether the incidence of fetal injury varied across incision lines.

17.5 Clinical Experience

Over the years, the authors have witnessed a number of difficult cesarean deliveries, performed by both trainees and experienced practitioners, and have been made aware of others where a traction injury occurred. With or without the use of forceps or a vacuum extractor, difficulty in delivering the fetal head was more likely in patients whose labor arrested. In contrast, difficulty in extracting either the anterior or posterior shoulder with traction (Figs 17.1 and 17.2) occurred with about the same frequency in primary and repeat cesarean deliveries. This type of soft tissue shoulder dystocia was easily resolved by enlarging a uterine, fascial, or skin incision that was inadequate, and only a few transient brachial plexus injuries were encountered. In one case, a reluctance to enlarge the uterine incision resulted in several failed attempts to deliver the anterior shoulder, before the "T" incision was finally made. Though all of the injuries resolved prior to hospital discharge, and the newborn records reflected transient brachial plexus injury, *none* of the maternal records were coded for shoulder dystocia or a traumatic delivery. In addition, *none* of the operative reports noted the brachial plexus injury present at birth, and only the case requiring a "T" incision noted any difficulty in delivery of the shoulders.

17.6 Conclusion

Soft tissue shoulder dystocia can occur at the time of cesarean section. Brachial plexus palsy can occur if excessive traction is applied to the infant's head.

Acknowledgments The authors greatly appreciate the contributions of Brice Karsh, President, and Brian Evans, Cim. I., of High Impact Graphics (Englewood, Colorado) for their invaluable dedication and effort in helping to complete this chapter.

References

1. Alexander J, Levine K, Hauth J, et al., For the National Institute of Child Health and Human Development Maternal - Fetal Medicine Units Network. Fetal injury associated with cesarean delivery. *Obstet Gynecol* 2006;108:885–890.
2. Gherman RB, Goodwin TM, Ouzourian JG, Miller DA, Paul RH. Brachial plexus injury associated with cesarean section: An in utero injury? *Am J Obstet Gynecol* 1997;177:1162–1164.

Chapter 18
Delivery of the Nondiabetic Macrosomic Infant

Lisa Gittens-Williams

Summary The intrapartum management of the fetus with known or suspected macrosomia presents a considerable challenge to the clinician. Risks and complications are reviewed, and management is discussed.

Keywords: injury · macrosomia · ultrasound

Contents

18.1 Macrosomia 257
18.2 Complications.. 258
18.3 Macrosomia and Shoulder Dystocia 258
18.4 Ultrasound and Macrosomia 259
18.5 Obesity and Macrosomia 260
18.6 Previous Macrosomia.. 261
18.7 Labor Abnormalities 262
18.8 Elective Cesarean Section and Induction of Labor 262
18.9 Instrumental Delivery... 263
18.10 Management Recommendations 264
18.11 Conclusion 265

18.1 Macrosomia

Fetal macrosomia has historically been defined as birthweights in categories of >4,000 g, >4,500 g, or >5,000 g. Macrosomia has been associated with a variety of adverse perinatal outcomes including shoulder dystocia, brachial plexus injury, skeletal injury, meconium aspiration, asphyxia, and fetal death. The American College of Obstetricians and Gynecologists (ACOG) defines macrosomia as a fetal weight of >4,500 g [1]. In the United States, 10% of infants have a birthweight of 4,000 g or more, and 1.5% weigh at least 4,500 g [2]. More than 12% of pregnant women gained 46 lb or more in 2000; only 9.1% experienced

L. Gittens-Williams
Associate Professor, Department of Obstetrics, Gynecology & Women's Health,
New Jersey Medical School, Newark, New Jersey, USA

J.A. O'Leary (ed.), *Shoulder Dystocia and Birth Injury,*
DOI 10.1007/978-1-59745-473-5_18, © Humana Press, a part of Springer
Science+Business Media, LLC 2009

this degree of weight gain a decade prior [2]. These trends parallel the increases in nationwide obesity; excessive birthweight is associated with maternal obesity and maternal weight gain. Risks, complications, and delivery management of the macrosomic fetus will be reviewed. This discussion will be limited to the nondiabetic mother, with the understanding that infants of diabetic mothers, regardless of their birthweight, will have increased risks of birth-related injuries.

18.2 Complications

Complications associated with delivery of the macrosomic fetus include an increased risk for cesarean section and an increase in maternal and neonatal morbidity. Operative and traumatic deliveries are increased, and there is increase in the frequency of shoulder dystocia [3,4]. Perineal injury is increased when compared with delivery of normal-weight infants and was seen in 1 of 20 macrosomic vaginal deliveries in one series [5]. In an observational study, it was noted that macrosomic infants had up to five times the odds of having at least one of the following: shoulder dystocia, postpartum hemorrhage, transfusion, chorioamnionitis, or fourth degree laceration. Prolonged labor, postpartum hemorrhage, third and fourth degree lacerations, and infections are increased in women with macrosomic infants when compared with women with infants of normal weight [6].

18.3 Macrosomia and Shoulder Dystocia

An abundance of literature supports the relationships between fetal weight, shoulder dystocia, and brachial plexus injury. In an analysis of perinatal outcomes in macrosomic infants (>4,500 g) who were delivered vaginally over a 10-year period, Raio et al. [5] reported that the incidence of brachial plexus injury increased steadily from 0.8% in fetuses weighing 4,500 to 4,599 g to 2.86% in those weighing more than 5,000 g [5]. Maternal height additionally affected outcome in macrosomic fetuses, as brachial plexus injury increased from 2.1% in women taller than 180 cm to 35.1% in women shorted than 155 cm [5]. Other studies report that the incidence of shoulder dystocia ranges from 4.2% to 22% in infants with a birthweight >5,000 g [8,9].

Acker et al. reported that in a cohort of nondiabetic women, infants weighing >4,500 g experience shoulder dystocia 22% of the time. The shoulder dystocia rate in their general population was 2%. Among infants weighing <4,000 g, 1.1% experienced shoulder dystocia [10]. Sandmire reported a rate of shoulder dystocia of 9.4 in infants >4,500 g, and Nesbit reported a rate of 21% in infants of 4,750 to 5,000 g. There is some evidence to support that shoulder dystocia is increasing. Dandolu reported an increase in shoulder dystocia over two decades among patients identified from the Maryland

State database [12]. This increase may be associated with parallel increases in fetal birthweight over time [13].

Data clearly support higher rates of shoulder dystocia and brachial plexus injury as fetal weights increase. Although it is frequently mentioned in discussion about shoulder dystocia that most occur among infants of normal weight, more permanent injury occurs among infants that are >4,500 g. This distribution of injury should be considered when managing a macrosomic infant.

18.4 Ultrasound and Macrosomia

Traditionally, fetal weight has been estimated by the clinical assessment of fundal height and by uterine palpation in the form of the Leopold maneuvers, which also assesses fetal presentation. Weights can additionally be determined by ultrasound, or fetal weights can be predicted or estimated by the gravida. To reduced neonatal risks of birth trauma, particularly risks of shoulder dystocia, the clinician must accurately identify babies who will weigh >4,000 g so delivery plans can be optimized to reduce risks.

With the availability and use of ultrasound to assess fetal weight, sonography commonly supplements the clinical assessment of fetal weight. Several studies, however, report that clinical estimated fetal weight can reliably predict fetal birthweight. Chauhan et al. [14] reported that in more than half of the models for ultrasound prediction of fetal weight, the clinical predictions by physicians were as or more accurate. This was especially true when the fetal weights exceeded or were equal to 4,000 g [14,15]. The margin of error of ultrasound fetal weight prediction appears to be similar to that seen when fetal weight is clinically estimated. Chauhan additionally reported that pregnant women themselves were as accurate as ultrasound or the physician in clinical estimating of birthweights of their infants [16]. The patient's assessment or concerns about excessive fetal weight should not be ignored.

The ACOG reports that ultrasound has a sensitivity of 22% to 44% and a predictive value of 30% to 44% in predicting fetal weight [1]. This wide range of sensitivity has led to conclusions that macrosomia cannot be reliably predicted or diagnosed. Data that report about serial sonographic assessments of fetal weight suggest that this methodology more reliably predicts macrosomia. Biparietal diameter above 2 standard deviations on a growth curve as well as serial abdominal circumferences that are above the 90th percentile have reported sensitivities and specificities (100%, 98% and 84%, 100%) that are greater than those of estimated fetal weight alone [19]. If macrosomia is suspected or significant risk factors exist, serial sonography with careful attention to trends is in order as it improves prediction of macrosomia.

Because macrosomic infants deposit adipose in the abdomen and shoulders, other anthropomorphic measures have been suggested to predict macrosomia and shoulder dystocia. The fetal deposition of subcutaneous fat correlates well with birthweight. Several investigators have sought to identify patterns of fat deposition that would allow for prediction of macrosomia. Excessive abdominal growth alone or subcutaneous tissue thickness on both face and shoulders have been studied. The transthoracic diameter/biparietal diameter and abdominal circumference >35 cm have also been described. Although cutoff values for some macrosomic infants may overlap the values in the range reported for nonmacrosomic infants, reviewing additional parameters such as these may be useful when data are conflicting or when index of suspicion for macrosomia is high. Newer imaging techniques such as magnetic resonance imaging or three-dimensional ultrasound will likely contribute to the improvement of our ability to predict macrosomia.

18.5 Obesity and Macrosomia

Diabetes and prolonged pregnancy are well-established risk factors for macrosomia [10,20]; maternal obesity and increases in maternal weight gain are additional associated risk factors. The relationship between obesity and macrosomia is well recognized. Obesity is defined by the World Health Organization and the National Institutes of Health as a body mass index (BMI; {weight [kg]/height [in]} [2]) of 30 or greater. Obesity is further classified by BMI into class I (30 to 34.9), class II (35 to 39.9), and class III (>40) [21]. As obesity is a well-recognized risk factor for macrosomia, delivery management of the obese gravida will be reviewed here. Weiss reported that incidence of macrosomia, defined as a birthweight of >4,000 g, was 8.3% in the nonobese group, 13.3% in obese group and 14.6% among morbidly obese women [22].

Recent reports note an increase in mean birthweights in both North America and Europe, especially among infants >4,000 g [23,24]. This parallels a noted increase in prevalence of obesity in the United States. One third of adult women are reported to be obese [25]. Non-Hispanic Black women have the highest prevalence (48.8%) whereas non-Hispanic white women have the lowest (31%) [25].

Prepregnancy obesity is a significant risk factor for adverse outcome in early pregnancy and during labor and delivery. In addition, obesity in pregnancy is associated with an increased risk of hypertensive disorders, diabetes, chronic cardiac dysfunction, sleep apnea, and associated complications of metabolic syndrome [26,27]. Parturition is associated with increased risks of cesarean delivery, complications of anesthesia, wound disruption, and deep venous thrombosis. An increase in the cesarean section rate has been reported in obese women when compared with nonobese women, especially when the indication is for failure to progress [22,28–31].

Usha Kiran et al. reported that in a population data base of 60,167 deliveries, women with BMI >30 had an increase risk for postdates, cesarean section, macrosomia, shoulder dystocia, and failed instrumental delivery [32]. An increase in labor induction has also been reported in obese women [30].

The relationship between obesity and shoulder dystocia may be largely related to the increase in macrosomia seen in this group an unrelated to obesity alone. Robinson et al. reported that although macrosomia is the strongest predictor of shoulder dystocia, among obese women with fetuses of normal weight, the risk of shoulder dystocia is not increased [33]. Similar lack of association between obesity and shoulder dystocia was noted by Jensen et al., however, one possible reason for this finding is the increase in cesarean section generally noted in obese women, which may have reduced the number of subjects who would have had shoulder dystocia in this analysis [30].

Maternal pregravid weight has a strong correlation with birthweight [13]. Weight gain in pregnancy is also correlated with fetal weight. Abrams and Laros reported a correlation between maternal weight gain and birth weight in moderately overweight, ideal body weight, and underweight women [34]. In women weighing 135% of ideal weight for height, before conception, however, there was no correlation between weight gain in pregnancy and birthweight. Diabetes appears to be the greatest risk factor for having a large for gestational age infant (OR 4.4) compared with maternal obesity (OR 1.6). Because, however, the prevalence of obesity is far greater than the prevalence of diabetes, obesity alone is a more significant factor that contributes to increases in fetal birthweight [35].

From a cohort of 14,359 patients in Sweden, a strong correlation was noted between birth injury and both fetal macrosomia and maternal short stature. Using risk estimation curves, these investigators suggest that the rate of birth injury is greatest when the birthweight is higher and the maternal height shorter [36].

18.6 Previous Macrosomia

The management of patients who have previously delivered a macrosomic infant is of significant concern to the clinician, particularly if the delivery was complicated by neonatal or pelvic floor injury. Even in the absence of prior injury, the gravida may express concern about recurrent macrosomia if other labors were difficult or prolonged. To evaluate the outcome of the second delivery among nondiabetic women whose first fetus was macrosomic (>4,500 g), Mahoney et al. [37] reviewed a database of 13,020 pregnancies. In this cohort, macrosomia complicated 2.3% of all pregnancies and recurred up to one third of the time in the second pregnancy. The first macrosomic deliveries were associated with higher rates of operative delivery, anal sphincter injury, and shoulder dystocia when compared with nonmacrosomic deliveries. In the second pregnancy, more prelabor cesareans were performed in the macrosomic group (17.3%) compared with a control group (4.7%). Among those who had a successful vaginal delivery of a macrosomic infant and who attempted vaginal delivery the second time, the success rate was 99%. In patients who delivered the first baby by cesarean for macrosomia, there was a high risk (56%) for repeat intrapartum cesarean, whether macrosomia recurred or not. These data demonstrate that macrosomia (>4,500 g) recurs with high frequency and that patients with a prior macrosomic infant undergo elective section more frequently than do control women. The high success rate of vaginal delivery after prior macrosomic vaginal birth reported by the authors may have been because the patients at highest risk for failed delivery and complications were selected out to undergo elective cesarean section [37].

18.7 Labor Abnormalities

A relationship between abnormal labor patterns and fetal weight has been established. Both arrest disorders in women with large babies and prolongation of the second stage in obese women were associated with shoulder dystocia [10,38]. An increase in the incidence of labor abnormalities in infants >4,500 g was reported by Acker. In this study, such labor abnormalities were not seen among average-weight infants [39].

A consistent relationship between labor abnormalities and shoulder dystocia, however, has not always been noted. McFarland et al. compared labor abnormalities in shoulder dystocia and control groups and found no significant difference in labor abnormalities between the groups. When diabetic and macrosomic infants (>4,000 g) were analyzed separately, differences in labor abnormalities still were not identified when compared with controls. A higher incidence of prolonged second stage was seen among nulliparous women who had shoulder dystocia, suggesting that a prolonged labor may identify patients at risk for shoulder dystocia in this group [40].

Additionally, Strofenoyoh reported that duration of labor, percentage of prolonged labor, and mean duration of the second stage do not appear to be different among macrosomic infants (4,000 g or >) and those of normal (2,500 g to <4,000 g) weight [41]. Mehta et al. reported, however, that the combination of fetal macrosomia (birthweight >4,000 g) second stage >2 hours and the use of operative vaginal delivery was associated with shoulder dystocia in nulliparous women [42].

18.8 Elective Cesarean Section and Induction of Labor

Although numerous studies have focused on the debate concerning prophylactic cesarean section as a management option when macrosomia is suspected, the optimal management strategy remains undefined. There are researchers who support the benefit and safety of vaginal delivery in infants that weigh >4,500 g [8,9,43,44]. Although ACOG recommends consideration of cesarean delivery when fetal weight is estimated to be 5,000 g in a nondiabetic mother, the optimal management of these patients and the risks of vaginal delivery versus the benefits of elective cesarean section continues to be questioned. Nassar reported a statistically non-significant increase in birth injuries when infants weighing more than 4,500 g who were delivered vaginally were compared with similar-weight infants who were delivered by cesarean section (7.7% vs. 1.6%) [45]. When infants >4,000 g who were delivered vaginally were compared with infants of the same weight delivered by cesarean, among the vaginally delivered infants, asphyxia and long bone injury occurred more frequently, however sample size in this study was small [6]. In contrast, when delivery outcome was evaluated among infants weighing >4,000 g, and vaginal delivery and cesarean delivery were compared, newborn infant morbidity was low, but higher in the cesarean group for transient tachypnea, hypocalcemia; these reported complications are generally not permanent [46].

The absence of large, prospective randomized trials comparing risks and benefits of the various delivery methods in these patients precludes the development of a definitive management recommendation, however, a rise in maternal obesity and shoulder dystocia suggest that each case be individualized and a discussion held with the mother about the associated risks [6].

Because induction of labor is more common in postdate pregnancies and among diabetic pregnancies, it is difficult to determine whether induction alone creates an independent risk for shoulder dystocia in the macrosomic infant. McFarland et al. found that shoulder dystocia occurred more commonly when labor was induced but concluded that induction alone did not predispose to shoulder dystocia [40].

Induction of labor when macrosomia is suspected, however, has not been shown to reduce the incidence of shoulder dystocia among nondiabetic women. In a meta-analysis that included nine observational studies, women who experienced onset of labor had a lower incidence of cesarean section without any effect on the rate of shoulder dystocia [47]. Similar conclusions have been made by the Cochrane review, which confirms that induction of labor for suspected macrosomia in nondiabetic patients does not alter the risk of perinatal morbidity [46,49].

18.9 Instrumental Delivery

Multiple studies have reported that instrumental vaginal deliveries are associated with greater rate of shoulder dystocia when compared with unassisted births [50]. Among infants weighing 4,000 to 4,200 g, Nesbitt reported a rate of shoulder dystocia of 8.4% when the delivery was unassisted and 12.2% when operative vaginal intervention was used. In infants with weights >4,700 g, the rate of shoulder dystocia was 23.5% when the birth was unassisted and 34.8% when instrumental delivery occurred [51].

18.10 Management Recommendations

Identification of risks factors for macrosomia should occur during the prenatal visits. The high frequency with which macrosomia recurs in second or subsequent pregnancies should be remembered. A history of obesity or of prior macrosomic infants should be noted. Careful attention should be paid to birthweight of other infants and to labor course and outcome in other pregnancies. Details such as pelvic floor injury and rectal sphincter tear should be noted. Early diabetes screening may be indicated in some patients and should be repeated at 24 to 28 weeks if the initial screen is negative. The initial screen may be upon presentation or in the first trimester.

Maternal height and weight should be recorded and body mass index calculated. Obese patients ideally should be counseled regarding benefit of weight loss prior to conception. Data supporting safety of bariatric surgery for obese women and pregnancy outcomes is evolving, but this intervention appears to improve outcomes with respect to macrosomia and diabetes for the obese gravida [11,52]. Recommendations regarding pregnancy weight gain should be based on Institute of Medicine guidelines, which suggest weight gain of 25 to 35 lb in women of normal weight, 15 to 25 lb in overweight women, and 15 lb in obese women [53].

Throughout pregnancy, fundal height should be measured at regular intervals. Sonographic estimation of fetal weight should additionally be serially assessed, particularly when the woman is obese and fetal size cannot accurately be clinically determined. Data on the accuracy of ultrasound to predict fetal weight in an obese patient is conflicting, with some authors reporting that obesity, particularly above certain weight thresholds, impairs sonographic visualization of structures. Other authors report that when underweight, normal weight, overweight, and obese patients were compared, there was no difference in the ability of ultrasound to predict birthweight [54]. Serial assessments may provide more information in obese patients. Prior to onset of labor, careful evaluation of the pelvis with documentation of pelvic adequacy for the given fetus should be noted. When sonographic and clinical estimation of fetal weight appear to be discrepant, the larger fetal weight should be considered. Patients who are obese should understand the difficulty that may occur in estimating fetal weight, even by ultrasound. These patients should also be advised of other intrapartum complications that may occur including an increase risk for cesarean section. Other complications such as inability to obtain fetal heart and contraction pattern during labor and increased risks of shoulder dystocia, operative delivery, and transfusion should be reviewed with the patient [26]. Because of the increased operative morbidity associated with cesarean section among obese patients, delivery decisions must be individualized. Trial of labor is a reasonable option when fetal weight is determined to be in the normal range [11,33].

Until more reliable methods of assessing fetal weight are developed, the clinician is limited in his or her ability to accurately predict macrosomia; however, based on estimated fetal weights, and serial weight assessment, recommendations for cesarean delivery may be made when fetal weights exceed 5,000 g in a nondiabetic woman and exceed 4,500 g in a diabetic mother [1,26,44]. These recommendations, however, are based primarily on consensus and expert opinion rather than on large numbers of trials.

At known or suspected fetal weights of <5,000 g in a nondiabetic patient or 4,500 g in a diabetic pregnancy, decisions about vaginal delivery must be individualized and take into account pelvimetry, current fetal weight, comorbidities, maternal height, and prior obstetric history and involve a discussion with the mother about the risks of vaginal delivery at any given birthweight. Raio et al., based on their finding of greater risk of brachial plexus injury with increasing fetal weights, suggested that when fetal weights of >4,500 g are suspected, patients should be counseled about perinatal morbidity before decisions about the mode of delivery are undertaken [5]. Delivery and its attendant risks may be discussed with the gravida, and maternal concerns about fetal weight and mode of delivery should be noted. Data from Raio et al. suggest that the risks associated with macrosomia are not dependent upon estimated fetal weight alone, but rather that weight combined with other factors such as maternal height and type of delivery influence risk [5]. Although elective induction for presumed or impending macrosomia is not supported by the literature, should induction be necessary, risks, benefits, indications, and possibility of failure should be reviewed with the patient.

If spontaneous labor is allowed, labor management should proceed in the usual fashion with careful attention to the development of arrest and protraction disorder. If macrosomia is suspected antepartum or intrapartum, operative vaginal delivery should be avoided or used with caution. No labor pattern reliably predicts that the infant will be macrosomic or that shoulder dystocia will occur, however careful attention to normal time limits for the active phase and second stage of labor should occur. Evolving data regarding the contributing role of obesity, weight gain, and maternal height may more specifically modify these recommendations allowing for individualized patient management.

The obese gravida may also benefit from an antenatal anesthesia consult to evaluate for potential difficulties in catheter placement and airway management. She may additionally benefit from early placement of an epidural catheter without the administration of drugs, as difficulty in obtaining airway under emergent conditions may occur.

When faced with the possible delivery of a macrosomic infant, the operator and delivery team should review maneuvers to release shoulder dystocia described elsewhere in this text and be prepared to use these maneuvers as necessary.

18.11 Conclusion

Delivery of the known or suspected macrosomic infant involves careful attention to the evaluation of fetal weight and the assessment of adequacy of each individual fetus for the maternal pelvis. Sonographic and clinical estimations of fetal weight are both clinically useful. Maternal self-assessment of fetal weight among multiparous women is underused. When macrosomia is suspected, careful evaluation for risk factors and observation for related complication must take place. When estimated fetal weight exceeds 4,500 g in a diabetic mother or 5,000 g in a nondiabetic mother, elective cesarean section should be carefully considered as morbidity is highest above these birthweights. At estimated fetal weights below these values, management must be individualized. Among patients with a history of prior macrosomic birth, the frequency of recurrence should be noted.

References

1. American College of Obstetricians and Gynecologists. Practice Bulletin. Fetal macrosomia. No. 22. Washington, DC: ACOG; 2000.
2. Martin A, Hamilton B, Ventura S, Menacker F, Peck M. Births: Final data for 2000. *Natl Stat Rep* 2002;50:1–10.
3. American College of Obstetricians and Gynecologists. Practice Bulletin Shoulder dystocia. No. 40. Washington, DC: ACOG; 2002.
4. Boulet S, Alexander G, Salihu H, Pass M. Macrosomic births in the United States: Determinants, outcomes, and proposed grades of risk. *Am J Obstet Gynecol* 2003;188:1372–1378.
5. Raio L, Ghezzi E, DiNaro M, et al. Perinatal outcome of fetuses with a birth weight greater than 4500 grams: An analysis of 3356 cases. *Eur J Obstet Gynecol Reprod Biol* 2003;109:160–165.
6. Boulet Sl, Salihu H, Alexander G. Mode of delivery and birth outcomes of macrosomic infants. *Obstet Gynecol* 2004;24:622–629.
7. O'Leary J, Leonetti H. Shoulder dystocia: Prevention and treatment. *Am J Obstet Gynecol* 1990;162:5–9.
8. Dufur B, Vinatier D, Subtil D. Fetal macrosomia: Risk factors and outcome. A study of the outcome concerning 100 cases >4500 grams. *Eur J Obstet Gynecol Reprod Biol* 1998;77:51–59.
9. Mocanu E, Greene R, Byrne B. Obstetric and neonatal outcome of babies weighing more than 5.5 kg: An analysis by parity. *Eur J Obstet Gynecol Reprod Biol* 2000;92:229–233.
10. Acker D, Sachs B, Friedman E. Risk factors for shoulder dystocia. *Obstet Gynecol* 1985;66:762–768.
11. Sheiner E, Levy A, Silverberg D, et al. Pregnancy after bariatric surgery is not associated with adverse perinatal outcome. *Am J Obstet Gynecol* 2004;190:1335–1340.
12. Dandolu V, Lawrence L, Gaughan J, et al. Trends in the rate of shoulder dystocia over two decades. *J Mat Neonat Med* 2005;18:305–310.
13. Ross M, Beall M. Increases in the rate of shoulder dystocia. *J Mater-Fet Neo Med* 2006;19:315–316.
14. Chauhan S, Cowan B, Magann E, Bradford T, Roberts W, Morrison J. Intrapartum detection of a macrosomic fetus: Clinical versus 8 sonographic models. *Aust N Z J Obstet Gynecol* 1995;35:266.
15. Chauhan S, Grobman W, Gherman R, Chauhan V, Chang G, Magann E, Hendrix N. Suspicion and treatment of the macrosomic fetus: A review. *Am J Obstet Gynecol* 2005;193:332–346.
16. Chauhan S, Lutton P, Bailey K, Guerrieri J, Morrison J. Intrapartum: Clinical, sonographic, and parous patients' estimates of newborn birth weight. *Obstet Gynecol* 1992;79:956–958.
17. Delpapa D, Mueller-Heubach E. Pregnancy outcome following ultrasound diagnosis of macrosomia. *Obstet Gynecol* 1991;78:340–343.

18. Meshari A, DeSilva S, Rahman I. Fetal macrosomia: Maternal risks and fetal outcome. *Int J Gynaecol Obstet* 1990;32:215–222.
19. O'Reilly-Green C, Divon M. Sonographic and clinical methods in the diagnosis of macrosomia. *Clin Obstet Gynecol* 2000;43:309.
20. Chervenak J, Divon M, Hirsch J, Girz B, Langer O. Macrosomia in the postdate pregnancy: Is routine ultrasonographic screening indicated? *Am J Obstet Gynecol* 1989;161:753–756.
21. World Health Organization. Obesity: Preventing and managing the global epidemic. WHO Technical Report Series 2000;894-1-253. Geneva, Switzerland: World Health Organization.
22. Weiss J, Malone F, Emig D, et al. Obesity obstetric complications and cesarean delivery rate–a population-based screening study. FASTER Research Consortium. *Am J Obstet Gynecol* 2004;190:1091–1097.
23. Ananth C, Wen S. Trends in fetal growth among singleton gestations in the United States and Canada, 1985 through 1998. *Semin Perinatol* 2002;26:260–267.
24. Surkan P, Hsieh C, Johansson A, Dickman P, Cnattingius S. Reasons for increasing trends in large for gestational age births. *Obstet Gynecol* 2004;194:720–726.
25. Hedley A, Ogden C, Johnson C, Carroll M, Curtin L, Flegal K. Prevalence of overweight and obesity among US children, adolescents, and adults, 1999–2002. *JAMA* 2004; 291:2847–2850.
26. American College of Obstetricians and Gynecologists. Committee Opinion No. 314. Obesity in Pregnancy. Washington, DC: ACOG; 2005.
27. Catelano P. Management of obesity in pregnancy. *Obstet Gynecol* 2007;109:419–433.
28. Baeten J, Bukusi E, Lambe M. Pregnancy complications and outcomes among over-weight and obese nulliparous women. *Am J Pub Health* 2001;91:436–440.
29. Cedergren M. Maternal morbid obesity and the risk of adverse pregnancy outcome. *Obstet Gynecol* 2004;103:219–224.
30. Jensen D, Damm P, Sorensen B, Molsted-Pedersen L, Westergaard J, Ovesen P, Beck-Nielsen H. Pregnancy outcome and prepregnancy body mass index in 2459 glu-cose-tolerant Danish women. *Am J Obstet Gynecol* 2003;189:239–244.
31. Young T, Woodmansee B. Factors that are associated with cesarean delivery in a large private practice: The importance of pre-pregnancy body mass index and weight gain. *Am J Obstet Gynecol* 2002;187:312–318.
32. Usha Kiran T, Hemmadi S, Bethel J, Evans J. Outcome of pregnancy in a woman with an increased body mass index. *BJOG* 2005;112:768–772.
33. Robinson H, Tkatch S, Mayes D, Bott N, Okun N. Is maternal obesity a predictor of shoulder dystocia? *Obstet Gynecol* 2003;101:24–27.
34. Abrams B, Laros K. Prepregnancy weight, weight gain and birth weight. *Am J Obstet Gynecol* 1986;154:503–509.
35. Ehrenberg H, Mercer B, Catalano P. The influence of obesity and diabetes on the prevalence of macrosomia. *Am J Obstet Gynecol* 2004;191:964–968.
36. Gudmundsson S, Henningsson A, Lindqvist P. Correlation of birth injury with maternal height and birthweight. *BJOG* 2005;112:764–767.
37. Mahony R, Walsh C, Foley M, Daly M, O'Herlihy C. Outcome of second delivery after prior macrosomic infant in women with normal glucose tolerance. *Obstet Gynecol* 2006;107:557–862.
38. Al-Najashi S, Al-Suleiman S, El-Yahia A, Rahman M, Rahman J. Shoulder dystocia: A clinical study of 56 cases. *Aust N Z J Obstet Gynecol* 1989;29:129–132.
39. Acker D, Sachs B, Friedman E. Risk factors for shoulder dystocia in the average-weight infant. *Obstet Gynecol* 1986;67:614.
40. McFarland M, Hod M, Piper J, Xenakis E, Langer O. Are labor abnormalities more common in shoulder dystocia? *Am J Obstet Gynecol* 1995;173:1211–1214.
41. Strofenoyoh E, Seffah J. Prenatal, labor and delivery characteristics of mothers with macrosomic babies. *Int J Obstet Gynecol* 2006;93:49–50.

42. Mehta S, Bujold E, Blackwell S, Sorokin Y, Sokol R. Is abnormal labor associated with shoulder dystocia in nulliparous women? *Am J Obstet Gynecol* 2004;190:1604–1607.

43. Berard J, Dufour P, Vinatier D, Subtil D, Vanderstichele J, Monnier J, Puech F. Fetal macrosomia: Risk factors and outcome. A study of the outcome concerning 100 cases >4500 grams. *Euro J Obstet Gynecol* 1988;77:51–19.

44. Lipscomb K, Gregory K, Shaw K. The outcome of macrosomic infants weighing at least 4500 grams. Los Angeles County and University of Southern California experience. *Obstet Gynecol* 1995;85:558–564.

45. Nassar A, Usta I, Khalil A, Melmen Z, Nakad T, Abu Musa A. Fetal macrosomia (> or = 4500 grams): Perinatal outcome of 321 cases according to the mode of delivery. *J Perinatol* 2003;23:136–141.

46. Sandmire H, DeMott R. The Green Bay cesarean section study IV. The physician factor as a determinant of cesarean birth rates for the large fetus. *Am J Obstet Gynecol* 1996;174:1557–1564.

47. Sanchez-Ramos l, Bernstein S, Kaunitz A. Expectant management versus labor induction for suspected fetal macrosomia: A systematic review. *Obstet Gynecol* 2002;100:997–1002.

48. Irion O, Boulvain M. Induction of labour for suspected fetal macrosomia. Cochrane Database of Systematic Reviews 2007;1.

49. Gherman R, Chauhan S, Ouzounian J, Lerner H, Gonik B, Goodwin T. Shoulder dystocia: The unpreventable obstetric emergency with empiric management guidelines. *Am J Obstet Gynecol* 2006;195:657–672.

50. McFarland L, Raskin M, Daling J, Benedetti T. Erb/Duchenne's palsy: A consequence of fetal macrosomia and method of delivery. *Obstet Gynecol* 1986;68:784–788.

51. Nesbitt T, Gilbert W, Herrchen B. Shoulder dystocia and associated risk factors with macrosomic infants born in California. *Am J Obstet Gynecol* 1998;179:476–480.

52. Wittgrove A, Jester L, Wittgrove P, Clark G. Pregnancy following gastric bypass for morbid obesity. *Obes Surg* 1998;8:461–466.

53. Institute of Medicine. Nutritional status and weight gain. In: *Nutrition During Pregnancy*. Washington, DC: National Academy Press; 1990:27–2.

54. Field N, Piper J, Langer O. The effect of maternal obesity on the accuracy of fetal weight estimation. *Obstet Gynecol* 1995;86:102–107.

Chapter 19
The Midwifery View of Shoulder Dystocia

Judith S. Mercer and Debra A. Erickson-Owens

Summary Midwives and physicians face similar challenges. Preparedness is the key to success. Midwives often practice strategies unfamiliar to physicians. The Gaskin and somersault maneuvers are two examples.

Keywords: cord clamping · Gaskin · infant resuscitation · midwife-physician relationship · midwifery · nuchal cord · positions for birth · shoulder dystocia · somersault maneuver

Contents

19.1	Introduction	270
19.2	Management Issues	270
19.3	Labor and Birth Factors	271
19.4	Maternal Positions in Labor	271
19.5	Positions at Birth	272
19.6	The Gaskin "All-Fours" Maneuver	272
19.7	Running Start	273
19.8	Using Restitution to One's Advantage	273
19.9	Releasing the Anterior Shoulder	274
19.10	Suprapubic Not Fundal Pressure	274
19.11	Pushing	274
19.12	Avoid Assisted Delivery	274
19.13	Algorithms and Mnemonics	275
19.14	Is Routine Episiotomy Essential?	275
19.15	Safeguarding the Newborn	275
19.16	Delayed Cord Clamping	276
19.17	Cord Clamping Before Shoulder Delivery	276
19.18	Nuchal Cord Management	277
19.19	Education and Clinical Competency	278
19.20	Midwife and Physician Responsibilities	279
19.21	Legal Issues	280
19.22	Documentation	281
19.23	Conclusion	281

J.S. Mercer
Certified Nurse Midwife, Cranston, Rhode Island, USA

J.A. O'Leary (ed.), *Shoulder Dystocia and Birth Injury*,
DOI 10.1007/978-1-59745-473-5_19, © Humana Press, a part of Springer
Science+Business Media, LLC 2009

19.1 Introduction

Midwives share many of the same concerns and fears about shoulder dystocia as their physician colleagues. Shoulder dystocia is one of the leading causes of malpractice claims against midwives and obstetricians especially if fetal/ newborn injury such as brachial plexus injury or hypoxic damage has occurred. The purpose of this chapter is to present additional information about management of shoulder dystocia often used by midwives that may be beneficial to all providers and to discuss issues related to midwifery-physician relationships.

Shoulder dystocia can challenge even the most experienced midwife (or physician) as it frequently occurs without warning and is a birth emergency requiring quick recognition, preparedness, and well-rehearsed maneuvers. It requires a mental and physical readiness of the provider with the safety of mother and infant always a top priority. Midwifery practice in any setting—hospital, birth center, or home—must include ongoing maintenance of competence for management of intrapartum emergencies.

Although the basic maneuvers used to release shoulders during a shoulder dystocia are the same for midwives and physicians, midwives often incorporate additional techniques not considered "mainstream" such as changing the birth position to "all-fours." Midwives offer a complementary perspective in the management of shoulder dystocia. Some important midwifery strategies in the management of shoulder dystocia include avoiding supine position for late labor and birth; eliminating fundal pressure as part of practice; discouraging use of vacuum extraction when risk factors are known; protecting the infant against potential hypoxic damage by using the somersault maneuver to avoid cutting of a nuchal cord; and neonatal resuscitation performed at the perineum with an intact cord and/or milking the cord immediately after birth to rapidly accelerate placental transfusion to correct hypovolemia. Maternal and infant morbidity and medicolegal issues may be reduced with the application of appropriate management skills and the recording of the shoulder dystocia by accurate and comprehensive documentation.

Ultimately, the goals for all providers dealing with shoulder dystocia include safe-guarding maternal and newborn health, avoiding undue harm, and promoting a positive and satisfying birth experience in spite of this intrapartum complication. Practice drills in shoulder dystocia management are recommended for all staff participating in birth care. The importance of relationship and trust with laboring women, nursing staff, and physician colleagues is essential for communication, collaboration, and successful resolution of shoulder dystocia.

19.2 Management Issues

The well-known methods for management of shoulder dystocia such as suprapubic pressure, McRoberts, Woods screw and Rubin maneuvers, delivery of the posterior arm, and cephalic replacement are all presented in other chapters within this book. In this chapter, maneuvers less well-known but very effective are introduced. Also, a paradigm shift in management is offered for the care of an infant who has been distressed by shoulder dystocia.

19.3 Labor and Birth Factors

Certain intrapartum factors may put the laboring woman at greater risk for shoulder dystocia. These factors include (1) maternal positioning, such as supine or low semi-Fowler, which reduces blood flow to the uterus and thereby reduces strength of contractions; (2) application of a vacuum extractor or use of the Ritgen maneuver to facilitate birth; (3) closed glottal pushing, which can diminish fetal oxygenation; (4) fundal pressure, which can lodge the fetal shoulder behind the symphysis; and (5) "rushing the shoulders" after birth, which interferes with spontaneous restitution (Table 19.1). The following discussion addresses the issues and prevention strategies that midwives and others may consider to avert or resolve shoulder dystocia while minimizing damage to the woman and infant.

19.4 Maternal Positions in Labor

In a classic 1950 study, Caldeyro-Barcia documented that laboring women in the supine position had prolonged, less powerful contractions compared with women in a side-lying position [1]. When women in the supine position were placed on their sides, the contractions became shorter and stronger. Caldeyro-Barcia theorized that uterine circulation is better in a side-lying position and therefore contractions are more effective. Strong uterine contractions are essential to move a large fetus down the birth canal. The strength of contractions has a significant impact on the cardinal mechanisms of labor-flexion, descent, engagement, internal rotation, extension, restitution. Good contractions are essential to birth the large infant—maternal and provider efforts are secondary. Women in a side-lying position can be encouraged to push without difficulty by assisting them to pull up the top knee into the abdomen and applying counter pressure to the bottom of the feet. Hands and knees or squatting positions are equally effective in avoiding uterine pressure on the great vessels. Frequent change of maternal position is important for comfort and for the best possible uterine circulation. Avoiding long periods of supine or semi-Fowler positioning is strongly recommended to optimize uterine perfusion.

Table 19.1 Items to Avoid During Intrapartum Care

Prolonged supine or semi-Fowler position
Use of vacuum extractor if risk factors for shoulder dystocia
Ritgen maneuver
Closed-glottal pushing
Fundal pressure
Rushing the shoulders

19.5 Positions at Birth

Most midwives are comfortable in assisting women at birth in alternative positions such as squatting, standing, side-lying, or all-fours [2]. Ideally, all obstetric providers should be comfortable with different birthing positions. Birth positions can be an important strategy in shoulder dystocia prevention and management. Midwives and physicians not yet comfortable with alternative positions should begin to introduce a variety of positions into their day-to-day clinical practice preferably well before an alternative position is needed for the first time when a shoulder dystocia occurs.

Birth positioning can make a difference. As discussed above, lithotomy position, with or without the use of stirrups, decreases the effectiveness of the uterine contractions and restricts the posterior movement of the sacrum. Most obstetric texts provide illustrations of shoulder dystocia maneuvers with the woman in the lithotomy position. Although preferred and more convenient for many providers, this position may not be advantageous in releasing tight shoulders during a shoulder dystocia. Upright positioning, such as squatting and standing, can widen the transverse diameter of the pelvis and increase uterine contraction effectiveness. The squatting position can modify the pubic bone angle and encourage a "rolling" of the shoulder from out under the symphysis pubis [3]. Encouraging a woman at risk for shoulder dystocia to remain in hands and knees throughout the birth can be used as a preventative strategy.

The birth provider working with women who have minimal analgesia/anesthesia—at home, in a birth center, or in hospital—has an advantage because the laboring woman can more easily assume positions such as squatting, hands and knees, and so forth, to assist in the rotation and delivery of the infant. The mother is aware of sensations that guide her in positioning her pelvis and body to effectively push. She adjusts the "planes and angles" of her pelvis intuitively (A. Bailes, personal communication, 2007). Providers working in hospital are more likely to care for women who have their pain managed by intravenous opioids or epidural analgesia, which interferes with sensation and mobility. Dense epidurals may contribute to, complicate, and prolong shoulder dystocia. A side-lying position during second stage may be the best option to ensure adequate powers and decrease a risk of shoulder dystocia [4].

19.6 The Gaskin "All-Fours" Maneuver

The Gaskin maneuver, or all-fours maneuver, is an important approach in the release of a tight shoulder. The woman is simply turned from her current position to a position on her hands and knees. It can be used at the onset when a shoulder dystocia is identified or can be used as a measure of last resort. Midwives often use it from the onset. The maneuver is frequently criticized as being disorienting for the provider, time consuming, and difficult when the laboring woman is attached to monitoring equipment and intravenous lines. However, it has been demonstrated to be highly effective in releasing the tight shoulder (83% of the time) with minimal maternal and infant morbidity [3,5–7]. Even a woman with an epidural can be placed in all-fours, with assistance, in a reasonable amount of time [7].

19.7 Running Start

The "running start" position is another technique useful in releasing a tight shoulder. This technique maximizes the pelvic mobility that helps to dislodge a shoulder dystocia. The birthing woman is assisted into a hands and knees position. She lifts the knee of one leg up under her chest and places her foot down flat on the bed. This can assist with dislodging the "stuck" shoulder to facilitate birth [3].

19.8 Using Restitution to One's Advantage

Often, providers forget the mechanisms of labor and attempt to deliver the shoulders immediately after the head is born. Frequently, this is done without a contraction. Without restitution, the fetus' shoulders are usually in the anterior-posterior diameter behind the symphysis. Waiting for the spontaneous delivery of the shoulders rather than using traction before the shoulders have rotated is encouraged. This "waiting for the shoulders," or not rushing the shoulders, allows the restitution of the head and the normal rotation of the infant's shoulders to an oblique diameter that actually enhances delivery through completion of the normal cardinal movements [8]. Provider anxiety and fear of shoulder dystocia can cause one to attempt to rush and thereby interfere in the completion of these usual movements. This expectant approach to the delivery of the shoulders can avoid a hurried delivery with a subsequent dystocia and can reduce the risk of excessive force on the infant's neck during delivery.

In Europe, it is routine to deliver the infant's head and then wait for the next contraction to facilitate restitution and deliver the shoulders [9]. The diagnosis of shoulder dystocia is not made until after this second contraction. This is in direct contrast with the practice in the United States. Supporting the normal mechanisms of labor can allow spontaneous restitution. Not rushing the delivery of the shoulders is unfamiliar to many U.S. providers, but the practice may reduce risk of lodging the shoulder behind the symphysis and using excessive force.

19.9 Releasing the Anterior Shoulder

A variation on the previous technique is an attempt to release the anterior shoulder from under the symphysis with the same contraction that delivers the head. This technique uses uterine and maternal powers to slip the anterior shoulder under the symphysis just after the head delivers but during the same contraction. Once the provider feels that the shoulder is released, she or he can relax and wait for the next contraction to complete the birth so that uterine and maternal efforts can assist with full delivery of the large shoulders and body.

19.10 Suprapubic Not Fundal Pressure

Although "suprapubic" pressure is a highly valued technique in the management of shoulder dystocia, "fundal" pressure is not considered helpful. Fundal pressure increases the risk for an impacted anterior shoulder and prevents rotation of the shoulders from the anterior-posterior diameter to an oblique diameter needed for the fetus to birth. It should be avoided during the time of birth [10].

19.11 Pushing

Closed glottal pushing can exhaust the mother and may act in the same manner as fundal pressure by wedging the shoulder behind the symphysis. Most importantly, over time, it increases acidosis in the fetus and may contribute to a depressed fetus [11]. Long sessions of closed glottal pushing are not advised.

19.12 Avoid Assisted Delivery

Instrument delivery such as by vacuum or forceps has a long-standing association with shoulder dystocia [6]. When a vacuum or forceps delivery is used, it results in the delivery of the head without any rotation of the shoulders into an oblique diameter. Shoulders often stay in the anterior-posterior diameter forcing the anterior shoulder to wedge behind the symphysis.

Vacuum extraction is a selective advanced midwifery skill that a number of experienced midwives incorporate into their practice. Midwives as well as other obstetric providers must be cautioned of the increased risk of shoulder dystocia with the use of vacuum extraction. Strict adherence to vacuum extractor protocols should be followed.

The Ritgen maneuver, used to hasten extension and delivery of the head, may interfere with the usual rotation of the shoulders into an oblique diameter. This increases the risk of lodging the anterior shoulder behind the symphysis. Midwives rarely use this maneuver.

19.13 Algorithms and Mnemonics

Well-developed algorithms and mnemonics, which assist the provider to effectively manage a shoulder dystocia, have been described elsewhere in this book. Additional algorithms and mnemonics can be found in other sources such as *Varney's Midwifery* and the Advanced Life Support in Obstetrics Course Syllabus [2,12,13]. Memorized steps and algorithms assist the midwife or physician to remain current and clinically competent when or if confronted with a shoulder dystocia.

19.14 Is Routine Episiotomy Essential?

Routine episiotomy is controversial. Midwives prefer not to perform an episiotomy routinely with shoulder dystocia but are concerned about the legal ramifications. Commonly, the recommendation of prophylactic episiotomy for anticipation of a shoulder dystocia has been required to avoid allegations of malpractice. However, shoulder dystocia is a bony tissue, not a soft tissue, dilemma. The only advantage of episiotomy is it creates additional room for manipulation such as reaching for the infant's posterior arm. Currently, there is no evidence that supports prophylactic cutting of an episiotomy [6].

19.15 Safeguarding the Newborn

An infant who has experienced shoulder dystocia is frequently pale and limp with poor Apgar scores. Most often, the umbilical cord is clamped immediately and the newborn is rushed to the warmer for resuscitation. The infant may be depressed and floppy; appearing shocky and cyanotic. An infant with these symptoms frequently needs volume expansion. Volume expansion is readily available in any setting if the placental circulation is not interrupted by immediate cord clamping. Although most people interpret neonatal resuscitation guidelines to mean that the cord must be cut immediately, a full appropriate resuscitation can be done at the mother's perineum with the cord intact. Placental function does not cease in the first 2 minutes after birth and can help to support the infant's recovery through extrauterine resuscitation. This idea is supported by the EXIT procedure used during fetal surgery [14]. During the EXIT procedure used for fetal surgery, the uterus is opened, the fetus is partially removed, and life support is provided by the placenta. This method has been used to sustain an infant for more than 45 minutes. Our understanding of the EXIT procedure helps us to realize that at birth, even 2 minutes of life support from the placenta can benefit the newborn by facilitating the establishment of respirations and promoting adequate blood flow to vital organs.

19.16 Delayed Cord Clamping

Clamping the cord immediately after birth results in a 25% reduction in the infant's blood volume and a 50% reduction in red cell volume [15]. The most recent meta-analysis of delayed versus immediate cord clamping indicates that infants who experience immediate clamping have more anemia of infancy at 6 months of age compared with infants who have delayed clamping [16]. There has been no reported increase in symptomatic polycythemia or hyperbilirubine-mia in more than 1,000 infants with delayed cord clamping. A number of studies have related anemia of infancy, infants when treated with iron, with less favorable neurodevelopmental and behavioral outcomes up to the age of 19 years [17].

Shoulder dystocia, with or without the presence of a nuchal cord, can be especially dangerous for a newborn as it places an infant at particular risk for hypovolemia [18]. The squeeze of a tight fit through the birth canal may cause more fetal blood than usual to be extruded into the placenta due to pressure on the cord and on the body. The umbilical vein is a large, thin-walled, floppy, low-pressure structure that is easily subject to compression. The thicker-walled, muscular, high-pressure umbilical arteries are not so easily compressed. The impact of compression is significant for the infant and may account for the poor condition of these infants at birth—worse than what would be anticipated from a few minutes of hypoxia [19]. Rapid cutting of the cord to move these infants to a warmer to facilitate resuscitation may be a harmful intervention.

19.17 Cord Clamping Before Shoulder Delivery

Several case reports demonstrate neonatal anemia and hypovolemia with tight nuchal cords at birth [20,21]. The usual occurrence of shoulder dystocia is approximately 0.5% to 1.7% of all births, whereas nuchal cords occur in 20% to 33%; both phenomena are often unpredictable [22]. Case reports suggest that cutting a nuchal cord prior to the birth of the shoulders may increase an infant's risk of asphyxia and even death if there is a severe shoulder dystocia [22,23]. Iffy described several cases of cerebral palsy associated with a nuchal cord cut before delivery of the shoulders with a subsequent shoulder dystocia. In some of these cases, birth was delayed as little as 3 minutes [22]. All fetuses were considered healthy prior to the onset of labor. The infants were all born with low Apgar scores and developed signs of hypoxic-ischemic encephalopathy. The authors highly advise to not cut the nuchal cord prior to completion of the delivery whenever possible.

A recent integrated review of the literature by Mercer et al. found an increased risk to the newborn when the nuchal cord was clamped prior to the delivery of the shoulders [24].

Flamm reported the birth of an infant where he almost cut the nuchal cord before he was assured that the infant would be born [23]. He was able to slip the cord over the head. However, he was unable to deliver the baby vaginally. He used the Zavanelli maneuver to replace the head. The infant was born by cesarean section and had Apgar scores of 3 [1], 7 [5], and 9 [10]. Had he prematurely ligated the nuchal cord, the infant would not have survived.

19.18 Nuchal Cord Management

Nuchal cords can be managed without cutting them. There are several options. The first is to slip the cord over the head or down around the shoulders and slide the baby through the cord. The other option is the somersault maneuver, first described by Schorn and Blanco [25]. It involves delivering the baby slowly and bringing the head, as it is born, toward the mother's thigh. The baby is kept tucked near the perineum so that the body rolls out and the feet are away from the mother with the head still up toward the introitus (Fig. 19.1) [24]. Leaving the cord intact and using the somersault maneuver is recommended especially if shoulder dystocia is suspected. During the somersault maneuver,

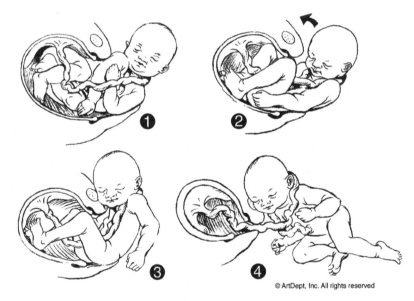

Fig. 19.1 Somersault maneuver. Involves holding the infant's head flexed and guiding it upward or sideways toward the pubic bone or thigh, so the baby does a "somersault," ending with the infant's feet toward the mother's knees and the head still at the perineum. (1) Once the nuchal cord is discovered, the anterior and posterior shoulders are slowly delivered under control without manipulating the cord. (2) As the shoulders are delivered, the head is flexed so that the face of the baby is pushed toward the maternal thigh. (3)The baby's head is kept next to the perineum while the body is delivered and "somersaults" out. (4) The umbilical cord is then unwrapped, and the usual management ensues

the infant's head is kept near the perineum as the body delivers so that little traction is exerted on the cord.

With either of the above options, it is particularly important to avoid cutting the nuchal cord immediately after the birth, no matter how depressed the infant appears. The dynamics of cord compression will likely result in an increased transfer of blood to the placenta. Pale color and poor tone indicate infant hypovolemia. A delay in cord clamping is needed for the blood volume to equalize after birth and assist with stabilizing the infant's transition to neonatal life. Resuscitation at the perineum allows the infant to regain the blood trapped in the placenta and can be accomplished using all the proper tenets of neonatal resuscitation.

If one must cut the cord immediately at birth, milking the cord first is a safe option that can help the infant restore blood volume after shoulder dystocia or shoulder dystocia with a nuchal cord [26]. This is done by rapidly milking (or stripping) the cord two to four times from the introitus to the infant's umbilicus prior to cutting the cord.

While the above techniques may seem radical to many providers who have only seen routine hospital birth, practicing midwives in all birth settings have been using these techniques for many years with excellent success [27].

19.19 Education and Clinical Competency

The backbone of midwifery practice is to "be prepared" for intrapartum emergencies such as shoulder dystocia. Midwives are well prepared during their basic educational programs to identify risk factors and to anticipate, recognize, and manage shoulder dystocia [28]. Sustaining clinical competency after graduation is essential as even the most experienced midwives will only see a few cases of "true" shoulder dystocia during their careers. Use of a mnemonic, such as HELPERR (Table 19.2), can be a useful tool for triggering the memorized steps of shoulder dystocia management at a time when a calm demeanor and highly competent care is essential [12]

Shoulder dystocia rehearsals or drills can confirm competency in shoulder dystocia management, similar to that of mock CPR drills. According to Crofts

Table 19.2 Example of a Shoulder Dystocia Mnemonic: HELPERR [12,13]

H: Call for help
E: Evaluate for episiotomy
L: Legs (the McRoberts maneuver)
P: Suprapubic pressure
E: Enter—internal maneuvers (Rubin, Woods screw, reverse Woods screw)
R: Remove the posterior arm
R: Roll the patient (all-fours or Gaskin maneuver)

and colleagues, regularly scheduled shoulder dystocia drills among all obstetric staff, including midwives and physicians, can improve emergency response, performance, and reduce the risk of excessive force and injury [29].

19.20 Midwife and Physician Responsibilities

Midwives independently manage the care of women during normal pregnancy, childbirth, and postpartum [28]. and work "within a healthcare system which provides for consultation, collaborative management or referral as indicated by the health status of the woman" [30]. When a problem such as shoulder dystocia is anticipated, a midwife may consult with a physician about a woman's ongoing care. The consultation may result in a decision for the midwife to retain independent management of the woman or a decision may be made to collaboratively manage the woman's care with the physician. Collaborative management implies shared responsibility for the care. A third option may be when the midwife and physician decide that the woman needs physician management for her care such as when a cesarean section is clearly indicated.

An established midwife-physician relationship that includes trust, mutual respect, and professional responsibility and accountability will enhance safety and performance when a shoulder dystocia is anticipated or encountered [31]. Evidence-based practice guidelines, used by a number of midwifery practices, can be jointly agreed upon between the midwife and physician and are helpful in guiding appropriate consultation to enhance safety and improve the outcomes of shoulder dystocia.

In hospital settings, midwives consult with a physician when a shoulder dystocia is anticipated, recognized, or when assistance is needed. Appropriate consultation includes the identification of risk factors and determination of whether the physician's presence before or during a shoulder dystocia is needed. Timely arrival of medical staff (obstetric and pediatric) and a well-prepared nursing staff is extremely useful in orchestrating a successful shoulder dystocia management.

In settings outside the hospital, the midwife may transfer a woman's care to a hospital practice prior to labor if risk factors suggest the woman is at high risk for a shoulder dystocia. If anticipated during labor, a woman can also be transferred to a hospital practice assuming safe transport is possible. Transfer during labor necessitates the importance of good communication and collaboration with the other providers in order for the laboring woman to have a seamless continuity of care.

However, shoulder dystocia is an unpredictable event more than 50% of the time. An unanticipated shoulder dystocia can be managed by the midwife in or out of the hospital setting.

In the case of an unexpected shoulder dystocia, the midwife requests that the staff summon the physician (obstetric and pediatric) while completing the appropriate management maneuvers. In and out of hospital setting, the midwife and ancillary staff are prepared to manage a dystocia and initiate a full neonatal resuscitation as necessary.

19.21 Legal Issues

Shoulder dystocia is a poorly predicted event and an intrapartum emergency with potentially very serious consequences for the woman and her newborn. Midwives, as well as their physician colleagues, are vulnerable to malpractice allegations in spite of correctly identifying the emergency and managing the shoulder dystocia effectively. Concerns about vicarious liability occasionally surface when a midwife-physician team manages a shoulder dystocia. Who is ultimately deemed to be responsible? The understanding of vicarious liability can often be confusing and frequently misinterpreted.

Some physicians fear they are responsible not only for their actions but also for the midwife's actions during the management of a shoulder dystocia. However, as midwives are licensed as independent practitioners to manage birth, it is redundant to hold a physician responsible for the midwife's actions. By definition, vicarious liability is known as "the liability of an employer for an employee's actions." [32]. This is often the case in clinical practice. Many midwives and physicians maintain an arrangement through guidelines and collaborative practice agreements but not an employer-employee relationship. A collaborative practice agreement is an example of a nonemployment relationship. Although all members of the health care team may be at risk for malpractice subsequent to a shoulder dystocia, physicians are not liable for the actions of the midwife or any other team member when there is not an employer-employee relationship. The reader is referred to an update by Joseph Booth [32] for further reading on vicarious liability.

Jevitt reports the four most common malpractice allegations related to the level of physician involvement in the management of shoulder dystocia [6]. These allegations represent examples of a midwife's failure to appropriately consult with a physician (1) when there is recognition of prenatal risk factors that suggest a planned cesarean birth might be warranted; (2) when multiple risk factors for shoulder dystocia accumulate during the intrapartum period; (3) when one anticipates a shoulder dystocia; or (4) when assistance is needed once a shoulder dystocia is identified. These examples emphasize the importance of appropriate consultation and good communication between midwife and physician [6]. However, these allegations reflect physician involvement in the hospital setting. Jevitt did not report on any cases involving out-of-hospital settings.

Table 19.3 Shoulder Dystocia: Generic Outline for Documentation [6,33]

Time and date
Position of vertex at delivery
Position and position changes of mother
Restitution to what position—which shoulder was anterior?
Time of delivery of the head
Time of delivery of the body
Who was present or who was called to the birth
Describe maneuvers used to deliver infant and the sequence and time in which they were done
Evidence of nuchal cord
Newborn weight and Apgar scores
Quality of newborn movement in the extremities (especially arms)
Disposition of the newborn
Any maternal injuries and condition

Note: Read documentation by other medical personnel (nurses' notes, pediatrician's note, etc.) and reconcile any discrepancies between the notes as soon as possible.

19.22 Documentation

Documentation is extremely important when addressing the issues surrounding shoulder dystocia. As Jevitt notes, "documentation … becomes the best defense." [6]. Written documentation records the midwife's actions: recognition and identification of risk factors, assessment, management, and consultation with the physician. During the autepartum period, the midwife should document the following: previous history of shoulder dystocia, height, prepregnancy weight, initial weight, and total weight gain, body mass index, diabetic screening, fundal height measurement particularly if size is greater than dates, and estimated fetal weight (EFW). Intrapartum documentation should include any risk factors associated with shoulder dystocia plus EFW, labor progress, and assessment of fetal descent through the pelvis. The birth and management of the shoulder dystocia must be documented as accurately as possible. A generic outline for documenting a shoulder dystocia is offered in Table 19.3 [6,33]. The outline is inclusive and guides the midwife in writing a thorough, accurate, and honest account of the management of the shoulder dystocia.

19.23 Conclusion

Midwives and physicians face similar challenges when confronted with a shoulder dystocia. Each provider is responsible for the conduct of his or her own professional practice when managing a shoulder dystocia. This highly litigious area of birth care requires each midwife and physician to be highly competent and prepared. Preparedness is key to the management of shoulder dystocia. Readiness for this often unpredictable event can be enhanced by continuing education, memorization of algorithms and mnemonics, and interval practice drills involving all staff in any birth setting.

Midwives offer practice strategies for shoulder dystocia that may or may not be familiar to their physician colleagues. These can include preventative or management techniques intended to safeguard the mother and the infant in order to avoid undue harm. Strategies can focus on avoiding factors that contribute to poor uterine contractions or labor and birth positions that reduce pelvic diameters. The Gaskin all-fours maneuver can open the pelvis and reduce a tight shoulder with good success. The somersault maneuver can optimize an infant's blood volume by avoiding the immediate cutting and clamping of a nuchal cord. Neonatal resuscitation at the perineum is optimized by an intact umbilical cord in the first few minutes of life.

Complete, thorough, and consistent documentation is an essential part of good care and the best defense against malpractice claims. Good teamwork between the midwives and physicians and use of the additional ideas and tools presented here will provide support for providers when confronted with a shoulder dystocia.

References

1. Caldeyro-Barcia R, Alvarez H, Reynolds S. A better understanding of uterine contractility through simultaneous recording with an internal and a seven channel external method. *Surg Gynecol Bostet* 1950;91:641–646.
2. Varney H, Kriebs J, Gegor C. *Varney's Midwifery*. 4th ed. Boston: Jones and Bartlett Publishers; 2004.
3. Tully G. Shoulder dystocia. *Midwifery Today E-News* 2005;7(3). Retrieved from http://www.midwiferytoday.com/enews/enews0723.asp#main
4. Nixon S, Avery M, Savik K. Outcomes of macrosomic infants in a nurse-midwifery service. *J Nurse Midwifery* 1998;43:280–286.
5. Simbruner G, Moulopoulos S [Blood volume determination in the newborn using blood of adults as an indicator (author's trans)]. *Padiatr Padol* 1977;12:235–244.
6. Jevitt C. Shoulder dystocia: etiology, common risk factors, and management. *J Midwifery Womens Health* 2005;50:485–497.
7. Bruner J, Drummond S, Meenan A, Gaskin I. All-fours maneuver for reducing shoulder dystocia during labor. *J Reprod Med* 1998;43:439–443.
8. Mortimore VR, McNabb M. A six-year retrospective analysis of shoulder dystocia and delivery of the shoulders. *Midwifery* 1998;14(3):162–173.
9. Iffy L, Varadi V, Papp E. Untoward neonatal sequelae deriving from cutting of the umbilical cord before delivery. *Med Law* 2001;20:627–634.
10. Walsh L. Midwifery. *Community-Based Care During the Childbearing Year*. 1st ed. Philadelphia: W.B. Saunders; 2001.
11. Roberts J. The "push" for evidence: Management of the second state. *J Midwifery Womens Health* 2002;47:2–15.
12. Baxley E, Gobbo R. Shoulder dystocia. *Am Fam Physician* 2004;69:1707–1714.
13. Ailsworth K, Anderson J, Atwood L, Bailey R, Canavan T. Advanced life support in Obstetrics Course Syllabus. Leawood, KS: American Academy of Family Physicians; 2000.

14. Bouchard S, Johnson M, Flake A, et al. The EXIT procedure: Experience and outcome in 31 cases. *J Pediatr Surg* 2002;37:418–426.
15. Yao A, Moinian M, Lind J. Distribution of blood between infant and placenta after birth. *Lancet* 1969;2:871–873.
16. Hutton E, Hassan E. Late vs early clamping of the umbilical cord in full-term neonates: Systematic review and meta-analysis of controlled trials. *JAMA* 2007;297:1241–1252.
17. Lozoff B, Beard J, Connor J, Barbara F, Georgieff M, Schallert T. Long-lasting neural and behavioral effects of iron deficiency in infancy. *Nutr Rev* 2006;64:S34–43; discussion S72–91.
18. Mercer J, Skovgaard R, Erickson-Owens D. Cardiac asystole at birth: Is hypovolemic shock the cause? Unpublished manuscript; 2007
19. Hope P, Breslin S, Lamont L, et al. Fatal shoulder dystocia: A review of 56 cases reported to the Confidential Enquiry into stillbirths and deaths in infancy. *Br J Obstet Gynaecol* 1998;105:1256–1261.
20. Cashore W, Usher R. Hypovolemia resulting from a tight nuchal cord at birth. *Pediatr Res* 1973;7:399.
21. Shepherd A, Richardson C, Brown J. Nuchal cord as a cause of neonatal anemia. *Am J Dis Child* 1985;139:71–73.
22. Iffy L, Varadi V. Cerebral palsy following cutting of the nuchal cord before delivery. *Med law* 1994;13:323–330.
23. Flamm B. Tight nuchal cord and shoulder dystocia: A potentially catastrophic combination. *Obstet Gynecol* 1999;94:853.
24. Mercer J, Skovgaard R, Peareara-Eaves J, Bowman T. Nuchal cord management and nurse-midwifery practice. *J Midwifery Womens Health* 2005;50:373–379.
25. Schorn M, Blanco J. Management of the nuchal cord. *J Nurse Midwifery* 1991;36:131–132.
26. Erickson-Owens D, A review of the literature on milking of the umbilical cord at birth. Unpublished dissertation proposal. University of Rhode Island; 2008
27. Mercer J, Nelson C, Skovgaard R. Umbilical cord clamping: Beliefs and practices of American nurse-midwives. *J Midwif Women Health* 2000;45:58–66.
28. Core Competencies for Basic Midwifery Practice. American College of Nurse-Midwives; 2002. Available at www.midwife.org. Accessed May 24, 2007.
29. Crofts J, Bartlett C, Ellis D, Hunt L, Fox R, Draycott T. Training for shoulder dystocia: A trial of simulation using low-fidelity and high-fidelity mannequins. *Obstet Gynecol* 2006;108:1477–1485.
30. Collaborative Management in Midwifery Practice for Medical, Gynecological and Obstetrical Conditions. American College of Nurse-Midwives; 1997. Available at www.midwife.org. Accessed May 24, 2007.
31. Joint Statement of Practice Relations Between Obstetrician/Gynecologists and Certified Nurse-Midwives/Certified Midwives. American College of Nurse-Midwives; 2002. Available at www.midwife.org. Accessed May 24, 2007.
32. Booth J. An update on vicarious liability for certified nurse-midwives/certified midwives. *J Midwifery Womens Health* 2007;52:153–157.
33. Mashburn J. Identification and management of shoulder dystocia. *J Nurse Midwifery* 1988;33:225–231.

Chapter 20
Recent Research: Relevant and Reliable

James A. O'Leary

The purpose of this chapter is to bring the reader up to date by briefly abstracting recent key clinical investigations.

1. Comparing mechanical fetal response during descent.

   Quantifiable muscle response occurs in routine and shoulder dystocia deliveries. Posterior brachial plexus stretching is significantly longer for routine deliveries than either unilateral or bilateral shoulder dystocia births [1].

2. Fetal manipulation for management of shoulder dystocia [2].

   It is readily apparent that relevant permanent obstetric brachial plexus injuries remain the near exclusive domain of shoulder dystocia births [2].

The following comments and speculations are proved false [2]:

(a) that the risk of injury cannot be reduced;
(b) that no maneuver has been proved superior to another or guaranteed to work in all circumstances;
(c) that the choice and sequence of specific shoulder dystocia maneuvers beyond the McRoberts maneuver should be left to the discretion of the birth attendant;
(d) that the predominant concern during shoulder dystocia is its expedient resolution, by whatever means necessary, to avoid central nervous system damage or even death.

Traction to the head should not be greater than normal during shoulder dystocia maneuvers or even *not* used at all [2].

Upward traction on the posterior shoulder was demonstrated in a 1916 illustration and appears in several editions of *Williams Obstetrics* with a cautionary statement about injury [2].

J.A. O'Leary
Professor Obstetrics & Gynecology (retired), University of South Florida, Tampa, Florida, USA

J.A. O'Leary (ed.), *Shoulder Dystocia and Birth Injury*,
DOI 10.1007/978-1-59745-473-5_20, © Humana Press, a part of Springer
Science+Business Media, LLC 2009

The Barnum posterior arm delivery when used as an initial approach is associated with lower injury rates [2].

The rate of brachial plexus injury has almost doubled in the past 15 years. This trend has developed over the past 25 years, the McRoberts' maneuver time frame [2].

Uterine forces may be the cause of 15% strain on the brachial plexus, well below the 50% elastic limit of fetal nerves [2].

3. Comparing the McRoberts and Rubin maneuvers for shoulder dystocia [3].

This study was undertaken to objectively compare delivery traction force, fetal neck rotation, and brachial plexus elongation after three different initial shoulder dystocia maneuvers: McRoberts, anterior Rubin, and posterior Rubin [3].

In a laboratory model of initial maneuvers for shoulder dystocia, the anterior Rubin maneuver requires the least traction for delivery and produces the least amount of brachial plexus tension. Further study is needed to validate these results clinically.

4. After shoulder dystocia: Managing the subsequent pregnancy and delivery [4].

Among risk factors for shoulder dystocia, a prior history of delivery complicated by shoulder dystocia is the single greatest risk factor for shoulder dystocia occurrence, with odds ratios 7 to 10 times that of the general population. Recurrence rates have been reported to be as high as 16%. Intervention efforts directed at the particular subgroup of women with a prior history of shoulder dystocia can concentrate on potentially modifiable risk factors and individualized management strategies that can minimize recurrence and the associated significant morbidities and mortality [4].

5. Risk factors for brachial plexus injury with and without shoulder dystocia [5].

Non–shoulder dystocia brachial plexus palsy is uncommon and mechanistically different from shoulder dystocia injuries [5].

6. The role for epislotomy [6].
7. The largest report of the pattern and degree of forces applied by obstetricians and midwives during simulated shoulder dystocia has recently been reported [7].

These data provide cause for concern with wide variation of both the number of pulls undertaken, and traction used, before shoulder dystocia was recognized. Some practitioners were using very high forces before commencing any resolution maneuvers: 20 (18%) applied a force greater than 100N prior to performing a maneuver.

There was great variation in the pattern and degree of traction used once shoulder dystocia was diagnosed, even among senior practitioners. It is of particular concern that forces that may cause damage were applied during two thirds of simulations!

The authors found there was wide variation in the rate at which force was applied. This is particularly noteworthy because increasing the rate of the applied force may increase the susceptibility of the brachial plexus to injury. The rate of force application may be as important as the maximum applied force in the etiology of brachial plexus injury.

Those practitioners who achieved delivery did so with a maximum force of less than 100 N (normal) in only 22% of cases, whereas 27% of the participants applied more than 150 N and 6% more than 200 N [7].

Although episiotomy may be needed to facilitate fetal manipulation for the management of severe shoulder dystocia, the addition of episiotomy does not otherwise confer any increased benefit over performance of fetal manipulation alone. If fetal manipulation can be performed without episiotomy, severe perineal trauma can be averted without increasing the risk of brachial plexus palsy [6].

References

1. Allen R, Cha S, Kranker L, Johnson T, Gurewitsch E. Comparing mechanical fetal response during descent, crowning, and restitution among deliveries with and without shoulder dystocia. *Am J Obstet Gynecol* 2007;196:539.E1–539.E5.
2. Gurewitsch E, Allen R. Fetal manipulation for management of shoulder dystocia. *Fetal Maternal Med Rev* 2006;17:239–280.
3. Gurewitsch E, Kim E, Yang J, Outland K, McDonald M, Allen R. Comparing McRoberts' and Rubin's maneuvers for initial management of shoulder dystocia: An objective evaluation. *Am J Obstet Gynecol* 2005;192:153–160.
4. Gurewitsch E, Johnson T, Allen R. After shoulder dystocia: Managing the subsequent pregnancy and delivery. *Sem Perinatol* 2007;31:185–195.
5. Gurewitsch E, Johnson E, Hanzehzadeh S, Allen R. Risk factors for brachial plexus injury with and without shoulder dystocia. *Am J Obstet Gynecol* 2006;194:486–492.
6. Gurewitsch E, Donithan M, Stallings S, Moore P, Agarwai S, Allen L, Allen R. Epislotomy versus fetal manipulation in managing severe shoulder dystocia: A comparison of outcomes. *Am J Obstet Gynecol* 2004;191:911–916.
7. Crofts J, Ellis D, James M, Hunt L, Fox R, Draycott T. Pattern and degree of forces applied during simulation of shoulder dystocia. *Am J Obstet Gynecol* 2007;197:e1–e6.

Chapter 21
Observations on the Etiology of Brachial Plexus Birth Palsy Based on Radiographic, Intraoperative, and Histologic Findings

Stephen M. Russell, Israel Alfonso, and John A.I. Grossman

Summary The objective of this chapter is to describe and discuss the radiographic, intraoperative, and histologic findings that are present after brachial plexus birth injury. This review is based on the authors' clinical and operative experiences and a survey of the peer-reviewed literature. Together our findings provide evidence that in the vast majority of cases of brachial plexus birth palsy are secondary to a forceful traction injury affecting the brachial plexus that occurs when the child is born.

Keywords Birth palsy · brachial plexus · nerve injury · neuroma · shoulder dystocia

Contents

21.1   Introduction   289
21.2   Radiographic Findings in Brachial Plexus Birth Palsy   290
21.3   Operative Findings in Brachial Plexus Birth Palsy.   290
21.4   Histologic Findings in Brachial Plexus Birth Palsy   293
21.5   Conclusion   293

21.1 Introduction

Brachial plexus birth palsy occurs when the forces stretching the brachial plexus overwhelm the ability of the brachial plexus to resist them. In many cases, brachial plexus birth palsy occurs when vaginal delivery is complicated by shoulder dystocia, because greater than usual forces are often placed on the infant during delivery [1]. Despite evidence that birth brachial plexus injury is most commonly an acute traumatic event that occurs during delivery, a recent review by Pitt and Vredeveld [2] highlights the continued disagreement as to the causation of birth brachial plexus injury, with some authors contending that

S.M. Russell
Department of Neurosurgery, NYU Medical Center, 550 First Avenue, NY, NY

J.A. O'Leary, *Shoulder Dystocia and Birth Injury*,
DOI 10.1007/978-1-59745-473-5_21, © Humana Press, a part of Springer
Science+Business Media, LLC 2009

a significant percentage of these injuries may be secondary to prenatal compression [3]. We acknowledge that prenatal conditions affecting the upper extremity may infrequently contribute to brachial plexus birth palsy. However, these cases can often be identified at birth by the presence of shoulder girdle atrophy, musculoskeletal deformities, or ear deformation. The latter subset of patients represents a distinct group of brachial plexus birth palsy [4,5] and will not be discussed further. The management of shoulder dystocia, its pathophysiologic relationship to brachial plexus birth palsy, and the risk factors for birth palsy will not be addressed in this review; discussion regarding these issues can be found in other reports [6–8] and in other chapters in this book. In this chapter, we review the preoperative radiographic findings and describe surgical observations and histologic findings regarding the causation of brachial plexus birth injury.

21.2 Radiographic Findings in Brachial Plexus Birth Palsy

Infants with significant neurologic deficits related to a brachial plexus birth injury that do not show early signs of recovery during the first few months of life are evaluated with magnetic resonance imaging (MRI) of the brachial plexus and cervical spine. Because of its sensitivity to edema and high resolution of anatomic structures, an appropriately performed MRI documents a number of findings that confirm the acute, traumatic nature of brachial plexus birth palsy (Fig. 21.1A, B) [9]. These findings include spinal rootlet avulsion, spinal cord hemorrhage secondary to rootlet avulsion, pseudomeningoceles from ruptured nerve root sleeves, marked edema of the spinal nerves and brachial plexus elements in the paraspinal and subclavicular space, traumatic neuromas, hemorrhage and swelling of torn scalene musculature, fracture or dislocation of the clavicle, and glenohumeral pathology [9–12]. The incidence and extent of these findings often correlate with the severity of neurologic injury. Abbott et al. [10] documented traumatic scar tissue and neuromas in all 15 patients with birth brachial plexus injury that were evaluated with MRI, and Medina et al. [9] correlated rootlet avulsion and brachial plexus neuromas with intraoperative observation and electrophysiology. MRI performed months to years after birth palsy reveals additional findings that support the traumatic nature of birth palsy: scarring of the scalene musculature, neuroma formation in the spinal nerves and plexal elements, and muscle edema [13].

21.3 Operative Findings in Brachial Plexus Birth Palsy

An acute traction mechanism as the etiology of brachial plexus birth palsy is strongly supported by the operative findings in a series of 100 consecutive primary microsurgical nerve reconstruction procedures performed in infants by the senior author (JG; unpublished data). This cohort demonstrated typical

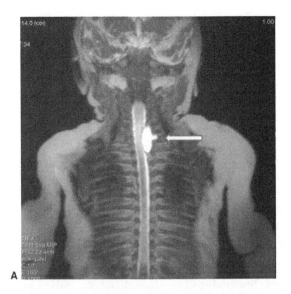

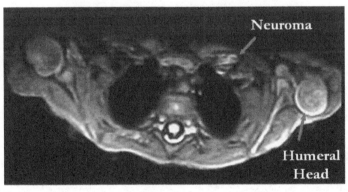

Fig. 21.1 Preoperative MRI in an infant with a brachial plexus birth palsy. (A) pseudome-ningocele (arrow). (B) Traumatic neuroma affecting the brachial plexus. Note typical glenohumeral abnormality in this patient

demographics, including the distribution of injury (Table 21.1), a near even gender distribution, average birth weight of 9 lb 1 oz, and 46% of newborns with a history of shoulder dystocia reported by the parents. At surgical exploration, marked disruption and scarring of the anterior scalene was a constant finding (100%). A neuroma mostly affecting the C5 and C6 spinal nerves and the upper trunk was also present in all patients (Fig. 21.2). Frequently, the brachial plexus neuroma was found to be contiguous with

Table 21.1 Distribution of Brachial Plexus Birth
Injury (N = 100)

Location of Injury	No. of Patients
C5/C6	46
C5/C6/C7	34
Global C5-T1	20

the heavily scarred scalene musculature. In more severely affected infants,
portions of the brachial plexus were completely ruptured in the supraclavi-
cular region, with the distal portion retracted below the clavicle. In most
severe injuries, the neuroma included elements of the middle and lower
plexus.

These pathologic findings, consistent with traction injury, provide
evidence of the traumatic etiology of brachial plexus birth palsy. Furthermore, these intraoperative observations are similar to those seen in adults
who undergo brachial plexus reconstruction after known traumatic
injuries.

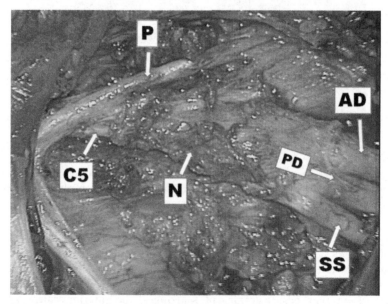

Fig. 21.2 Intraoperative view demonstrating typical upper trunk neuroma (N). Note zone of
injury extending from C5 across the upper trunk onto the divisions. Much fibrotic scalene
muscle has been removed or released. AD, anterior division; PD, posterior division; P, phrenic
nerve; SS, suprascapular nerve

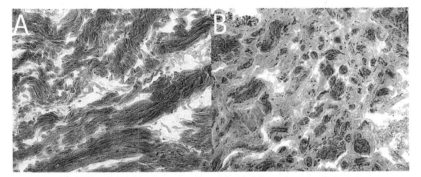

Fig. 21.3 Histologic sections (magnification X20) from a child with brachial plexus birth palsy using a Trichrome stain. Fibrotic and collagen tissues stain blue-green. Viable nerve fibers stain red. (A) Near normal nerve with minimal fibrosis. (B) A neuroma revealing extensive fibrosis and an overall reduction in the number of nerve fibers. (Courtesy of Dr. Panna Desai, New York University School of Medicine.)

21.4 Histologic Findings in Brachial Plexus Birth Palsy

For infants who have nonconducting neuromas or ruptured nerves, the neuroma is often resected and interposition nerve grafts placed, often in combination with nerve transfers. The resected neuromas are routinely sent for frozen-section histologic analysis to aid in maximizing the quality of repair. At surgery, it is often difficult to determine if a proximal nerve element remains viable as a donor for graft reconstruction. Therefore, as part of the intraoperative evaluation of these nerves, the neuroma is resected back until the proximal nerve stump appears to have a microscopically normal, or near-normal, fascicular structure. Serial frozen-sections are obtained of the nerve until an acceptable degree of fascicular organization and myelination are observed. These histologic results are also consistent with traction injury (Fig. 21.3). Findings include robust collagen deposition consistent with scar tissue and sporadic bundles of axons with thin layers of myelination (i.e., neuroma). Most of these axons demonstrate poor, or no, fascicular organization. Normal [14] structural boundaries like the epi- and perineurium are absent or indistinct, with aberrant axons often found regenerating outside these structures when present. A clear anatomic plane of separation between scarred scalene muscle and brachial plexus is frequently absent. These histopathologic findings are similar to those seen in adults with known traction injuries of the brachial plexus.

21.5 Conclusion

Brachial plexus birth palsy is usually secondary to traction injury. Radiographic abnormalities, intraoperative observations, and histologic analysis all support an acute traumatic etiology.

Acknowledgments The authors acknowledge Ilker Yaylali, MD, PhD, for assistance in data retrieval and analysis and Herbert Valencia, RN, for preparation of intraoperative figures.

References

1. Allen RH. On the mechanical aspects of shoulder dystocia and birth injury. *Clin Obstet Gynecol* 2007;50:607–623.
2. Pitt M, Vredeveld JW. The role of electromyography in the management of the brachial plexus palsy of the newborn. *Clin Neurophysiol* 2005;16:1756–1761.
3. Koenigsberger MR. Brachial plexus palsy at birth: intrauterine or due to delivery trauma? [abstract] *Ann Neurol* 1980;8:228.
4. Alfonso I, Dias-Arca G, Alfonso DT, Shuhaiber HH, Papazian O, Price AE, Grossman JAI. Fetal deformations: a risk factor for obstetrical brachial plexus palsy? *Pediatr Neurol* 2006;35(4):246–249.
5. Alfonso I, Alfonso DT, Price AE, Grossman JAI. Cortical dysplasia and obstetrical brachial plexus palsy. *J Child Neurol* 2008 (in press).
6. Gurewitsch ED. Optimizing shoulder dystocia management to prevent birth injury. *Clin Obstet Gynecol* 2007;50:592–606.
7. Gurewitsch ED, Johnson E, Hamzehzadeh S, Allen RH. Risk factors for brachial plexus injury with and without shoulder dystocia. *Am J Obstet Gynecol* 2006;194:486–492.
8. Hudic I, Fatusic Z, Sinanovic O, Skokic F. Etiological risk factors for brachial plexus palsy. *J Matern Fetal Neonatal Med* 2006;19:655–661.
9. Medina LS, Yaylali I, Zurakowski D, Ruiz J, Altman NR, Grossman JA. Diagnostic performance of MRI and MR myelography in infants with a brachial plexus birth injury. *Pediatr Radiol* 2006;6:1295–1299.
10. Abbott R, Abbott M, Alzate J, Lefton D. Magnetic resonance imaging of obstetrical brachial plexus injuries. *Childs Nerv Syst* 2004;20:720–725.
11. Birchansky S, Altman N. Imaging the brachial plexus and peripheral nerves in infants and children. *Semin Pediatr Neurol* 2000;7:15–25.
12. Francel PC, Koby M, Park TS, et al. Fast spin-echo magnetic resonance imaging for radiological assessment of neonatal brachial plexus injury. *J Neurosurg* 1995;83:461–466.
13. Bahm J, Wein B, Alhares G, Dogan C, Radermacher K, Schuind F. Assessment and treatment of glenohumeral joint deformities in children suffering from upper obstetric brachial plexus palsy. *J Pediatr Orthop Br* 2007;16:243–251.
14. Chen L, Gao SC, Gu YD, Hu SN, Xu L, Huang YG. Histopthologuc study of the neuroma-in-continuity in obstetric brachial plexux palsy. *Plast Reconstr Surg* 2008;121:2046–2054.

Index

A

A DOPE, 6, 15
Abdominal
  rescue, 126
  ultrasound for measurements, 37–38
  See also Gunn-Zavanelli-O'Leary
    maneuver
AGA (appropriate for gestational age)
  ultrasound and
    abdominal measurements, 38
    diabetes measurements, 39
    serial measurements, 41
    See also LGA (large for
     gestational age)
Age, *see under* Maternal
All-fours maneuver, *see* Gaskin "all-fours"
  maneuver
Android pelvis, 63
Antenatal risk factors
  SD-related fetal injuries, 212
Antepartum risk factors, 15
  excessive weight gain, 27–28
  fundal height, 29
  gestational diabetes and borderline
    diabetes, 16–19
  obesity, 26–27
  overt, 20–23
  postdate pregnancy, 23–25
  SD, 230
  See also Intrapartum risk factors;
    Preconceptual risk factors
Anterior
  Rubin maneuver, 96
  shoulder release, midwifery view
    of SD, 274
Anthropoid pelvis, 63
  engagement and, 74
  See also Pelvimetry
Avulsion, 130–131
  pathophysiology, 134
  SD-related birth injuries, 203–204

  See also Brachial plexus injuries (BPI);
    Neuromas
Axonotmesis
  pathophysiology, 133–134
  See also Avulsion; Neuromas

B

Barnum maneuver
  for moderate dystocia (grade II), 96–97
  posterior arm delivery
    recent research in, 286
    SD management aspects, 196
Birth injuries, *see* Infant injuries
Birthweight, *see under* Maternal
Bony dystocia
  after restitution, 187
  due to failure of restitution, 188–189
  See also Soft tissue dystocia
Bony pelvis, *see* Pelvimetry
Borderline diabetes, 16
  See also Gestational diabetes
Brachial plexus injuries (BPI), 129
  at cesarean section, 249–255
    clinical experience, 255
    discussion, 253–254
    mechanism, 250–253
  causation, 138–141, 147–161, 228–229
  classification
    avulsion, 130–131
    intermediate type, 131
    lower type (Klumpke palsy), 131
    neurapraxia, 131
    neuromas, 131
    total plexus injuries, 131
    upper plexus injury (Erb palsy), 131
  clinical presentation
    Erb-type upper-plexus patients, 135
    Klumpke patients, 135–136
    total plexus patients, 136
  CNS injury and, 136
  in utero causation, 147–161

Brachial plexus (*cont.*)
  incidence and prognosis, 132–133
  mechanism of labor and injury, 141
  mortality and morbidity, 136–138
  palsy (BPP), 289, 290–293
  pathophysiology
    avulsions, 134
    axonotmesis, 133–134
    neurapraxia, 133–134
    neuroma, 134
    neurotmesis, 133–134
  peripheral nerve anatomy, 134–135
  recent research in, 286–287
  shoulder dystocia and, 138–141
  vulnerable fetuses, 135
  See also Macrosomia; Traction
Brachial plexus palsy (BPP), 289
  histologic findings in, 293
  operative findings in, 290–292
  radiographic findings in, 290

C
Caput
  formation, 76
  succedaneum, 73
  See also Disproportion
Causation, 138–141
  BPI, 202–204, 228–229
  in utero, 147–161
  SD-related birth injuries, 169, 205
    avulsion, 203–204
    BPI causation aspects, 202–204
    clinical background, 169
    clinical interpretation, 173–175
    data analysis, 173
    database, 170–172
    in utero, 203
    rupture, 203–204
    See also Brachial plexus injuries
      (BPI)
Cephalic replacement
  Gunn-Zavanelli-O'Leary maneuver,
    119–120
    abdominal rescue, 126
    discussion, 124–126
    initial clinical experience, 120–121
    severe SD and, 119–120
    survey, 122–124
    technique and results, 121–122
    undeliverable dystocia (grade IV)
      and, 98
Cephalopelvic disproportion, 71
  assessment, 77–78

  See also Failure to progress (FTP);
    Pelvimetry
Cesarean section
  BPI at, 249–255
    clinical experience, 255
    discussion, 253–254
    mechanism, 250–253
  disproportion and, 72–73
  incision, 250–251, 255
  injuries, 141, 250
  nondiabetic macrosomic infant delivery
    and, 262–263
  See also Delivery; Infant injuries;
    Maneuvers
Clamping, *see* Cord clamping
Clinical pelvimetry, 60–61
CNS injuries
  SD-related birth injuries (causation
    analysis)
    clinical interpretation, 174
    data analysis, 173
    database, 170
    See also Brachial plexus injuries
      (BPI)
Computed tomography, 41–42
  See also Ultrasound
Contraction
  fundal dominance (uterine injury) and,
    157–158
  intraabdominal forces and, 159
  See also Delivery; In utero causation;
    Labor; Traction
Cord clamping
  before shoulder delivery, 276
  delayed, 276
  Nuchal cord management and, 277–278
  See also Delivery; Shoulder dystocia (SD)
CPD, true, 82

D
Deflexion
  disproportion and, 76
  See also Hyperflexion
Delivery, 89–104
  childbirth in America and abroad,
    217–219
  cord clamping before shoulder delivery,
    276
  current practice, 90–91
  dystocia and, 99–101
    fundal pressure, 99
    initial techniques, 92
    mild dystocia (grade I), 93–94

moderate dystocia (grade II), 94–97
severe dystocia (grade III), 97–98
time factor, 101–103
treatment, 91–92
undeliverable dystocia (grade IV,
cephalic replacement), 98
instrument
forceps delivery, 53–54, 274
vacuum extractions, 53–54, 274
midwifery view of SD
anterior shoulder release, 274
avoid assisted delivery, 274
Gaskin "all-fours" maneuver,
272–273
pushing, 274
restitution use, 273
running start position, 273
suprapubic not fundal pressure, 274
nondiabetic macrosomic infant,
257–263
cesarean section, 262
instrumental delivery, 263
management recommendations,
264–265
pelvimetry and, 63
posterior arm (Barnum maneuver), 196
SD
at cesarean section, 249–255
at vaginal delivery, 186
SD-related fetal injuries and
delivery method considerations,
219–221
two-step deliveries, 215–218
teaching tools, 55–57
techniques
Gunn-Zavanelli-O'Leary maneuver,
119–126
Mazzanti maneuver, 111–112
McRoberts maneuver, 107–115
types
cesarean section, 249–255
midpelvic, 53–54
vaginal, 186
See also Cesarean section; Delivery;
Infant injuries; Maneuvers
Diabetes
borderline, 16
gestational, 8, 16–19
infants of diabetic mothers
(IDMs), 20
overt, 20–23
ultrasound measurements, 39–40
See also Obesity

Disproportion, 71
caput and deflexion, 76
engagement and, 73–74
fundal height and, 79–80
intrapartum reevaluation and, 75–76
labor
active labor management, 85–86
evaluation and, 84–85
trial of labor, 80–81
molding and, 81–84
Muller-Hillis maneuver and, 78–79
signs and symptoms, 72–73
Disproportionate propulsion theory
(DPT), 154
See also In utero causation
DOPE, see A DOPE
Dunn and Engle study, 159

E
Engagement
disproportion and, 73–74
Engineering research
in utero BPI causation, 156
traction and, 156
Episiotomy
for SD management, 190
midwifery view of SD, 275
recent research in, 287
Erb palsy, 131, 135
in utero causation (Gherman theory),
152–153
risk factors, 230
See also Brachial plexus injuries (BPI);
Klumpke palsy
Estimated fetal weight (EFW), 50
Excessive weight gain, 27
antepartum risk factor, 27–28
See also Obesity

F
Failure to progress (FTP), 77
See also Cephalopelvic disproportion
Fetal
abdominal cirumference (AC), 38
injuries during cesarean section, 251
clinical experience, 255
discussion, 253, 254
incidence, 250
mechanism, 250
maternal fetal medicine, 227
risk factors (SD), 232
size, disproportion and, 72
ultrasound for estimating

Fetal (*cont.*)
    fetal growth, 34
    fetal weight, 36
  weight
    estimated (EFW), 50
    ultrasound for estimating, 36
    See also Risk factors
Flat pelvis, 61
Forceps delivery, 53–54
  midwifery view of SD, 274
  See also Vacuum delivery
Fundal dominance (uterine injury)
  differentiation of uterine activity,
    157–158
  See also In utero causation
Fundal height
  antepartum risk factor, 29
  disproportion and, 79–80
Fundal pressure
  delivery techniques and, 99
  See also Suprapubic pressure

G
Gaskin "all-fours" maneuver
    SD management aspects, 198–199
  midwifery view, 272–273
Gestational age
  appropriate for (AGA), 38–39, 41
  large for, *see* LGA (large for gestational
    age)
Gestational diabetes
  antepartum risk factor, 16–19
  borderline diabetes and, 16
  defined, 16
  identification, 16–18
  maternal obesity and, 8, 11
  3-hour GTT
    abnormal screen, normal, 19
    one abnormal value, 18–19
    See also Overt diabetes
Gherman theory, 151–153
  traction and, 151–152
  See also In utero causation
Gonik theory, 153–154
Growth rates, ultrasound for, 42
GTT (3-hour)
  abnormal screen, normal 3-hour GTT, 19
  one abnormal value on, 18–19
  See also Gestational diabetes
Gunn-Zavanelli-O'Leary maneuver,
    119–120
  abdominal rescue, 126
  discussion, 124–126
  initial clinical experience, 120–121
  severe shoulder dystocia and, 119–120
  survey, 122–124
  SD management aspects, 199
  technique and results, 121–122
Gynecoid pelvis, 63

H
Head measurements, ultrasound for, 36
Heery maneuver, 98
Height
  fundal, 29, 79–80
  maternal (preconceptual risk factor), 7–8
HELPERR mnemonic, 278
  See also Shoulder dystocia (SD)
Hibbard maneuver, 96
Hip hyperflexion
  for SD management, 190
  See also McRoberts maneuver
Hyperflexion
  hip and thigh, 190
  See also Deflexion

I
ICD-9 code, 228
Impaction mechanism
  shoulder, 64–66
  See also Pelvimetry
In utero causation, 147–161
  controversies concerning etiology,
    148–150
  discussion
    Dunn and Engle study, 159
    Jennett study, 160
    Koenigsberger study, 159
  intraabdominal forces, 159
  Johns Hopkins rebuttal, 154–155
  research
    engineering research, 156
    Gherman theory, 151–153
    Gonik theory, 153
    Jennett theory, 150–151
    Sandmire theory, 154
  SD-related birth injuries, 203
  uterine injury
    fundal dominance, 157
    uterine activity differentiation,
      157–158
    See also Brachial plexus injuries
      (BPI); Labor
Incision
  J, 250–251
  T, 250–251, 255

uterine, fascial, and/or skin, 250
See also Cesarean section
Infant injuries
    BPI, *see* Brachial plexus injuries (BPI)
    cesarean injuries, 141
    classification (BPI)
        avulsion, 130–131
        intermediate type, 131
        lower type (Klumpke palsy), 131
        neurapraxia, 131
        neuromas, 131
        total plexus injuries, 131
        upper plexus injury (Erb palsy), 131
    fetal injuries (SD-related), 209–221
        childbirth in America and abroad,
            217–219
        delivery method considerations,
            219–221
        diagnosis, 214–217
        etiology and prevention, 219
        risk factors, 211–214
Infants of diabetic mothers (IDMs), 20
Initial exam
    intrapartum risk factor, 50
Injury, *see* Infant injuries
Instrument delivery
    midwifery view of SD, 274
    nondiabetic macrosomic infant delivery
        and, 263
    type
        forceps delivery, 53–54, 274
        vacuum extractions, 53–54, 274
Intermediate type plexus injury, 131
Intraabdominal forces
    contraction and, 159–160
    See also In utero causation
Intrapartum risk factors, 49
    disproportion and, 75–76
    initial exam, 50
    labor as end point, 51
    legal implications, 243
    midpelvic delivery, 53–54
    oxytocin, 52–53
    prior history, 51–52
    SD-related fetal injuries, 213–214, 230
    teaching tools, delivery, 55–57
    See also Antepartum risk factors;
        Preconceptual risk factors

J
J incision, 250–251
Jennett theory, 150–151
    in utero causation and, 160

traction and, 150
Johns Hopkins rebuttal, 154–155

K
Klumpke palsy, 131, 135–136
    See also Erb palsy
Koenigsberger study, 159

L
Labor
    brachial plexus injury and mechanism
        for, 141
    childbirth in America and abroad,
        217–219
    disproportion aspects
        active labor management, 85–86
        labor evaluation and, 84–85
        trial of labor practice, 80–81
    exam and pelvimetry, 66–67
    induction in nondiabetic macrosomic
        infant delivery, 262–263
    intrapartum risk factor, 51
    midwifery view of SD
        labor factors, 271
        maternal positions in labor, 271
        positions at birth, 272
    pelvimetry and, 63
    risk factors and SD, 232–233
    See also In utero causation
LeftOcciput Trauma (LOT) position, 95
Legal implications
    midwife and, 280
    shoulder dystocia-related, 231, 241–243
LGA (large for gestational age)
    maternal birthweight and, 4
    SD-related fetal injuries and
        antenatal risk factors, 212
        preconceptual risk factors, 211
    ultrasound and
        abdominal measurements, 37–38
        diabetes measurements, 39
        serial measurements, 41
        See also AGA (appropriate for
            gestational age); Causation
Lithotomy position, 272
Litigation, *see* Legal implications
Lower plexus injury, 131, 135–136
    See also Brachial plexus injuries (BPI)

M
Macrosomia
    antenatal risk factors, 212
    complications, 258

Macrosomia (*cont.*)
  fetal, 257
  maternal factors
    age, 6–7
    obesity, 10
  McRoberts maneuver and, 110
  nondiabetic macrosomic infant
      delivery, 257
    elective cesarean section and
        induction of labor, 262–263
    instrumental delivery, 263
    macrosomia and obesity, 260–261
    macrosomia and shoulder dystocia,
        258–259
    macrosomia and ultrasound, 259–260
    management recommendations,
        264–265
    previous macrosomia, 261–262
  SD-related fetal injuries and, 212
  ultrasound
    for early macrosomia detection,
        35–36
    in nondiabetic macrosomic infant
        delivery, 259–260
    See also Brachial plexus injuries (BPI);
        Causation
Maneuvers
  Barnum, 96–97
  Gunn-Zavanelli-O'Leary, 119–126, 199
  Heery, 98
  Hibbard, 96
  Mazzanti, 111–112
  McRoberts, 93–94, 107–115,
      235–236
  midwifery view positions at birth
    Gaskin "all-fours" maneuver,
        272–273
    running start position, 273
    side-lying, 272
    squatting, 272
    standing, 272
  Muller-Hillis, 78–79
  Ritgen, 274
  Rubin, 94–96, 194–196
  SD clinical management, 234–237
    Barnum maneuver (posterior arm
        delivery), 196
    Gaskin (all-fours), 198–199
    Gunn-Zavanelli-O'Leary, 199
    McRoberts maneuver, 235–237
    Zavanelli maneuver, 236
  Woods screw, 94–95, 193–194
  See also Delivery; Labor

Maternal
  age
    A DOPE and, 6
    advanced, 6
    macrosomia and, 6, 7
    preconceptual risk factor and, 5–7
  birthweight
    LGA aspects, 4
    macrosomia and, 5
    preconceptual risk factor and, 4
  fetal medicine, 227–244
  height, 7–8
  obesity, 8–11
    gestational diabetes and, 8, 11
    macrosomia and, 10
  weight
    excessive weight gain, 27
    gain and infant's birthweight, 27–28
Mazzanti maneuver
  McRoberts maneuver combined
      with, 112
  suprapubic pressure and, 111–112
McRoberts maneuver, 107
  clinical case experience, 114–115
  delivery, 112
  effects of, 113
  for mild dystocia (grade I), 93–94
  improper, 114
  literature review, 108–109
  Mazzanti maneuver combined with, 112
  recent research in, 285
  research aspects, 113, 286
  SD clinical management, 190–192,
      235–237
  technique, 109–111
    for macrosomia, 110
    for shoulder dystocia, 109
  thighs hyperflexion in, 109, 114, 190
Midpelvic delivery
  intrapartum risk factor, 53–54
Midwifery view, *see under* Shoulder
      dystocia (SD)
Mild dystocia (grade I), 93–94
Moderate dystocia (grade II)
  Barnum maneuver for, 96–97
  Hibbard maneuver for, 96
  Rubin maneuver for, 94–96
  Woods screw maneuver for, 94–95
Molding, 76
  disproportion and, 81–84
  score, 83
MRI, 290
Muller-Hillis maneuver, 78–79

N

Neurapraxia, 131
  pathophysiology, 133–134
  See also Brachial plexus injuries (BPI)
Neuromas, 131
  histologic findings in, 293
  operative findings in, 292
  pathophysiology, 134
  See also Avulsion
Neurotmesis, 133–134
  SD-related birth injuries (BPI causation aspects), 203–204
Nondiabetic macrosomic infant delivery, 257–263
  cesarean section, 262
  instrumental delivery, 263
  management recommendations, 264–265
Nuchal cord management, 277–278
  See also Cord clamping

O

Obesity
  antepartum risk factor, 26–27
  excessive weight gain, 27–28
  maternal (preconceptual risk factor), 8–11
  nondiabetic macrosomic infant delivery and, 260–261
  ultrasound measurements, 40–41
Operative delivery, *see* Instrument delivery
Operative injuries, *see* Infant injuries
Overt diabetes
  antepartum risk factor, 20–23
  IDM and, 20
  incidence, 20–21
  treatment, 21–23
  See also Gestational diabetes
Oxytocin
  intrapartum risk factor, 52–53

P

Pelvic inadequacy
  intrapartum risk factors, 213
  preconceptual risk factors, 211
Pelvimetry, 59
  clinical, 60–61
  flat pelvis, 61
  labor and delivery mechanism
    android pelvis, 63
    anthropoid pelvis, 63
    gynecoid pelvis, 63
    posterior pelvis, 63

labor exam, 66–67
  prenatal assessment, 61–62
  shoulder dystocia issues, 63–64
  shoulder impaction mechanism, 64–66
  See also Cephalopelvic disproportion
Peripheral nerve
  anatomy, 134–135
  See also Brachial plexus injuries (BPI)
Pivoting, 91
Plexus injury, *see* Brachial plexus injuries (BPI)
Positions at birth, *see* Maneuvers
Postdate pregnancy
  antepartum risk factor, 23–25
Posterior arm delivery (Barnum maneuver), 196
Posterior pelvis, 63
Posterior Rubin maneuver, 95–96
Preconceptual risk factors, 3
  maternal
    age, 5–7
    birthweight, 4
    height, 7–8
    obesity, 8–11
    obesity and diabetes, 11
    SD-related fetal injuries, 211
    See also Antepartum risk factors; Intrapartum risk factors
Pregnancy
  prepregnancy risk, 15
  postdate, 23–25
  See also Risk factors
Prenatal assessment
  pelvimetry and, 61–62
Prenatal legal implications
  shoulder dystocia, 243
Pulling, 91
Pushing, 91, 274

R

Radiographic findings (BPI), 290
Recurrent SD, *see under* Shoulder dystocia (SD)
Restitution
  bony dystocia after, 187
  bony dystocia due to failure of, 188–189
  midwifery view of SD, 273
  soft tissue dystocia after, 186
Right Occiput Trauma (ROT) position, 95
Risk factors
  antenatal, 212
  antepartum, 15–29
  intrapartum, 49, 213–214

Risk factors (*cont.*)
  preconceptual, 3–11, 211
  shoulder dystocia
    fetal, 232
    labor, 232–233
Ritgen maneuver, 274
Rotational maneuvers
  Rubin's, 194–196
  Woods', 193–194
Rubin maneuver
  anterior, 96
  for moderate dystocia (grade II), 94–96
  posterior, 95–96
  recent research in, 286
  SD management aspects, 194–196
Running start position, 273
Rupture, *see* Neurotmesis

S
Sandmire theory, 154
Severe dystocia (grade III), 97–98
Shoulder dystocia (SD)
  brachial plexus injury
    at cesarean section, 249–255
    causation, 138–141
  classification
    bony dystocia after restitution, 187
    bony dystocia due to failure of
      restitution, 188–189
    SD at cesarean section, 249–255
    SD at vaginal delivery, 186
    soft tissue dystocia after restitution,
      186
  clinical management, 234–237
    McRoberts maneuver, 235–237
    squatting, 237
    symphysiotomy, 236
    Zavanelli maneuver, 236
  current practice of delivery and, 90–91
  defining standard of care, 238–240
    nursing staff responsibilities, 240
    physician responsibilities, 239–240
  delivery techniques and, 89–103
  documentation, 237
  fetal risk factors, 232
  fundal pressure aspects, 99
  Gunn-Zavanelli-O'Leary maneuver,
    119–120
  in utero BPI causation and, 148–150
  incidence and etiology, 229, 231
  initial techniques, 92
  Johns Hopkins rebuttal, 154–155
  labor risk factors, 232–233

  legal implications, 231, 241–243
    intrapartum, 243
    prenatal, 243
  management, 190–192
    all-fours maneuver (Gaskin), 198–199
    diagnosis and management pitfalls,
      240–241
    delivery of posterior arm (Barnum
      maneuver), 196
    episiotomy, 190
    Gunn-Zavanelli-O'Leary Maneuver,
      199
    McRoberts position effects, 190–192
    Rubin's rotational maneuvers,
      194–196
    suprapubic pressure, 192–193
    Woods' rotational maneuvers,
      193–194
  McRoberts maneuver and, 109, 190–192
  mechanism, 231
  midwifery view, 269–281
    algorithms and mnemonics, 275
    anterior shoulder release, 274
    avoid assisted delivery, 274
    cord clamping before shoulder
      delivery, 276–278
    delayed cord clamping, 276
    documentation, 281
    education and clinical competency,
      278–279
    episiotomy, 275
    Gaskin "all-fours" maneuver,
      272–273
    labor and birth factors, 271
    legal issues, 280
    management issues, 270
    maternal positions in labor, 271
    midwife and physician
      responsibilities, 279–280
    newborn safeguarding, 275
    positions at birth, 272
    pushing, 274
    restitution use, 273
    running start position, 273
    suprapubic not fundal pressure, 274
  mild dystocia (grade I), 93–94
  moderate dystocia (grade II), 94–97
  nondiabetic macrosomic infant delivery
    and, 258–259
  pelvimetry and, 63–64
  prediction models, 233–234
  recent research in, 285–287
  recurrent, 163–167

defeatist attitude, 164
mathematical calculations, 164–165
predictability, 166–167
prior knowledge, 165
related birth injuries
avulsion, 203–204
BPI causation aspects, 202–205
definition and incidence, 181–185
in utero causation, 203
management, 190–199
modern-day classification, 185–190
rupture, 203–204
related birth injuries (causation analysis),
predisposing factors for, 169–175
clinical background, 169
clinical interpretation, 173–175
data analysis, 173
database, 170–172
related fetal injuries, 209
antenatal risk factors, 212
childbirth in America and abroad, 217
diagnosis, 214–217
intrapartum risk factors, 213–214
preconceptual risk factors, 211
preventive medicine and, 210
two-step deliveries, 215–218
risk factors, 230
severe dystocia (grade III), 97–98
standard of care for
defining of, 238
nursing staff responsibilities, 240
physician responsibilities, 239–240
time factor and, 101–103
traction injury and BPI, 229–230
treatment, 91–92
pivoting, 91
pulling, 91
pushing, 91
ultrasound in, 33–34
undeliverable dystocia (grade IV,
cephalic replacement), 98
See also Infant injuries; Macrosomia;
Risk factors
Shoulder impaction mechanism, 64–66
See also Pelvimetry
Shoulder ratios, 43
Side-lying position, 272
midwifery view of SD, 272
See also Maneuvers
Soft tissue dystocia
after restitution, 186–187
ultrasound for, 42–43
See also Bony dystocia

Squatting, 272
SD clinical management, 237
See also Delivery
Standing, 272
midwifery view of SD, 272
See also Side-lying position
Suprapubic pressure
Mazzanti maneuver and, 111–112
McRoberts maneuver, 112
midwifery view of SD, 274
SD management aspects,
192–193
See also Fundal pressure
Symphysiotomy, 236

T
T incision, 250–251, 255
Thigh hyperflexion, 114
for SD management, 190
thighs hyperflexion, 110
See also McRoberts maneuver
3-hour GTT, see GTT (3-hour)
Tissue thickness
soft, 42–43
See also Ultrasound
Total plexus injury, 131, 136
Traction, 147
engineering research, 156
Gherman theory, 151–152
Gonik theory, 154
injuries, 229
during cesarean section, 255
operative findings in, 290, 292
Jennett theory, 150
Johns Hopkins rebuttal, 155
recent research in, 285–286
SD-related birth injuries, 181–185
See also Brachial plexus injuries (BPI);
In utero causation
Trial of labor practice, 80–81
Two-step deliveries, 215–218

U
Ultrasound
early macrosomia detection, 35–36
for abdominal measurements,
37–38
for diabetes, 39–40
for fetal weight estimation, 36
for head measurements, 36
for obesity, 40–41
growth rates investigation, 42
in shoulder dystocia, 33–34

Ultrasound (*cont.*)
    nondiabetic macrosomic infant delivery
        and, 259–260
    serial measurements, 41
    shoulder ratios evaluation, 43
    soft tissue thickness evaluation,
        42–43
Undeliverable dystocia (grade IV, cephalic
    replacement), 98
Upper plexus injury, 131
Uterine injury
    fundal dominance,
        157–158
    See also In utero causation

V
Vaccum delivery, 53–54
    midwifery view of SD, 274
    vacuum extractions, 54
    See also Forceps delivery
Vaginal delivery
    SD at, 186
    See also Cesarean section

W
Weight
    birth
        maternal weight gain and, 27–28
        preconceptual risk factor and, 4
    fetal
        estimated (EFW), 50
        ultrasound for estimating, 36
    maternal weight gain
        excessive, 27
        infant's birthweight and, 27–28
        See also Obesity
Woods maneuver
    for moderate dystocia (grade II),
        94–95
    rotational maneuvers, 193–194
    SD management aspects, 193–194

Z
Zavanelli maneuver, 119–120
    SD clinical management, 236
    See also Gunn-Zavanelli-O'Leary
        maneuver

Made in the USA
Monee, IL
12 November 2020